Hematology in Practice

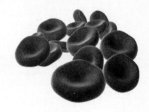

Betty Ciesla, MS, MT(ASCP)SH
Faculty, Medical Technology Program
Morgan State University
Baltimore, Maryland
Assistant Professor
Villa Julie College
Stevenson, Maryland

F. A. DAVIS COMPANY • Philadelphia

F. A. Davis Company
1915 Arch Street
Philadelphia, PA 19103
www.fadavis.com

Printed in the United States of America

Last digit indicates print number: 10 9 8 7 6 5 4 3 2 1

Acquisitions Editor: Christa Fratantoro
Manager of Content Development: Deborah Thorp
Developmental Editor: Keith Donnellan
Art and Design Manager: Carolyn O'Brien

As new scientific information becomes available through basic and clinical research, recommended treatments and drug therapies undergo changes. The author(s) and publisher have done everything possible to make this book accurate, up to date, and in accord with accepted standards at the time of publication. The author(s), editors, and publisher are not responsible for errors or omissions or for consequences from application of the book, and make no warranty, expressed or implied, in regard to the contents of the book. Any practice described in this book should be applied by the reader in accordance with professional standards of care used in regard to the unique circumstances that may apply in each situation. The reader is advised always to check product information (package inserts) for changes and new information regarding dose and contraindications before administering any drug. Caution is especially urged when using new or infrequently ordered drugs.

Library of Congress Cataloging-in-Publication Data

Ciesla, Betty.
  Hematology in practice / Betty Ciesla.
   p. ; cm.
  Includes bibliographical references.
  ISBN-13: 978-0-8036-1526-7
  ISBN-10: 0-8036-1526-4
1. Blood—Diseases. 2. Hematology. I. Title.
[DNLM: 1. Hematologic Diseases. 2. Case Reports. 3. Hematologic Tests—methods. WH 120 C569h 2007]
  RB145.C5444 2007
  616.1'5—dc22   2006028917

For my daughters, who changed my life

For my husband, whom I cherish

For my mother and sisters, who challenged my imagination

Preface

In its most fundamental form, hematology is the study of blood in health and in disease. Blood is the window to the body; it is the predictor of vitality and long life. In ancient times, blood was worshipped. Men were bled to obtain a cure and blood was studied for its mystical powers. It was an elevated body fluid. The discipline of hematology was an outgrowth of this fascination with blood. As we practice it in the clinical laboratory today, this discipline encompasses skill, art, and instinct.

Hematology is about relationships; the relationships of the bone marrow to the systemic circulation, the relationship of the plasma environment to the red cell life span and the relationship of hemoglobin to the red cell. In this textbook, you, the student, are a vital part of this relationship. I have queried many students over my two decades of teaching and asked them what it is they want to see in a textbook. I have asked, What helps? What gets in the way? What makes you feel more comfortable? Students answered honestly and in great detail, and I even managed to have one of my students review each chapter, so that the student perspective would not be minimized.

Hematology is a difficult subject to master because it forces students to think in an unnatural way. Educators are always asking why, well before students can cross the intellectual bridge between the marrow and the peripheral smear. Many students begin a hematology course with little foundation in blood cell morphology, physiology, or medical terminology. With this is mind, I have built several helpful strategies within this text. Each chapter contains readable text that engages the students to learn, master, and then apply the critical concepts in hematology. Medical terminology is absorbed through a designated Word Key section, defining terms to which student may not have been exposed. End of chapter summaries and multiple levels of case studies illustrate the key principles of each chapter. Additionally, there are unique troubleshooting cases in each chapter which encourage each student to role play as a working professional to develop and refine problem solving skills in practice. An Instructor's Resource Disk is available to adopting educators. The CD includes a Brownstone electronic test generator, a PowerPoint presentation with lecture points, and a searchable Image Ancillary.

I hope that this text travels with you as you continue your career in the laboratory professions and I hope that the information motivates you and arouses your intellectual curiosity. Two year and four year students can benefit from the chosen topics within the text and perhaps it may even find a home on the shelves of working laboratories nationally and internationally. I welcome your comments (bciesla@jewel.morgan.edu) and encourage you to assist me in creating a memorable textbook.

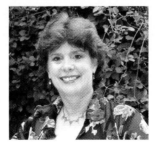

Betty Ciesla, MS, MT (ASCP)SH

Contributors

Barbara Caldwell, MS, MT(ASCP)SH
Manager, Clinical Laboratory Services
Montgomery General Hospital
Olney, Maryland

Donna D. Castellone, MS, MT(ASCP)SH
Technical Specialist, Department of Special
Coagulation
New York Presbyterian/Weill Cornell Medical Center
New York, New York

Betty Ciesla, MS, MT(ASCP)SH
Faculty, Medical Technology Program
Morgan State University
Baltimore, Maryland
Assistant Professor, MLT Program
Villa Julie College
Stevenson, Maryland

Kathleen Finnegan, MS, MT(ASCP)SH
Clinical Assistant Professor
School of Health Technology and Management
Department of Clinical Laboratory Sciences
Stony Brook University
Stony Brook, New York

Lori Lentowski, BS MT(ASCP)
St. Joseph Medical Center
Towson, Maryland

Mitra Taghizadeh, MS, MT(ASCP)
Assistant Professor
Department of Medical and Research Technology
University of Maryland School of Medicine
Baltimore, Maryland

Reviewers

Hassan Aziz, PhD, CLS(NCA)
Department Head
Medical Technology
Armstrong Atlantic State University
Savannah, Georgia

Linda Collins, MS, MT(ASCP)
Instructor
Medical Laboratory
Delaware Tech
Georgetown, Delaware

Sharon T. Columbus, MEd, MT(ASCP)
Program Coordinator
Medical Laboratory Technology
Clinton Community College
Plattsburgh, New York

Susan Conforti, MS, MT(ASCP)SBB
Chairperson, Program Director
Medical Laboratory Technology
Farmingdale State University
Farmingdale, New York

Sandra Cook, MS, MT(ASCP)
Coordinator, Adjunct Instructor
Clinical Laboratory Science
Ferris State University
Big Rapids, Michigan

Kozy Corsaut, MS, MT(ASCP), CLS(NCA)
Program Director, Associate Professor
Medical Laboratory Technology
Stark State College
North Canton, Ohio

Veronica Dominguez, MEd, MT-NCA
Program Coordinator
Medical Laboratory Technology
El Paso Community College
El Paso, Texas

Andrea G. Gordon, MEd, MT(ASCP)SH
Program Director
Clinical Laboratory Science
New Hampshire Community Technical College
Concord, New Hampshire

Cindy Handley, PhD, MT(ASCP)
Instructor
Medical Laboratory Technology
Seward County Community College
Liberal, Kansas

Debbie Heinritz, MT(ASCP), CLS(NCA)
Instructor
Clinical Laboratory Science
Northeast Wisconsin Technical College
Green Bay, Wisconsin

Sheryl Herring, MSA, BS, MT(ASCP)
Program Coordinator, Assistant Professor
Clinical Laboratory Technology
Louisiana State University
Alexandria, Louisiana

Judy A. Horton, DA, MT(ASCP)
Interim Dean
Allied Health
Northern Virginia Community College
Springfield, Virginia

Jeanne M. Isabel, MSEd, MT(ASCP), CLSpH(NCA)
Associate Professor
Clinical Laboratory Sciences
Northern Illinois University
DeKalb, Illinois

Arthur Keehnle, MS, MT(ASC), CLS(NCA)
Program Director
Medical Laboratory Technology
Beaufort County Community College
Washington, North Carolina

Susan J. LeClair, PhD, CLS(NCA)
Chancellor Professor
Medical Laboratory Science
University of Massachusetts
Dartmouth, Massachusetts

Sandra Paynter, MT(ASCP)(AMT)
Coordinator
Medical Laboratory
Maria Parham Medical Center
Henderson, North Carolina

Terry Piatz, MS, MT(ASCP)
Program Director, Assistant Professor
Medical Laboratory Technology
Presentation College
Aberdeen, South Dakota

Kelly Ryan AAS, MLT(ASCP)
Student
Villa Julie College
Stevenson, Maryland

Yasmen Simonian, PhD, MT(ASCP), CLS(NCA)
Department Chair, Professor
Clinical Laboratory Sciences
Weber State University
Ogden, Utah

Lauren Strader, MEd, MT(ASCP)
Program Director, Department Chair
Medical Laboratory Technology
North Georgia Technical College
Clarkesville, Georgia

Kathleen Wagner, MT(ASCP)
Adjunct Faculty
Clinical Laboratory Technology
Elgin Community College
Elgin, Illinois

Acknowledgments

Writing a textbook is a collaborative exercise, and it takes a collective group of supportive individuals to bring a project to completion. I consider myself extremely fortunate to have Christa Fratantoro of F. A. Davis and Keith Donnellan of Dovetail Content Solutions to guide me through this writing endeavor. Their patience, counsel, good humor, and psychology were invaluable. I am indebted to Dr. Diane Wilson of Morgan State University, who gave me the time and encouragement to pursue and complete this project. I am humbled by her gentle spirit and deeply grateful for her friendship. A special note of thanks goes to my talented contributors, whose manuscripts came in on time and in good form. Without them, this text would have been much less complete. With regard to the procedures chapter, Kathy Finnegan and Joyce Feinberg offered me much needed help within an extremely short time frame and I am so grateful. And many thanks to Candi Grayson and Dr. Robert Palermo from Greater Baltimore Medical Center for providing the expertise to shoot the digital selections. I appreciate the efforts of Lori Lentowski and St. Joseph Hospital in Baltimore, Maryland, in augmenting the case study and procedures sections. In addition, thanks to Kelly Ryan who was my student reviewer and author of the PowerPoint section.

Contents

PART I BASIC HEMATOLOGY PRINCIPLES

CHAPTER 1
Introduction to Hematology and Basic Laboratory Practices, 3

Betty Ciesla

Introduction to Hematology, 4

The Microscope, 4
Significant Parts of the Microscope, 4
Care of the Microscope, 5
Corrective Actions in Light Microscopy, 6
Innovations in Microscopy, 6

Standard Precautions, 6
Personal Protective Equipment, 6
Safety Features Other Than Personal
  Protective Equipment, 7
Chemical and Environmental Hazards, 8

**Basic Concepts of Quality Assurance
  Plans in the Hematology Laboratory, 8**
Quality Control Monitoring in the
  Hematology Laboratory, 9
Normal, or Reference, Intervals, 9
Delta Checks, 10
Reflex Testing, 10
Preanalytic Variables, 10
Postanalytic Variables, 10
Critical Results, 11

CHAPTER 2
From Hematopoiesis to the Complete Blood Count, 15

Betty Ciesla

**Hematopoiesis: The Origin of Cell
  Development, 16**

**The Spleen as an Indicator Organ of
  Hematopoietic Health, 17**
The Functions of the Spleen, 17
Potential Risks of Splenectomy, 17

**The Bone Marrow and the
  Myeloid:Erythroid Ratio, 18**

Alterations in the M:E Ratio, 18
The Role of Stem Cells and Cytokines, 18
Erythropoietin, 20
The Role of the Laboratory Professional in
  the Bone Marrow Procedure, 21
Bone Marrow Procedure, 21
Bone Marrow Report, 21
The Complete Blood Count, 22
The Morphological Classification of the
  Anemias, 23
Calculating Red Cell Indices and Their
  Role in Sample Integrity, 25
The Value of the Red Cell Distribution
  Width, 25
Critical Values, 26
The Clinical Approach to Anemias, 26
The Value of the Reticulocyte Count, 26

CHAPTER 3
Red Blood Cell Production, Function, and Relevant Red Cell Morphology, 33

Betty Ciesla

Basic Red Cell Production, 34

Red Cell Maturation, 34

Red Cell Terminology, 34

Maturation Stages of the Red Cell, 35
Pronormoblast, 35
Basophilic Normoblast, 36
Polychromatophilic Normoblast, 36
Orthochromic Normoblast-Nucleated
  (nRBC), 36
Reticulocyte, 36
Mature Red Cell, 36

**Red Blood Cell Membrane Development
  and Function, 37**
Composition of Lipids in the Interior and
  Exterior Layers, 37
Composition of Proteins in the Lipid
  Bilayers, 38
The Cytoskeleton, 38

Red Cell Metabolism, 38
Abnormal Red Cell Morphology, 39
  Variations in Red Cell Size, 39
  Variations in Red Cell Color, 41
  Variations in Red Cell Shape, 41
Red Cell Inclusions, 43

CHAPTER 4
Hemoglobin Function and Principles of Hemolysis, 51
  Betty Ciesla

  Hemoglobin Structure and Synthesis, 52
    Types of Hemoglobin, 52
    Hemoglobin Function, 53
    Abnormal Hemoglobins, 54
  The Hemolytic Process, 55
    Types of Hemolysis, 55
    Laboratory Evidence of Hemolysis, 56
    The Physiology of Hemolysis, 57
  Terminology Relevant to the Hemolytic Anemias, 58

PART II   RED CELL DISORDERS

CHAPTER 5
The Microcytic Anemias, 65
  Betty Ciesla

  Iron Intake and Iron Absorption, 66
  Iron Storage and Recycled Iron, 66
  Iron Deficiency Anemia, 68
    Pathophysiology and Symptoms, 68
    Tests Used to Diagnose Iron Deficiency, 68
    Causes of Iron Deficiency, 70
    Treatment for Iron Deficiency, 70
  Anemia of Chronic Disease and Inflammation: Pathophysiology, Diagnosis, and Treatment, 70
  Anemias Related to Iron Overload Conditions, the Sideroblastic Anemias, 71

Hereditary Hemochromatosis, 72
The Thalassemia Syndromes, 74
  Brief History and Demographics, 74
  The Pathophysiology of the Thalassemias, 75
  The Alpha Thalassemias, 75
  Beta Thalassemia Major: Cooley's Anemia, Mediterranean Fever, 77
  Thalassemias Intermedia and Beta Thalassemia Trait, 79

CHAPTER 6
The Macrocytic Anemias, 85
  Betty Ciesla

  The Macrocytic Anemias and the Megaloblastic Process, 86
  The Red Cell Precursors in Megaloblastic Anemia, 86
  Ineffective Erythropoiesis in Megaloblastic Anemia, 86
  Vitamin B_{12} and Folic Acid: Their Role in DNA Synthesis, 87
  Nutritional Requirements, Transport, and Metabolism of Vitamin B_{12} and Folic Acid, 87
  Incorporating Vitamin B_{12} Into the Bone Marrow, 88
  Clinical Features of Patients With Megaloblastic Anemia, 88
  Hematological Features of Megaloblastic Anemias, 88
  Pernicious Anemia as a Subset of Megaloblastic Anemias, 89
  Vitamin B_{12} and Folic Acid Deficiency, 89
  Laboratory Diagnosis of Megaloblastic Anemias, 90
  Treatment and Response of Individuals With Megaloblastic Anemia, 90
  Macrocytic Anemias That Are Not Megaloblastic, 91

CHAPTER 7

Normochromic Anemias, Biochemical and Membrane Disorders, and Miscellaneous Red Cell Disorders, 97

Betty Ciesla

The Role of the Spleen in Red Cell Membrane Disorders, 98
Hereditary Spherocytosis, 98
The Genetics and Pathophysiology of Hereditary Spherocytosis, 98
Clinical Presentation in Hereditary Spherocytosis, 98
Laboratory Diagnosis of Hereditary Spherocytosis, 100
Treatment and Management of Hereditary Spherocytosis, 100
Hereditary Elliptocytosis, 100
Common Hereditary Elliptocytosis, 101
Southeast Asian Ovalocytosis, 101
Spherocytic Hereditary Elliptocytosis, 101
Hereditary Pyropoikilocytosis, 101
Hereditary Stomatocytosis and Hereditary Xerocytosis, 102
Glucose-6-Phosphate Dehydrogenase Deficiency, 102
The Genetics of Glucose-6-Phosphate Dehydrogenase Deficiency, 102
Clinical Manifestations of Glucose-6-Phosphate Dehydrogenase Deficiency, 103
Diagnosis of Glucose-6-Phosphate Dehydrogenase Deficiency, 105
Pyruvate Kinase Deficiency, 105
Miscellaneous Red Cell Disorders, 105
Aplastic Anemia, 105
Fanconi's Anemia, 105
Diamond-Blackfan Anemia, 106
Paroxysmal Nocturnal Hemoglobinuria, 106
Cold Agglutinin Syndrome, 107
Paroxysmal Cold Hemoglobinuria, 108

CHAPTER 8

The Normochromic Anemias Due to Hemoglobinopathies, 113

Betty Ciesla

General Description of the Hemoglobinopathies, 114
Sickle Cell Anemia, 114
Genetics and Incidence of Sickle Cell Anemia, 114
Pathophysiology of the Sickling Process, 115
Clinical Considerations for Sickle Cell Anemia, 115
Disease Management and Prognosis, 117
Laboratory Diagnosis, 117
Sickle Cell Trait, 120
Hemoglobin C Disease and Trait and Hemoglobin SC, 120
Variant Hemoglobins of Note, 121
Hemoglobin S-beta Thalassemia, 121
Hemoglobin E, 121
Hemoglobin D_{Punjab}/Hemoglobin G_{phila}, 122
Hemoglobin O_{Arab}, 122

PART III   WHITE CELL DISORDERS

CHAPTER 9

Leukopoiesis and Leukopoietic Function, 129

Betty Ciesla

Leukopoiesis, 130
Stages of Leukocyte Maturation, 130
Features of Cell Identification, 130
Myeloblast, 130
Promyelocyte (Progranulocyte), 131
Myelocyte, 131
Metamyelocyte, 131
Band, 132
Segmented Neutrophil, 132
Eosinophils and Basophils, 132
The Agranular Cell Series, 133

Lymphocyte Origin and Function, 134
Lymphocyte Populations, 136
The Travel Path of Lymphocytes, 136
Lymphocytes and the Development of
  Immunocompetency, 137
The Response of Lymphocytes to Antigenic
  Stimulation, 137
Lymphocyte Cell Markers and the Cluster
  Designation (CD), 137
**Leukocyte Count From the Complete
  Blood Cell Count to the Differential,
  137**
Manual Differential Versus Differential
  Scan, 138
Relative Versus Absolute Values, 139

CHAPTER 10
**Abnormalities of White Cells: Quantitative,
Qualitative, and the Lipid Storage Diseases,
143**
Betty Ciesla

**Introduction to the White Cell Disorders,
  144**
**Quantitative Changes in the White Cells,
  144**
Conditions With Increased Neutrophils,
  144
Conditions With Increased Eosinophils,
  144
Conditions With Increased Basophils, 144
Conditions With Increased Monocytes,
  144
Specific Terminology Relating to
  Quantitative White Cell Changes, 144
Stages of White Cell Phagocytosis, 145
Qualitative Defects of White Cells, 145
Toxic Changes in White Cells, 146
Nuclear Abnormalities: Hypersegmentation,
  148
Hereditary White Cell Disorders, 149
May-Hegglin Anomaly, 149
Alder's Anomaly (Alder-Reilly Anomaly),
  149

Pelger-Huët Anomaly, 149
Chediak-Higashi Syndrome, 149
**Reactive Lymphocytosis in Common
  Disease States, 150**
Other Sources of Reactive Lymphocytosis,
  150
**The Effect of Human Immunodeficiency
  Virus/Acquired Immune Deficiency
  Syndrome on Hematology Parameters,
  151**
Lipid Storage Diseases (Briefly), 152
Common Features of a Few of the Lipid
  Storage Diseases, 152
Bone Marrow Cells in Lipid Storage
  Disorders, 152
**Bacteria and Other Unexpected White
  Cell Changes, 153**

CHAPTER 11
Acute Leukemias, 159
Barbara Caldwell

Definition of Leukemia, 160
**Comparing Acute and Chronic Leukemia,
  160**
Leukemia History, 160
Acute Myeloid Leukemia, 161
Epidemiology, 161
Clinical Features, 162
Laboratory Features, 163
Classifications, 166
Acute Lymphoblastic Leukemia, 175
Epidemiology, 175
Clinical Features, 175
Classifications, 176
Prognosis in Acute Lymphoblastic
  Leukemia, 179

CHAPTER 12
Chronic Myeloproliferative Disorders, 187
Kathy Finnegan

Chronic Myelogenous Leukemia, 189
Disease Overview, 189
Pathophysiology, 189

Clinical Features and Symptoms, 189
Peripheral Blood and Bone Marrow, 190
Diagnosis, 191
Treatment, 191
Prognosis, 191
Chronic Neutrophilic Leukemia, 192
Chronic Eosinophilic Leukemia, 192
Polycythemia Vera, 192
Disease Overview, 192
Pathophysiology, 192
Clinical Features and Symptoms, 192
Peripheral Blood and Bone Marrow
   Findings, 192
Diagnosis, 193
Treatment, 193
Prognosis, 194
Myelofibrosis With Myeloid
   Metaplasia, 194
Disease Overview, 194
Pathophysiology, 194
Clinical Features and Symptoms, 195
Peripheral Blood and Bone Marrow
   Findings, 195
Diagnosis, 195
Treatment, 195
Prognosis, 196
Essential Thrombocythemia, 196
Disease Overview, 196
Pathophysiology, 196
Clinical Features and Symptoms, 196
Peripheral Blood and Bone Marrow
   Findings, 197
Diagnosis, 197
Treatment, 197
Prognosis, 198

CHAPTER 13
Lymphoproliferative Disorders and Related
Plasma Cell Disorders, 205
   Betty Ciesla

Lymphoid Malignancies, 206
   Chronic Lymphocytic Leukemia, 206
   Hairy Cell Leukemia, 207

Sézary Syndrome, 208
Prolymphocytic Leukemia, 208
Hodgkin's and Non-Hodgkin's Lymphoma
   (Briefly), 208
Plasma Cell Disorders, 209
Normal Plasma Cell Structure and
   Function, 209
Multiple Myeloma, 210
Waldenström's Macroglobulinemia, 214

CHAPTER 14
The Myelodysplastic Syndromes, 219
   Betty Ciesla

Pathophysiology, 220
Chromosomal Abnormalities, 220
Common Features and Clinical
   Symptoms, 220
How to Recognize Dysplasia, 220
Classification of the Myelodysplastic
   Syndromes, 221
Specific Features of the World Health
   Organization Classification, 221
Prognostic Factors and Clinical
   Management, 222

PART IV   **HEMOSTASIS AND DISORDERS**
OF COAGULATION

CHAPTER 15
Overview of Hemostasis and Platelet
Physiology, 229
   Donna Castellone

History of Blood Coagulation, 230
Overview of Coagulation, 230
Vascular System, 231
Overview, 231
Mechanism of Vasoconstriction, 231
The Endothelium, 231
Events Following Vascular Injury, 231
Primary Hemostasis, 232
Platelets: An Introduction, 232
Platelet Development, 232

Platelet Structure and Biochemistry, 232
Platelet Function and Kinetics, 233
Platelet Aggregation Principle, 234
Secondary Hemostasis, 235
Classification of Coagulation Factors, 235
Physiological Coagulation (In Vivo), 237
Laboratory Model of Coagulation, 237
Extrinsic Pathway, 237
Intrinsic System, 238
Activated Partial Thromboplastin
Time, 238
Common Pathway, 238
Formation of Thrombin, 238
Feedback Inhibition, 239
Fibrinolysis, 239
Coagulation Inhibitors, 240
Kinin System, 240
Complement System, 240

CHAPTER 16
Quantitative and Qualitative Platelet Disorders, 245

Betty Ciesla

Quantitative Disorders of Platelets, 246
Thrombocytopenia Related to Sample
Integrity/Preanalytic Variables, 246
Thrombocytopenia Related to Decreased
Production, 246
Thrombocytopenia Related to Altered
Distribution of Platelets, 246
Thrombocytopenia Related to the Immune
Effect of Specific Drugs or Antibody
Formation, 246
Thrombocytopenia Related to Consumption
of Platelets, 247
Thrombocytosis, 249
**Inherited Qualitative Disorders of
Platelets, 249**
Disorders of Adhesion, 249
Platelet Release Defects, 251
Acquired Defects of Platelet Function, 251
**Vascular Disorders Leading to Platelet
Dysfunction, 252**

CHAPTER 17
Defects of Plasma Clotting Factors, 257

Betty Ciesla

**Evaluation of a Bleeding Disorder and
Types of Bleeding, 258**
The Classic Hemophilias, 258
The Factor VIII Molecule, 258
Symptoms in the Hemophilia A Patient,
258
Laboratory Diagnosis of Hemophilia
Patients, 260
Treatment for Hemophilia A Patients, 261
Quality of Life Issues for Hemophilia A
Patients, 261
Hemophilia B or Christmas Disease, 262
Congenital Factor Deficiencies With
Bleeding Manifestations, 262
Congenital Factor Deficiencies Where
Bleeding Is Mild or Absent, 262
Factor XIII Deficiency, 263
Bleeding Secondary to a Chronic Disease
Process, 263
The Role of Vitamin K in Hemostasis, 263
Vitamin K Deficiency and Subsequent
Treatment, 264

CHAPTER 18
**Fibrinogen, Thrombin, and the Fibrinolytic
System, 269**

Betty Ciesla

**The Role of Fibrinogen in Hemostasis,
270**
Disorders of Fibrinogen, 270
Afibrinogenemia, 270
Hypofibrinogenemia, 270
Dysfibrinogenemia, 271
**The Unique Role of Thrombin in
Hemostasis, 271**
Physiological Activators of Fibrinolysis, 272
Naturally Occurring Inhibitors of
Fibrinolysis, 272
Measurable Products of the Fibrinolytic
System, 273

Disseminated Intravascular Coagulation, 274

The Mechanism of Acute Disseminated Intravascular Coagulation, 274

Clinical Symptoms and Laboratory Results in Acute Disseminated Intravascular Coagulation, 275

Treatment in Acute Disseminated Intravascular Coagulation, 276

CHAPTER 19
Introduction to Thrombosis and Anticoagulant Therapy, 281

Mitra Taghizadeh

Physiological and Pathological Thrombosis, 282

Pathogenesis of Thrombosis, 282

Vascular Injury, 282

Platelet Abnormalities, 282

Coagulation Abnormalities, 283

Fibrinolytic Abnormalities, 283

Antithrombotic Factors (Coagulation Inhibitors), 283

Thrombotic Disorders, 284

Inherited Thrombotic Disorders, 284

Acquired Thrombotic Disorders, 286

Laboratory Diagnosis for Thrombotic Disorders, 288

Anticoagulant Therapy, 288

Antiplatelet Drugs, 288

Anticoagulant Drugs, 289

Thrombolytic Drugs, 289

PART V   LABORATORY PROCEDURES

CHAPTER 20
Basic Procedures in a Hematology Laboratory, 297

Lori Lentowski and Betty Ciesla

Microhematocrit, 298

Principle, 298

Reagents and Equipment, 298

Specimen Collection and Storage, 299

Quality Control, 299

Procedure, 299

Interpretation, 299

Calculating Red Blood Cell Indices, 300

Normal Average Values, 300

Modified Westergren Sedimentation Rate, 300

Principle, 300

Reagents and Equipment, 301

Specimen Collection and Storage, 301

Quality Control, 301

Procedure, 301

Normal Ranges, 301

Limitations, 301

Conditions Associated With…, 302

Manual Reticulocyte Procedure, 302

Principle, 302

Reagents and Equipment, 302

Specimen Collection and Storage, 302

Quality Control, 302

Procedure, 302

Normal Values, 302

Conditions Associated With…, 302

Limitations, 303

Reticulocyte Procedure With Miller Eye Disc, 303

Principle, 303

Reagents and Equipment, 303

Specimen Collection and Storage, 303

Quality Control, 303

Procedure, 303

Normal Values, 304

Conditions Associated With…, 304

Limitations, 304

Peripheral Smear Procedure, 304

Principle, 304

Reagents and Equipment, 304

Specimen Collection and Storage, 304

Quality Control, 304

Procedure, 304

Limitations, 305

Performing a Manual Differential and Assessing Red Blood Cell Morphology, 305

Principle, 305

Reagents and Equipment, 305

Specimen Collection and Storage, 305

Quality Control, 305

Procedure, 306

Unopette White Blood Cell/Platelet Count, 309

Principle, 309

Reagents and Equipment, 310

Specimen Collection and Storage, 310

Quality Control, 310

Procedure, 310

Cell Counts and Calculations, 311

Normal Values, 311

Limitations, 312

Sickle Cell Procedure, 312

Principle, 312

Reagents and Equipment, 312

Specimen Collection and Storage, 312

Quality Control, 312

Procedure, 312

Interpretation of Results and Result Reporting, 312

Limitations, 312

Cerebrospinal Fluid/Body Fluid Cell Count and Differential, 313

Principle, 313

Reagents and Equipment, 313

Specimen Collection and Storage, 313

Quality Control, 314

Procedure, 314

Prothrombin Time and Activated Partial Thromboplastin Time: Automated Procedure, 315

Principle, 315

Reagents and Equipment, 315

Specimen Collection and Storage, 316

Quality Control, 316

Procedure, 316

Results, 317

Limitations, 317

Qualitative D-Dimer Test, 318

Principle, 318

Reagents and Equipment, 319

Specimen Collection and Storage, 319

Quality Control, 319

Procedure, 319

Interpretation, 320

Results, 320

Limitations, 320

An Approach to Interpreting Automated Hematology Data, 320

Principle, 321

Instruments, 322

Flow Cytometry: The Basics in Hematology Interpretation, 326

Overview, 327

Principles, 327

Data Interpretation: One Role for the Medical Technologist, 327

Flow Cytometry Case Studies, 328

Answers to Chapter Review Questions, 331

Index, 337

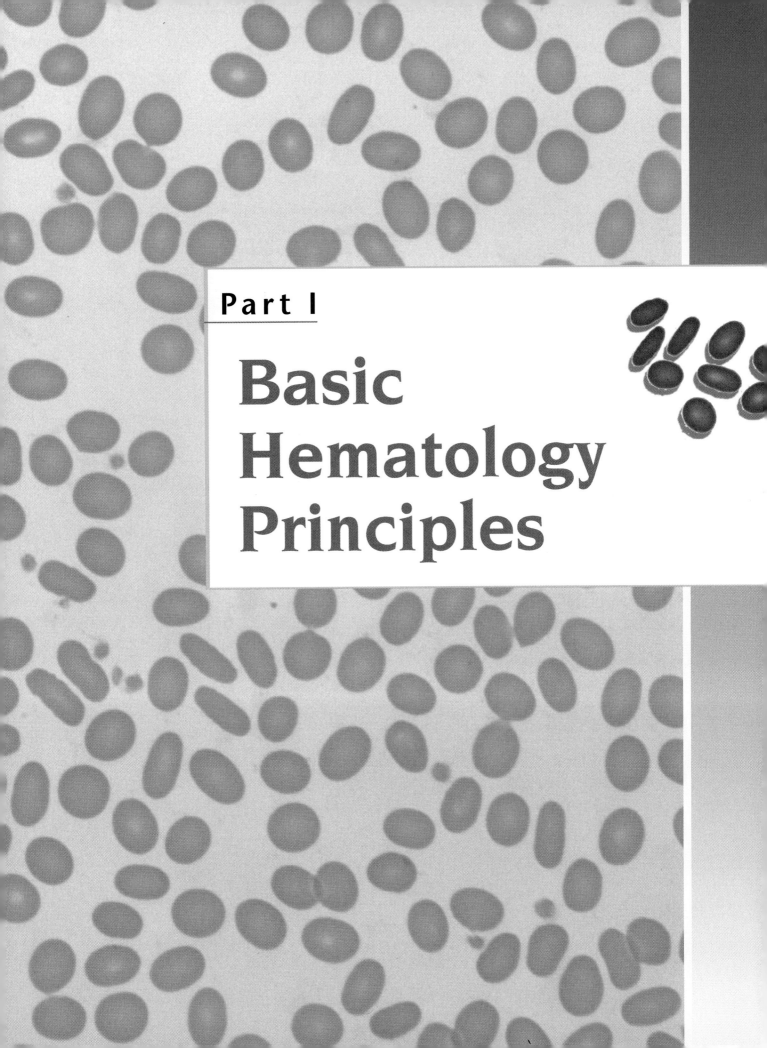

Part I

Basic Hematology Principles

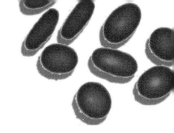

1

Introduction to Hematology and Basic Laboratory Practice

Betty Ciesla

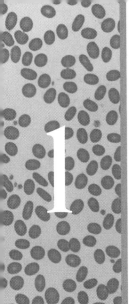

Introduction to Hematology

The Microscope

Significant Parts of the Microscope

Care of the Microscope

Corrective Actions in Light Microscopy

Innovations in Microscopy

Standard Precautions

Personal Protective Equipment

Safety Features Other Than Personal Protective Equipment

Chemical and Environmental Hazards

Basic Concepts of Quality Assurance Plans in the Hematology Laboratory

Quality Control Monitoring in the Hematology Laboratory

Normal, or Reference, Intervals

Delta Checks

Reflex Testing

Preanalytic Variables

Postanalytic Variables

Critical Results

Objectives

After completing this chapter, the student will be able to:

1. Describe the significance of the field of hematology in relation to sickness and health.

2. List the basic parts of the compound microscope.

3. Discuss the function and magnification of each of the microscope objectives.

4. Identify appropriate corrective actions when encountering routine problems with the operation of a microscope.

5. Define *standard precautions* as related to biological hazards.

6. Describe safe work practices for personal protective equipment and disposal of biological hazards.

7. Describe the components of quality assurance in the hematology laboratory.

8. Define the terms *preanalytic and postanalytic variables, delta checks, accuracy, precision, reproducibility,* and *reference intervals.*

9. Formulate a plan of action based on the troubleshooting scenarios presented within the text.

In its most fundamental form, hematology is the study of blood in health and in pathological conditions. Blood is the window to the body; it is a predictor of vitality, of long life. In ancient times, blood was worshipped. Men were bled to obtain a cure, and blood was studied for its mystical powers. It was an elevated bodily fluid. The discipline of hematology was an outgrowth of this fascination with blood. As we practice it in the clinical laboratory today, this discipline encompasses skill, art, and instinct. For those of us who are passionate about this subject, it is the art of hematology that so intrigues us. To view a peripheral smear and to have the knowledge not only to correctly identify the patient's hematological condition but also to predict how the bone marrow may have contributed to that condition is an awesome feeling. Hematology is about relationships: the relationship of the bone marrow to the systemic circulation, the relationship of the plasma environment to the red cell life span, and the relationship of the hemoglobin to the red cell. For most students, hematology is a difficult subject to master because it forces students to think in an unnatural way. Instructors are always asking, Why? Why does this cell appear in the peripheral smear? What relationship does it have to the bone marrow? How was it formed? Many students begin a hematology course with little foundation in blood cell morphology. They have no real grasp of medical terminology and few facts concerning blood diseases. They are not equipped to answer Why? As instructors, our goal is to guide the student toward an appreciation of his or her role as a clinical laboratorian in hematology. Certainly we can help the student to develop the morphological and analytic skills necessary for adept practice in the hematology laboratory. Yet, to be truly notable in this field, keen instincts concerning a set of results, a particular cell, or a patient history play a defining role.

Blood has always been a fascinating subject for authors, poets, scholars, and scientists. References to blood appear in hieroglyphics, in the Bible, in ancient pottery, and in literature. Hippocrates laid the foundation for hematology with his theory of the body's four humors—blood, phlegm, black bile, and yellow bile—and his concept that all blood ailments resulted from a disorder in the balance of these humors. Unfortunately, these principles remained unchallenged for 1400 years! Gradually, men of science such as Galen, Harvey, van Leeuwenhoek, Virchow, and Ehrlich were able to elevate hematology into a discipline of medicine with basic morphological observations that can be traced to a distinct **pathophysiology.** It is to these men that we owe a huge debt of gratitude. Although they had little in the way of advanced technology, their inventions and observations helped describe and quantify cells, cellular structure, and function. Much of what has been learned concerning the etiology of hematological disease has been discovered since the 1920s, and therefore hematology, as a distinct branch of medicine, is in its early stages.[1]

THE MICROSCOPE

The microscope is an essential tool to the hematology laboratory professional. It is a piece of equipment that is stylistically simple in design, yet extraordinarily complex in its ability to magnify an image, provide visual details of that image, and make the image visible to the human eye.[2] Most commonly used today are compound microscopes, which use two lens systems to magnify the image. The ocular devices on the microscope provide an initial ×10 magnification, and then additional magnification is obtained through the use of three or four different powered objectives.[3] A light source is located within the microscope base. Light is beamed to the image directly, or filters are used that vary the wavelength. In addition, a diaphragm apparatus is usually located in the base of the microscope. Opening or closing the diaphragm can optimize or reduce the volume of light directed toward the image.[4] This is most useful when examining cellular structures in the nucleus that need more light to be properly visualized. Below is a *brief* description of the most significant parts of the microscope

Significant Parts of the Microscope

The *eyepieces,* or *oculars,* are located laterally to the microscope base (Fig. 1.1) and function as an additional magnification component to the objective magnification. Most microscopes are binocular and contain two eyepieces, each of which will magnify the diameter of an object placed on the stage to the power of the eyepiece, usually ×10.

The *objectives* of the compound microscope are ×10, ×40, or ×100. Often, a ×50 (oil) magnification will be incorporated. Each objective has three numbers inscribed on the objective: a magnification number, an aperture number (NA), and a tube length number. The NA refers to the resolution power of the objective, the ability of the objective to gather light. The higher the NA number, the higher is the resolution. Tube length refers to the distance from the eyepiece to the objective. Magnification refers to how large the image will appear, as well as how much of the viewing field will be observed. Objectives on modern microscopes are com-

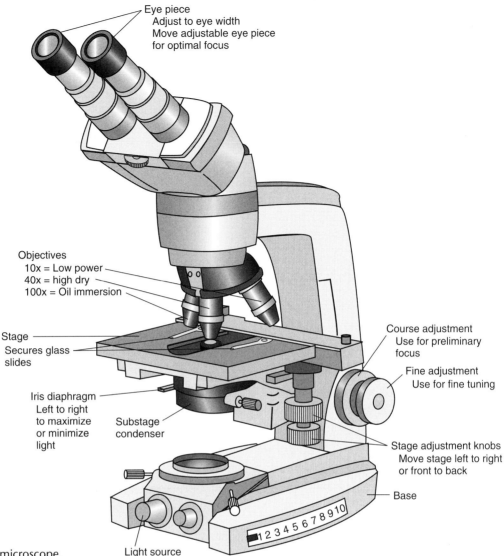

Eye piece
Adjust to eye width
Move adjustable eye piece
for optimal focus

Objectives
10x = Low power
40x = high dry
100x = Oil immersion

Stage
Secures glass
slides

Iris diaphragm
Left to right
to maximize
or minimize
light

Substage
condenser

Course adjustment
Use for preliminary
focus

Fine adjustment
Use for fine tuning

Stage adjustment knobs
Move stage left to right
or front to back

Base

Light source

Figure 1.1   Compound microscope.

posed of many lenses and prisms that produce an extremely high quality of optical performance.

The *iris diaphragm*, located below the microscope stage, increases or decreases light from the microscope light source. If the diaphragm is opened to its full capacity, the cell or structure is viewed with maximum light. If the diaphragm is minimally opened, the cell or structure is much less illuminated, which may be desirable depending on the source of the sample (i.e., hematological cells versus urine casts).

The *stage* is a flat surface with an opening created for light to pass through. Two flat metal clips have been mounted in which to secure the glass slide. Below the stage surface are two control knobs that move the slide in a horizontal or vertical fashion.

Coarse and *fine adjustment knobs* are located on either side of the microscope base. These adjustments

bring the image into focus through movement of the stage, which is either raised or lowered according to the level of focus needed.

Care of the Microscope

The microscope is an essential piece of equipment to the practice of hematology and must be handled with care and respect. Hematology instructors owe it to themselves to teach the care and maintenance of the microscope in hopes that these "best practices" can be adopted and practiced in the workplace. The microscope should be on a level, vibration-free surface. If it needs to be lifted from a storage cabinet to another location, the microscope must be secured on the bottom by one hand and held by the neck with the other hand. Additionally, users must be instructed on how to move objectives from one position to another without dragging non–oil objectives into oil from a slide left on the stage. The high-dry objectives must never be used with oil, only with coverslipped slides. Objectives are easily scratched or damaged by careless handlers; consequently, they must be cleaned with lens paper after each use. Oil objectives should be wiped free of oil when not in use, and eyepieces must be cleaned with lens paper from dust, dirt, or cosmetic debris with each viewing. Good microscopy habits should always be cultivated, practiced, and communicated. Microscopy guidelines should be posted in each area where microscopes are used. The guidelines should include

- General use of the microscope
- Instructions for transporting the microscope
- Instructions for proper cleaning of the microscope
- Storage guidelines that include proper position of microscope cording

Corrective Actions in Light Microscopy

Many of the problems that are encountered when using a microscope can be easily corrected by using common sense. Some of the most common "problems" in light microscopy are as follows:

- Image cannot be seen at any power—Try turning the slide over; perhaps the wrong side of the slide has been placed on the microscope stage.
- Fine details cannot be detected in immature cells—For immature cells, use the ×100 lens and open up both diaphragms to the maximum width, for maximum light.
- The ×40 objective is blurred—Try wiping off the ×100 lens; perhaps the ×100 lens was oil filled and was dragged across the slide.
- Dustlike particles appear on the slide but they are not large enough to be platelets—- Perhaps mascara has been left on the eyepiece; use lens cleaner to clean the eyepieces.

Innovations in Microscopy

Digital microscopy is gaining in popularity as a routine piece of equipment in hematology laboratories. Simply stated, these microscopes scan blood smears for cells, identify them, calculate a white blood cell differential count, and then store the cellular images of the cells for future review. Slides are then reviewed for red cell morphology and abnormalities by a trained operator.[5] The initial purchase cost is expensive, yet the speed, sensitivity, and reduced technologist time are making this an attractive option for larger laboratories.

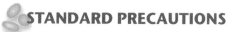 ## STANDARD PRECAUTIONS

The clinical laboratory presents an environment with many potential risks from biological hazards to chemical or fire hazards. Safety training has become a mandatory part of responsible employee practice, not only for employees themselves but also for their colleagues. Safety training sessions are an essential part of employee training. These sessions represent a lifeline toward optimal behavior should an employee encounter an unexpected hazard. Biological hazards constitute one of the more major risk areas, and this section focuses specifically on this area. Chemical and environmental hazards are briefly summarized. Most of the patient samples used in the hematology laboratory are derived from human body fluids (blood, organ or joint fluids, stools, urine, semen, etc.). Each of these is a potential source of bacterial, fungal, or viral infection; consequently, each sample is potentially hazardous. Laboratorians must protect themselves from contamination by observing practices that prevent direct contact with body fluids or a contaminated surface, contamination, or inhalation. In 1996, the Centers for Disease Control and Prevention issued a set of standard precautions aimed at creating a safe working environment for laboratory practice. These standard precautions combine principles of body substance isolation and universal precautions. The main features of standard precautions that relate to safe hematology laboratory practice include personal protective equipment (PPE) and safety features other than PPE.[6]

Personal Protective Equipment

PPE includes gloves, eye and face shields, countertop shields, and fluid-resistant gowns or laboratory coats.

Gloves

Gloves must be worn during any activity with potential for contact with bodily fluids. Gloves must be changed immediately if contaminated or damaged. When patient contact is initiated, gloves must be changed with each patient. Gloves are removed before exiting the laboratory for any purpose (Fig. 1.2).

Gowns and Laboratory Coats

Gowns and laboratory coats must be fluid resistant with long sleeves or wrist cuffs. They may not be worn outside of the laboratory and must be changed if con-

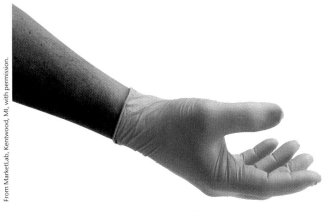

Figure 1.2 Gloves.

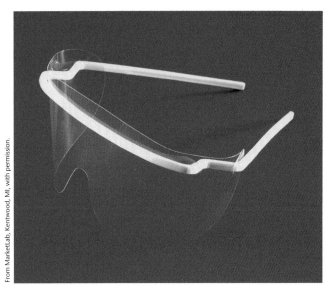

Figure 1.4 Eye protection.

taminated or torn. Disposable coats are treated as biohazardous material and discarded, whereas cloth coats are laundered by the hospital service.

Splash Shields (Face, Eye, Surface)

Goggles, face shields, masks, and Plexiglas countertop shields are used to minimize the risks of aerosol and specimen splashes. Although most automated instrumentation is cap piercing, there are many laboratory operations in which these precautions are vital to employee safety (Figs. 1.3 through 1.5; Table 1.1).

Safety Features Other Than Personal Protective Equipment

1. Handwashing is a basic yet most effective tool to prevent contamination. Soap and water must be used, and the handwashing procedure should include the wrists and at least a 10- to 15-second soap application. This soap application represents significantly more time than most individuals spend in handwashing. It cannot be stressed enough that proper handwashing using the recommended times is the first step in the decontamination **protocol.** Germicidal soaps are suggested. Hands must be washed with every patient contact, after gloves are removed, and if gloved or ungloved hands have been contaminated with a bodily fluid sample.

2. Care must be taken with contaminated sharps; needles, blades, pipettes, syringes, and glass

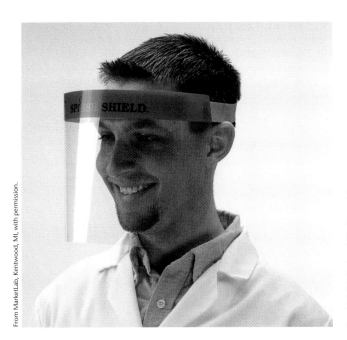

Figure 1.3 Face shield.

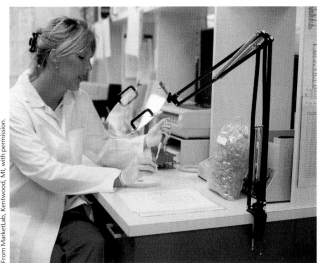

Figure 1.5 Biohazard shield with flexible arm.

Table 1.1 ● Personal Protective Equipment

- Gloves
- Fluid-resistant gowns
- Laboratory coats
- Goggles
- Face shield
- Mask
- Plexiglas countertop shield

slides must be placed in a leak-proof, puncture-proof, properly labeled biohazard container.

3. Mouth pipetting is never permitted, and other objects, such as pens, pencils, and so on, should be kept away from the mouth and mucous membranes.

4. Eating, drinking, and smoking in the laboratory area are strictly forbidden. Food or drink items should not be kept in the laboratory.

5. Notebooks, textbooks, and loose papers are not allowed in the laboratory work area.

6. Regarding issues of personal hygiene, long hair must be tied back, beards must be trimmed to no more than 1 inch in length, fingernails must be no longer than $1/4$ inch beyond the end of the finger, and with no jewelry ornamentation of the fingers.

7. Dangling jewelry (earrings or necklaces) is not allowed.

8. Cosmetics or lip balm cannot be applied.

Chemical and Environmental Hazards

The clinical laboratory is an area in which chemicals are handled and maintained. Clothing, body parts, and surface areas are all potential spill areas for hazardous chemicals. Each employee should understand and adhere to the chemical spill action plan. Additionally, employees who routinely handle chemicals should use goggles, avoid splashing, and stringently follow mixing guidelines. Environmental hazards are hazards such as fire hazards, electrical hazards, radioactive hazards, and physical hazards. The details of the corrective actions are listed next:

- Fire hazards—Be familiar with the fire evacuation route, fire blanket location, fire and extinguisher location.

- Electrical hazards—Be aware of frayed cords, unsafe practices such as wet hands on electrical sockets, and whether all electrical equipment is grounded.
- Radioactive hazards—There are areas in the laboratory where radioactive materials are used; persons in this area should wear a radioactive badge.
- Physical hazards—Dangling jewelry should be avoided, hair should be pulled back and contained, and close-toed shoes must be worn.

BASIC CONCEPTS OF QUALITY ASSURANCE PLANS IN THE HEMATOLOGY LABORATORY

Quality assurance is a comprehensive and systematic process that strives to ensure reliable patient results. This process includes every level of laboratory operation.[7] Phlebotomy services, competency testing, error analysis, standard protocols, PPE, quality control, and turnaround time are each a key factor in the quality assurance system (Table 1.2). From the time a sample arrives in the laboratory until the results are reported, a rigorous quality assurance system is the key feature in ensuring quality results. Each part of the quality assurance plan or process should be analyzed, monitored, and reconfigured as necessary to emphasize excellence at every outcome. Although many hospitals and research facilities have "quality" professionals who provide oversight for quality assurance plans for their facilities, an elemental understanding of terms related to the total quality assurance plan is required of all staff technologists and students.

Table 1.2 ● Short List of Quality Assurance Indicators

- Number of patient redraws
- Labeling errors
- Patient and specimens properly identified
- Critical values called
- Pass rate on competency testing
- Test cancellation
- Integrity of send-out samples
- Employee productivity
- Errors in data entry
- Testing turnaround times
- Delays due to equipment failures or maintenance
- Performance on proficiency testing

Quality control is a large part of the quality assurance program at most facilities. Students will be introduced to the term *quality control* early and often. It is an essential function in the clinical laboratory. The information that follows provides a brief overview of the quality control procedures used in promoting quality assurance in the hematology laboratory. It is not intended to be comprehensive but introduces terminology and concepts pertinent to the entry-level professional.

Quality Control Monitoring in the Hematology Laboratory

The analytical component, or the actual measurement of the analyte in body fluids, is monitored in the laboratory by quality control, a component of the laboratory quality assurance plan. Similar to the chemistry laboratory, the analytic method in the hematology laboratory primarily includes instrumentation and reagents. *Standards,* or *calibrators,* are solutions that have a known amount of an analyte and are used to calibrate the method. A standard, or calibrator, has one assigned, or fixed, value.[7] For example, the hemoglobin standard is 12 g/100 mL, meaning that there is exactly 12 g of hemoglobin in 100 mL of solution. Conversely, controls, or control materials, are used to monitor the performance of a method after calibration. Control materials are assayed concurrently with patient samples, and the analyte value for the controls is calculated from the calibration data in the same manner as the unknown or patient's results are calculated.[7]

Control materials are commercially available as stable or liquid materials that are analyzed concurrently with the unknown samples. The control material measured values are compared with their expected values or target range. Acceptance or rejection of the unknown (patient) sample results is dependent on this evaluation process.

A **statistical quality control system** is used to establish the target range. The procedure involves obtaining at least 20 control values for the analyte to be measured. Ideally, the repeated control results should be the same; however, there will always be variability in the assay. The concept of clustering of the data points about one value is known as central tendency. The mean, mode, and median are statistical parameters used to measure the central tendency. The mean is the arithmetic average of a group of data points; the mode is the value occurring most frequently; and the median is the middle value of a dataset. If the mean, mode, and the median are nearly the same for the control values, the data have a normal distribution.[7]

The standard deviation and coefficient of variation are a measure of the spread of the data within the distribution about the mean. Standard deviation is a precision measurement that describes the average "distance" of each data point from the mean in a normal distribution. This measurement is mathematically calculated for a group of numbers. If the measured control values follow a normal distribution curve, 68.6% of the measured values fall within the mean and one standard deviation (SD) from the mean, 95.5% falls within the mean and two standard deviations (2SD) from the mean, and 99.7% fall within the mean and three standard deviations (3SD) from the mean. The 95.5% confidence interval is the accepted limit for the clinical laboratory.

Coefficient of variation (CV) is the standard deviation expressed as a percentage. The lower the CV, the more precise are the data. The usual CV for laboratory results is less than 5%, which indicated that the distribution is tighter around the mean value.[8]

Clarifying *accuracy* and *precision* is usually a troublesome task as these terms are often used interchangeably. When a test result is accurate, it means that it has come closest to the correct value if the reference or correct value is known. In most cases, once a methodology has been established for a particular analysis, standard or reference material is run to establish a reference interval. Accuracy is defined as the best estimate of the result to the true value.[9]

Precision relates to reproducibility and repeatability of test samples using the same methodology. Theoretically, patient results should be repeatable if analyzed a number of times using the same method. If there is great variability of results around a target value, then the precision is compromised[8] (Fig. 1.6).

Normal, or Reference, Intervals

Normal, or reference, intervals are values that have been established for a particular analyte, method, or instrument and a particular patient population. To establish a reference interval, the size of the sample must be at least 25 and should represent healthy male and female adults as well as the pediatric population. Once the test samples have been analyzed under predetermined conditions, a set reference value is determined from which reference limits and reference intervals may be established according to statistical methods. Subsequent patient samples will be compared to the reference interval to determine if they are normal or outside of the reference interval.[10]

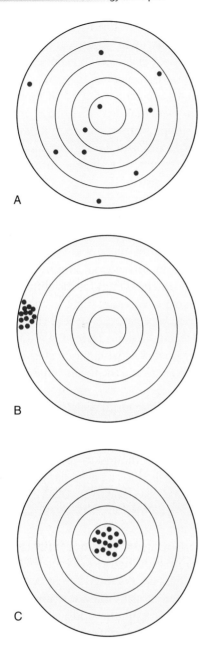

Figure 1.6 Is it accurate or precise? *(A)* Shots are neither accurate nor precise. *(B)* Shots are precise but miss the mark, not accurate. *(C)* Shots are accurate and precise.

Delta Checks

Delta checks are a function of the laboratory information system. This function allows the operator to perform a historical check on the sample from the previous results. If the variation in patient sample exceeds the established standard set for delta checks, a cause must be identified. Preanalytic problems, misidentified samples, analytical errors, or changes in the patient condition may contribute to erratic delta checks.

Reflex Testing

If automated complete blood count (CBC) results present a flagging signal, operations must be performed by the technologist to validate this sample. Usually flags are displayed next to a specific result. For example, an "H" indicates high results, while an "L" indicates low results. However, multiple flags may be generated for the entire CBC. Manual methods may be needed, or additional tests (e.g., adding a differential count or manual slide review) may need to be performed on the sample to present accurate test results. Technologists should be vigilant when hematological data are flagged, because it almost always means that the sample has some abnormality.

Preanalytic Variables

Preanalytic variables refer to any factors that may affect the sample before testing. Some issues to be considered are whether the sample was properly identified, properly collected in the correct **anticoagulant**, and delivered to the testing facility in a timely fashion. See Table 1.3 for a list of preanalytic variables.

Postanalytic Variables

This term refers to operations that ensure the integrity of sample results. Some examples are proper documentation of test results, timely reporting of results to a designated individual if a critical result was observed, and proper handling of samples that may involve calculations or dilutions. See Table 1.4 for postanalytic variables.

Table 1.3 ○ Preanalytic Variables

- Proper patient identification
- Properly labeled tubes
- Proper anticoagulant
- Proper mixing of sample
- Timely delivery to laboratory
- Tubes checked for clots
- Medications administered to the patient
- Previous blood transfusions
- Intravenous line contamination
- Blood sample properly collected (proper tube, proper anticoagulant)

Critical Results

Critical results are those results that exceed or are markedly decreased from the reference range or the patient's history of results. These results are usually flagged by the automated instrument. It is essential that either the physician or the appropriate designee be notified immediately by a member of the reporting laboratory, as many critical results involve immediate medical or patient care decisions.

Table 1.4 ● Postanalytic Variables

- Delta checks
- Results released
- Critical results called
- Reflex testing initiated
- Specimen check for clots

CONDENSED CASE

A purple top tube was received from the emergency department on a 24-year-old man with a possible gastrointestinal bleed. A hemoglobin and hematocrit were ordered. Once the sample was run through the automated instrumentation, a clot was detected. A redrawn sample was ordered and again the same thing occurred—a clotted sample. Name three reasons for a clotted sample.

Answer

Clotted samples may occur if (A) the phlebotomy was difficult, (B) the sample was not inverted at least eight times, or (C) the tube was expired.

Summary Points

- Hematology is the study of blood in health and disease.
- Morphological and analytical skills are needed in the practice of hematology.
- Compound microscopes have a two-lens system to magnify the image.
- The objectives of the microscope are ×10, ×40, and ×100; a ×50 oil immersion lens may be added.
- Proper care of the microscope is essential for maintaining microscopic quality.
- Standard precautions involve behaviors that prevent contact with bodily fluids, aerosol contamination, or contaminated surfaces.
- PPE includes gloves, eyewear, laboratory coats, face shields, and fluid-resistant gowns.
- Handwashing is the most important element of standard precautions.
- Quality assurance is a set of laboratory practices that ensure reliable outcomes for patient results.
- Quality control is part of the quality assurance plan and consists of standards, controls, normal distribution, and statistical parameters.
- Accuracy and precision are measured by the mean standard deviation around a set of data points.
- Patient identification is the essential first step in ensuring the quality of laboratory results.
- Preanalytic variables refer to events or circumstances that occur to the unknown sample before analysis.
- Postanalytic variables refer to laboratory practice after the sample has been analyzed.
- Critical results are those results that exceed or are markedly decreased from the reference interval.

CASE STUDY

A technologist in the hematology laboratory has been observed wearing blood-spattered gloves. Her colleagues in the laboratory are uncomfortable working with her, and they have confronted her on this issue. Her explanation for her behavior is that gloves are expensive and that frequent changing leads to excessive spending on gloves and other disposables. Her colleagues are concerned for their safety, and because they have been unsuccessful in changing her behavior, they consult the hematology supervisor for guidance. How should this employee be counseled?

(continued on following page)

(Continued)

Insights to the Case Study

The employee is jeopardizing the health of her co-workers because of her noncompliance. Standard laboratory precautions clearly state that she is to remove soiled or contaminated gloves and replace them with clean gloves. She should be counseled as such. Although her concern for the laboratory budget is commendable, issues of finances are under the auspices of administration and not a matter for her concern. The employee needs to review the safety manual, a mandatory document that she has already signed stating that she understands and will comply with all of the safety requirements of the laboratory.

Review Questions

1. Standard precautions involve
   a. behavior that prevents contact with virally infected patients.
   b. behavior that prevents direct contact with bodily fluids or contaminated surfaces.
   c. behavior that prevents contact with pediatric patients.
   d. behavior that prevents contact with terminally ill patients.

2. Which one of the following is considered personal protective equipment?
   a. Operating room attire
   b. Head nets
   c. Laboratory coats
   d. White shoes

3. What types of samples are used primarily in the clinical laboratory?
   a. Blood and bodily fluids
   b. Solid organs

   c. Bone
   d. Skin

4. Which setting(s) on the microscope is (are) used for focusing?
   a. Oculars
   b. Stage
   c. Diaphragm
   d. Coarse and fine adjustments

5. Which one of the following is a postanalytic factor?
   a. Calling results when a critical value is noticed
   b. Tube checked for clots
   c. Patient identification
   d. Sample mixing

6. The proper definition for a *standard* is
   a. materials used to monitor a method.
   b. normal distribution curve.
   c. a target range.
   d. solutions with a known amount of the analyte.

⊙ TROUBLESHOOTING

What Do I Do When the Results Fail the Delta Check?

A sample was received into the laboratory on a patient who has been admitted 70 hours earlier. Several results on the patient, a white man, had changed dramatically since the last CBC results were evaluated in the hematology laboratory. The results in questions are marked by an asterisk. Please refer to Chapter 2 for definitions of abbreviations.

Test	Saturday	Sunday	Unit of Measure	Reference Range
WBC	18.1*	13.7	$\times 10^9$/L	4.8 to 10.8
RBC	3.55*	4.94	$\times 10^{12}$/L	4.7 to 6.1
Hgb	11.4*	15.4	g/dL	14 to 18
Hct	32.1*	44.5	%	37 to 47

Test	Saturday	Sunday	Unit of Measure	Reference Range
MCV	90.3	90.1	fL	80 to 100
MCH	32.0	32.0	pg	27 to 31
MCHC	35.4	34.7	%	31 to 36
RDW	13.0	12.1	%	11.5 to 14.5
Platelets	152	261	$\times 10^3/\mu L$	150 to 350

The parameters that are marked with an asterisk (*) have failed the delta check. What can account for the variation in the patient's results in a 24-hour period? An investigation was begun. There are two likely possibilities. *Is there a medical explanation for the change in results, or is this a preanalytic variable (mislabeling; i.e., wrong patient results)?* The white blood cell count, red blood cell count, hemoglobin, and hematocrit have dramatically changed from Saturday to Sunday. A frequent explanation for this is blood transfusions being administered to the patient and causing an increment in red blood cell count, hemoglobin, and hematocrit. This patient had no transfusion history and the previous results do not indicate transfusion need; therefore, this is not considered a factor in the dramatically increased values. The technologist requested that the blood bank ABO type both samples. Both samples typed as O positive. No new information was obtained from this procedure. The laboratory then began another line of investigation. The floor was called and the laboratory was informed that the patient whose laboratory results were being called (the Sunday sample) had been discharged the previous day. The sample in question (the Sunday sample) was incorrectly identified. How could the mislabeling take place? The patient's name **had not** been removed from the room or from the computer system. The labeling had not taken place at the bedside, with voice confirmation by the patient. Instead, the sample had been labeled based on the room number alone. Due to the diligence of the laboratory staff, the mistakes were identified and any further adverse complications were prevented. The sample that the laboratory has received was actually the blood from the new patient who now occupied the room.

WORD KEY

Anticoagulant • Agent that prevents or delays blood coagulation

Pathophysiology • Study of how normal processes are altered by disease

Protocols • Formal ideas, plan, or scheme concerning patient care, bench work, administration, or research

References

1. Wintrobe M. Milestones on the path of progress. In: Wintrobe M, ed. Blood, Pure and Eloquent. New York: McGraw-Hill, 1980; 1–27.
2. Abramowitz M. Microscope: Basic and Beyond. Vol. 1. Melville, NY: Olympus America Inc, 2003; 1.25.
3. Wallace MA. Care and use of the microscope. In: Rodak B, ed. Hematology: Clinical Principles and Applications, 2nd ed. Philadelphia: WB Saunders, 2002; 32–34.
4. Strasinger SA, Di Lorenzo MS. Use of the microscope. In: Strasinger SA, Di Lorenzo MS, eds. Urinalysis and Body Fluids, 4th ed. Philadelphia: FA Davis, 2001; 73.
5. Patton M. Advances in microscopy. ADVANCE for Medical Laboratory Professionals 15:21–23, 2003.
6. Strasinger SA, Di Lorenzo MS. Safety in the clinical laboratory. In: Strasinger SA, Di Lorenzo MS, eds. Urinalysis and Bodily Fluids, 4th ed. Philadelphia: FA Davis, 2001; 2–5.
7. Koepke JA. Quality control and quality assurance. In Steine-Martin EA, Lotspeich-Steininger CA, Koepke JA, eds. Clinical Hematology: Principles, Procedures and Correlation, 2nd ed. Philadelphia: Lippincott, 1998; 567.
8. Finch SA. Safety in the hematology laboratory. In: Rodak BF, ed. Hematology: Clinical Principles and Applications, 2nd ed. Philadelphia: WB Saunders, 2003; 4–5.
9. Kellogg MD. Quality assurance. In: Anderson SK, Cockayne S, eds. Clinical Chemistry: Concepts and Applications. New York: McGraw-Hill, 2003; 47–49.
10. Sasse EA. Reference intervals and clinical decisions limits. In: Kaplan LA, Pesce AH, eds. Clinical Chemistry: Theory, Analysis and Correlations, 3rd ed. St. Louis: Mosby, 1996; 366–368.

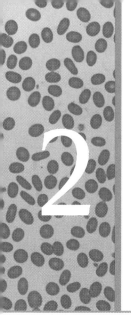

2

From Hematopoiesis to the Complete Blood Count

Betty Ciesla

Hematopoiesis: The Origin of Cell Development

The Spleen as an Indicator Organ of Hematopoietic Health
    The Functions of the Spleen
    Potential Risks of Splenectomy

The Bone Marrow and the Myeloid: Erythroid Ratio

Alterations in the M:E Ratio

The Role of Stem Cells and Cytokines

Erythropoietin

The Role of the Laboratory Professional in the Bone Marrow Procedure

Bone Marrow Procedure

Bone Marrow Report

The Complete Blood Count

The Morphological Classification of the Anemias

Calculating Red Cell Indices and Their Role in Sample Integrity

The Value of the Red Cell Distribution Width

Critical Values

The Clinical Approach to Anemias

The Value of the Reticulocyte Count

Objectives

After completing this chapter, the student will be able to:

1. Define the components of hematopoiesis.

2. Describe the organs used for hematopoiesis throughout fetal and adult life.

3. Define the microenvironment and the factors affecting differentiation of the pluripotent stem cell (PSC).

4. Discuss the four functions of the spleen.

5. Differentiate between intramedullary and extramedullary hematopoiesis.

6. Define the myeloid:erythroid ratio.

7. Review the bone marrow procedure, methods and materials, and the technologist's role in ensuring that bone marrow was recovered.

8. List the components of the complete blood count (CBC).

9. Calculate red blood indices.

10. Describe clinical conditions that cause valid shifts in the mean corpuscular volume.

11. Recognize normal and critical values in an automated CBC.

12. Describe ineffective and effective erythropoiesis.

13. Define the importance of correlation checks in a CBC.

14. Describe the clinical conditions that may produce polychromatophilic cells and elevate the reticulocyte count.

15. Define the morphological classification of anemias.

16. Summarize the symptoms of anemia.

HEMATOPOIESIS: THE ORIGIN OF CELL DEVELOPMENT

Hematopoiesis is defined as the production, development, differentiation, and maturation of all blood cells. Within these four functions is cellular machinery that outstrips most high-scale manufacturers in terms of production quotas, customs specifications, and quality of final product. When one considers that the bone marrow is able to produce 3 billion red cells, 1.5 billion white cells, and 2.5 billion platelets per day per body weight,[1] the enormity of this task in terms of output is almost incomprehensible. Within the basic bone marrow structure lies the mechanism to

1. constantly supply the peripheral circulation with mature cells.
2. mobilize the bone marrow to increase production if hematological conditions warrant.
3. compensate for decreased hematopoiesis by providing for hematopoietic sites outside of the bone marrow (non-bone marrow sites, the liver and spleen).

The bone marrow is extremely versatile and serves the body well by supplying life-giving cells with a multiplicity of functions. Various organs serve a role in hematopoiesis, and these organs differ from fetal to adult development. The yolk sac, liver, and spleen are the focal organs in fetal development. From 2 weeks until 2 months in fetal life, most erythropoiesis takes place in the fetal yolk sac. This period of development, the mesoblastic period, produces primitive erythroblasts and embryonic hemoglobins (Hgbs) such as Hgb Gower I and Gower II and Hgb Portland. These Hgbs are constructed as tetramers with two alpha chains combined with either epsilon or zeta chains. As embryonic Hgbs, they do not survive into adult life and do not participate in oxygen delivery. During the hepatic period, which continues from 2 through 7 months of fetal life, the liver and spleen take over the hematopoietic role (Fig. 2.1). White cells and megakaryocytes begin to appear in small numbers. The liver serves as an erythroid-producing organ primarily but also gives rise to fetal Hgb, which consists of alpha and gamma chains. The spleen, thymus, and lymph nodes also become hematopoietically active during this stage, producing red cells and lymphocytes; from 7 months until birth, the bone marrow assumes the primary role in hematopoiesis, a role that continues into adult life. Additionally, Hgb A, the majority adult Hgb (alpha 2, beta 2), begins to form. The full complement of Hgb A is not realized until 3 to 6 months postpartum, as gamma chains from hemoglobin F are diminished and beta chains are increased.

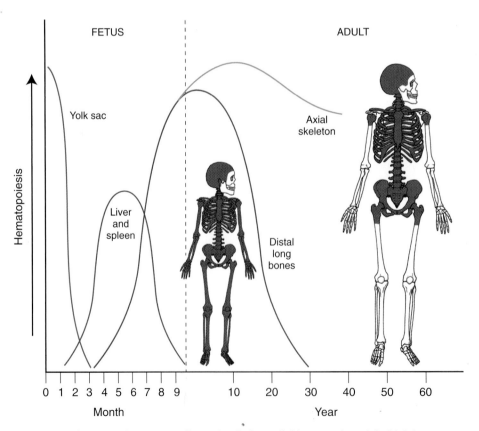

Figure 2.1   Marrow formation in fetus *(left)* versus the adult *(right)*

Hematopoiesis within the bone marrow is termed *intramedullary hematopoiesis*. The term *extramedullary hematopoiesis* describes hematopoiesis outside the bone marrow environment, primarily the liver and spleen. Because these organs play major roles in early fetal hematopoiesis, they retain their hematopoietic memory and capability. The liver and spleen can function as organs of hematopoiesis if needed in adult life. Several circumstances within the bone marrow (infiltration of leukemic cells, tumor, etc.) may diminish the marrow's normal hematopoietic capability and force these organs to once again perform as primary or fetal organs of hematopoiesis. If extramedullary hematopoiesis develops, the liver and spleen become enlarged, a condition known as **hepatosplenomegaly.** Physical evidence of hepatosplenomegaly will be an individual who looks puffy and protrusive in the left upper abdominal area. Hepatosplenomegaly is always an indicator that hematological health is compromised.

THE SPLEEN AS AN INDICATOR ORGAN OF HEMATOPOIETIC HEALTH

Few organs can match the versatility of the spleen. This small but forgotten organ is a powerhouse of prominent red cell activity such as filtration, production, and cellular immunity. Under normal circumstances, the organ cannot be felt or palpated on physical examination. This fist-shaped organ, located on the left side of the body under the rib cage, weighs about 8 ounces, is soft in texture, and receives 5% of the cardiac output per minute. The spleen, a blood-filled organ, consists of red pulp, white pulp, and the marginal zone. The function of the red pulp is primarily red cell filtration, whereas the white pulp deals with lymphocyte processing and the marginal zone with storage of white cells and platelets.

The Functions of the Spleen

There are four main tasks of the spleen that relate to red cell viability and the spleen's immunologic capability. The first function is the reservoir, or storage, function of the spleen. The spleen harbors one third of the circulating mass of platelets and one third of the granulocyte mass and may be able to mobilize platelets into the peripheral circulation as necessary. In the event of splenic rupture or trauma, large numbers of platelets may be spilled into the peripheral circulation. This event may predispose to unwanted clotting events, because platelets serve as catalysts for hemostasis. The second function of the spleen is the filtration function. The spleen has a unique inspection mechanism and examines each red cell and platelet for abnormalities and inclusions. Older red cells may lose their elasticity and deformability in the last days of their 120-day life span and are culled from the circulation by splenic phagocytes. Bilirubin, iron, and globin byproducts released through the culling process are recycled through the plasma and circulation.

Red cells that are filled with inclusions (Howell Jolly bodies, Heinz bodies, Pappenheimer bodies, etc.) are selectively reviewed and cleared. Inclusions are "pitted" and pulled from the red cell without destroying the cellular integrity, and red cells are left to continue their journey through the circulation.[2] Antibody-coated red cells have their antibodies removed and usually reappear in the peripheral circulation as spherocytes, a smaller, more compact red cell structure with a shortened life span. One of the least appreciated roles of the spleen is the immunologic role. As the largest secondary lymphoid organ, the spleen plays a valuable role in the promotion of phagocytic activity for encapsulated organisms such as *Haemophilus influenzae, Streptococcus pneumoniae,* or *Neisseria meningitidis.* The spleen provides opsonizing antibodies, substances that strip the capsule from the bacterial surface. Once this is accomplished, the unencapsulated bacteria is more vulnerable to the phagocytic **reticuloendothelial system (RES)**[3] and less able to mount an infection to the host system. Without a functioning spleen, this important function is negated and can lead to serious consequences, including fatality, for the infected individual. The final function of the spleen is its hematopoietic function, discussed earlier in this chapter.

Potential Risks of Splenectomy

Spleens that are enlarged, infarcted , or minimally functioning can cause difficulty for patients and these conditions are discussed in later chapters. Traditionally, the spleen was seen as an inconsequential organ, easily discarded and one that was not necessary to life function. While it is true that the splenectomy procedure may provide hematological benefit to patients who have problems with their spleen, it is equally true that individuals who do not have spleens have additional risks, as mentioned earlier. There have been reports in the literature of overwhelming postsplenectomy infections (OPSIs) that may occur years after the spleen has been removed. In most cases, these infections occur within 3 years, but they have been reported as long as 25 years after the splenectomy. Many individuals die from OPSIs or at the very least have multiorgan involvement. As an organ of the hematopoietic system, the spleen has

Table 2.1 ⊙ Functions of the Spleen

Hematopoietic function Can produce white cell, red cells, and platelets if necessary

Reservoir function One third of platelets and granulocytes are stored in the spleen

Filtration function Aging red cells are destroyed, spleen removes inclusion from red cells, if red cell membrane is less deformable or antibody-coated spleen presents a hostile environment leading to production of spherocytes

Immunologic function Opsonizing antibodies produced, trapping and processing antigens from encapsulated organs

immense capability and provides a high value and versatility (Table 2.1). If splenic removal is decided upon, the surgeon should leave some splenic tissue in place and carefully manage the asplenic patient; asplenic individuals represent a more vulnerable population.

THE BONE MARROW AND THE MYELOID:ERYTHROID RATIO

The bone marrow is one of the largest organs of the body, encompassing 3% to 6% of body weight and weighing 1500 g in the adult.[4] It is hard to conceptualize the bone marrow as an organ, because it is not a solid organ that one can easily touch, measure, or weigh. Because bone marrow tissue is spread throughout the body, one can visualize it only in that context. It is composed of yellow marrow, red marrow, and an intricate supply of nutrients and blood vessels. Within this structure are erythroid cells (red cells), myeloid cells (white cells), and megakaryocytes (platelets) in various stages of maturation, along with osteoclasts, stoma, and fatty tissue.[5] Mature cells enter the peripheral circulation via the bone marrow sinuses, a central structure lined with endothelial cells that provide passage for mature cells from extravascular sites to the circulation (Fig. 2.2). The cause and effect of hematological disease usually find root in the bone marrow, the central factory for production of all adult hematopoietic cells. In the first 18 years of life, bone marrow is spread throughout all of the major bones of the skeleton, especially the long bones. Gradually, as the body develops, the marrow is replaced by fat until the prime locations for bone marrow in the adult are the iliac crest, located in the pelvic area, and the sternum, located in the chest area. In terms of cellu-

larity, there is a unique ratio in the bone marrow termed the *myeloid:erythroid (M:E)* ratio. This numerical designation provides an approximation of the myeloid elements in the marrow and their precursor cells and the erythroid elements in the marrow and their precursor cells. The normal ratio of 3 to 4:1 reflects the relationship between production and life span of the various cell types. White cells have a much shorter life span than red cells, 6 to 10 hours for neutrophils as opposed to 120 days for erythrocytes,[5] and thus need to be produced at a much higher rate for normal hematopoiesis.

ALTERATIONS IN THE MYELOID:ERYTHROID RATIO

The M:E ratio is sensitive to hematological factors that may impair red cell life span, inhibit overall production, or cause dramatic increases in a particular cell line. Each of these conditions reflects bone marrow dynamics through alterations of the M:E ratio. Many observations in the peripheral smear can be traced back to the pathophysiological events at the level of bone marrow. A perfect example of this is the bone marrow's response to anemia. As anemia develops and becomes more severe, the patient becomes symptomatic and the kidney senses **hypoxia** due to a decreased Hgb level. Tissue hypoxia stimulates an increased release of erythropoietin (EPO), a red cell-stimulating hormone, from the kidney. EPO travels through the circulation and binds with a receptor on the youngest of bone marrow precursor cells, the pronormoblast. The bone marrow has the capacity to expand production six to eight times in response to an anemic event.[6] Consequently, the bone marrow delivers reticulocytes and nucleated red blood cells to the peripheral circulation prematurely if the kidney senses hypoxic stress. What will be observed in the peripheral blood smear is polychromasia (stress reticulocytes, large polychromatophilic red cells) and nucleated red cells. Both of these cell types indicate that the bone marrow is regenerating in response to an event. This dynamic represents the harmony between bone marrow and peripheral circulation.

THE ROLE OF STEM CELLS AND CYTOKINES

A unique feature to the bone marrow microenvironment is the presence of stem cells. These multipotential cells resemble lymphocytes and are available in the bone marrow in the ratio of one stem cell for every 1000 non-stem cell elements.[1] Stem cells were demonstrated in the classic experiment of Till and McCullugh in

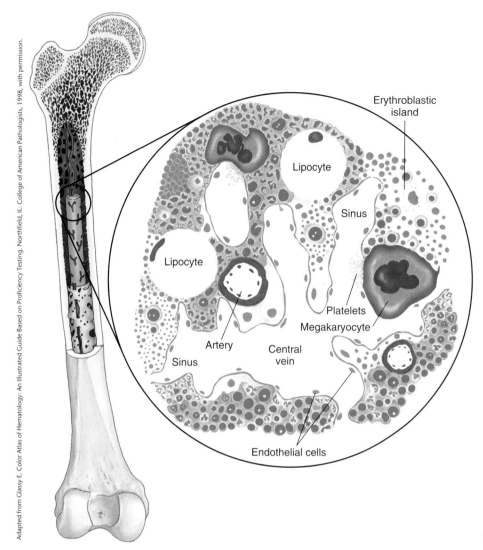

Figure 2.2 Internal structure of the bone marrow.

1961. These investigators irradiated the spleens and bone marrows of mice, rendering them acellular, and then injected them with bone marrow cells. Within days, colonies appeared on the spleens of the mice and were referred to as colony-forming units-spleen (CFU-S), with cells capable of regenerating into mature hematopoietic cells. In present-day terminology, CFU-S are the pluripotential stem cells (Fig. 2.3). Multipotential stem cells are capable of differentiation into nonlymphoid or lymphoid precursor committed cells.[7] Nonlymphoid committed cells will develop into the entire white cell, red cell, or megakaryocytic family (CFU-GEMM). The lymphocytic committed cell (LSC) will develop into T cells or B cells, which are of different origins. T cells are responsible for cellular immunity (cell-to-cell communication), whereas B cells are responsible for humoral immunity, the production of circulating antibodies directed by plasma cells. Each of these committed cells evolves into their adult form

through proliferation, differentiation, and maturation. Chemical signals such as cytokines and interleukins are uniquely responsible for promoting a specific lineage of cell. Most of these substances are glycoproteins that will target specific cell stages. They control replication, clonal or lineage selection and are responsible for maturation rate and growth inhibition of stem cells.[8] Many cytokines are available as pharmaceutical products. Recombinant technology has made it possible to purify and produce cytokines such as EPO, granulocyte-colony stimulating factor (G-CSF), and granulocyte-macrophage colony-stimulating factor (GM-CSF). These products are used to stimulate a specific cell production to yield therapeutic benefit for the patient. Specific conditions in which recombinant cytokines have been useful are as follows[9]:

1. Recovery from neutropenia resulting from **myelotoxic** therapy

2. Graft versus host disease after bone marrow transplant therapy
3. To increase white counts in patients with AIDS on antiretroviral therapy

An abbreviated list of cytokines and the cell lines they stimulate is included in Table 2.2.

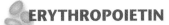

ERYTHROPOIETIN

Erythropoietin (EPO), a cytokine, is a hormone produced by the kidneys that functions as a targeted erythroid growth factor. This hormone has the ability to stimulate red cell production through a receptor on the pronormoblast, the youngest red cell precursor in the

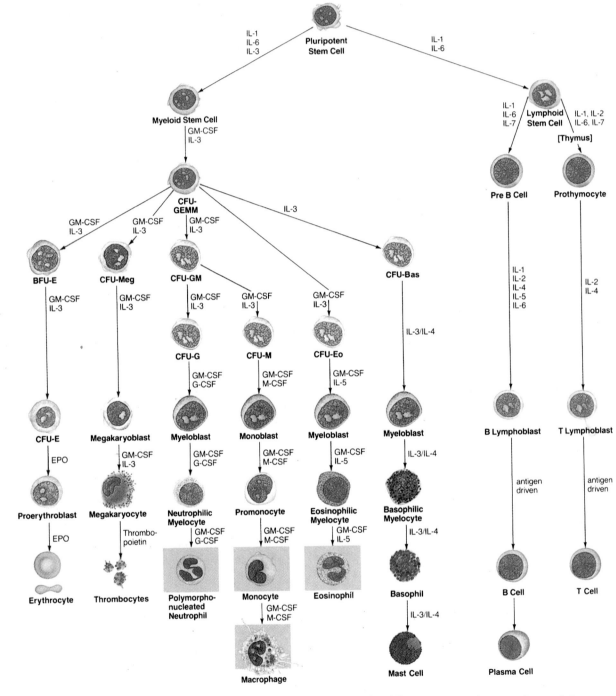

Figure 2.3   Blood cell formation from stem cells to mature cells. Notice the differentiation and maturation path from stem cells, through the CFU-GEMM to the LSC, terminating in mature cells into the peripheral circulation. IL, interleukin; CFU, colony-forming unit, GEMM, granulocyte, erythrocyte, monocyte, macrophage; LSC, lymphoid stem cell.

Table 2.2 ⊙ Abbreviated List of Cytokines and Growth Factors	
Cytokine	Cell Modifier
IL-2	T cells, B cells, NK cells
IL-3	Multilineage stimulating factor
IL-4	B cells, T cells, mast cells
IL-6	Stem cells, B cells
IL-7	Pre-B cells, T cells, early granulocytes
IL-11	Megakaryocytes
GM-CSF	Granulocytes, macrophages, fibroblasts, endothelial cells
EPO	Red cell progenitor cells

IL, interleukin; GM, granulocyte-monocyte; CSF, colony-stimulating factor; EPO, erythropoietin; NK, natural killer; fibroblast, connective tissue support cell; endothelial cells, lining cells of blood vessels.

bone marrow. EPO is secreted on a daily basis in small amounts and functions to balance red cell production.[10] If the body becomes anemic and Hgb levels decline, the kidney senses tissue hypoxia and secretes more EPO; consequently, red cell production is accelerated and younger red cells are released prematurely. Normal red cell maturation from the precursor cell the pronormoblast takes 5 days; with accelerated erythropoiesis, the maturation is decreased to 3 to 4 days. Human recombinant erythropoietin (r-HuEPO) is available as a pharmaceutical product and can be used for individuals experiencing renal disease, for individuals who have become anemic as a result of **chemotherapy**, or for individuals who refuse whole blood products on religious grounds.

THE ROLE OF THE LABORATORY PROFESSIONAL IN THE BONE MARROW PROCEDURE

Obtaining a bone marrow aspirate or biopsy is an invasive and potentially painful procedure, and for this reason, this procedure is carefully evaluated before proceeding. The technologist has multiple roles in the bone marrow aspirate and/or biopsy procedure. Fundamentally, the technologist acts as an assistant to the pathologist/hematologist in the preparation of materials for the procedure. Next, the technologist informs the pathologist/hematologist if the sample is acceptable or unacceptable. This judgment of the technologist determines whether the procedure is repeated or completed.

There are few anemias for which a bone marrow procedure is necessary for diagnostic purposes. However, diagnosing white cell disorders such as leukemia or lymphoma relies on a baseline bone marrow evaluation.

BONE MARROW PROCEDURE

In the adult patient, the iliac crest is the site of choice, and the patient is usually face down while the physician chooses an appropriate area. The area is anesthetized with local anesthesia for an appropriate amount of time and the physician proceeds to advance the aspirate needle with a twisting, downward motion[11] (Fig. 2.4). Once the needle has seeded into the marrow, its position is solid and not moveable. The stylus is removed and a syringe is placed at the end of the needle. With a quick motion, a small amount of bloody fluid (approximately 1 mL) and marrow spicule material is obtained. The technologist/technician assesses the sample for bone marrow, communicates to the physician whether marrow is observed, and then proceeds to prepare slides from the aspirate material, fishing out bone marrow spicules with a microbiologic loop or pipette. If a biopsy sample is requested, the cutting blade is introduced into the bore of the needle and advanced until the medullary cavity is entered. A very small core of bone, $^3/_4$ in., is obtained, and the biopsy sample is removed by inserting a stylus into the cutting blade and pushing the sample through the open end. The procedure is terminated as the physician withdraws the needle and applies pressure to the area. Touch preparation of the core biopsy is made by the technologist by gently applying the biopsy sample to several coverslips with the use of sterile tweezers. In the event that an aspirate cannot be obtained, this may present a viable option. The remaining aspirate and biopsy material are placed in a 5% Zenker's fixative and processed in the histology laboratory. The patient should remain in bed for the next hour so that pressure is applied to the aspirate location. Patients with decreased platelet counts may need to be monitored more closely and have pressure exerted on the biopsy site for longer periods once the procedure is completed.

BONE MARROW REPORT

Once the slides from the biopsy and/or aspirate material are stained, the physician will evaluate the bone marrow for overall cellularity, M:E ratio (300 to 500 cells are scanned), maturation of each cell line, marrow-to-fat ratio, and presence of abnormal or tumor cells. The

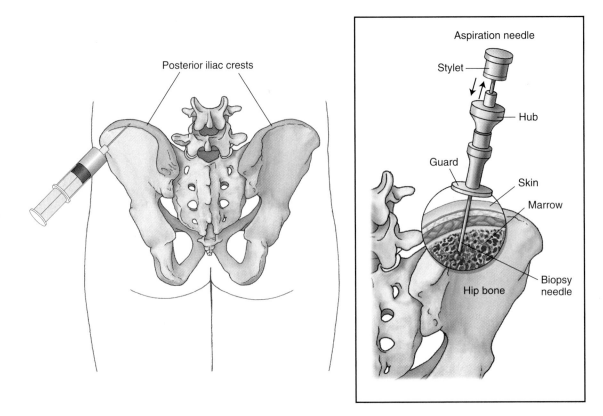

Figure 2.4 Bone marrow aspiration.

bone marrow iron store will be evaluated by the use of Prussian blue stain, and the marrow architecture will be observed for abnormalities in the stromal structure (necrosis, fibrosis, etc.).[12] These results combined with the patient's complete blood count (CBC) will enable the physician to reach a diagnosis. A copy of a sample bone marrow report is included in Figure 2.5.

THE COMPLETE BLOOD COUNT

The complete blood count (CBC) is one of the most frequently ordered and most time-honored laboratory tests in the hematology laboratory. This evaluation consists of nine components and offers the clinician a variety of hematological data to interpret and review that directly relate to the health of the bone marrow, represented by the numbers and types of cells in the peripheral circulation. The nine components of the CBC (Fig. 2.6) are the white blood cell count (WBC), red blood cell count (RBC), Hgb, hematocrit (Hct), mean corpuscular volume (MCV), mean corpuscular Hgb (MCH), mean corpuscular Hgb content (MCHC), platelet count, and red cell distribution width (RDW). Depending on the type of automated instrumentation used, some of these parameters are directly read from the instrument and

some are calculated. Generally, most automated instruments directly read the WBC, RBC, Hgb, and MCV. The Hct is a calculated parameter. Correlation checks between the Hgb and Hct are a significant part of quality assurance for the CBC and are known as the "rule of three." The formulas for correlation checks/rule of three are as follows: $Hgb \times 3 = Hct \pm 3$ and $RBC \times 3 = Hgb$. As a matter of practice, each operator of any automated instrumentation should be able to quickly and accurately establish a correlation check for each sample. Failure to fall within the correlation check is usually the first indicator of preanalytic error and may indicate corrective actions such as reviewing a peripheral smear, tracing the origin of the samples, or other investigation. Additionally, each instrument presents a pictorial representation of the hematological data registered as either a histogram or a scatterplot, and most now offer an automated reticulocyte count. This is discussed in the Procedure section. Table 2.3 presents normal values for a CBC from the adult, and Table 2.4 gives selected red cell values for the newborn. These data are also presented on the inside cover of this text.

Not all data on the CBC are viewed with equal importance or usefulness. Indeed, in an informal study at the University of Cleveland conducted by Dr. Linda Sandhaus (Director, Core Laboratory for Hematology,

Patient :   Pathology No. :

Med. Record No. :   **405004**   Date Collected :   2/4/04
Sex : F   Age :   70   Date Received :   2/5/04
Date of Birth :   6/10/33   Physicians :
Location: General Hospital

Specimen(s): . Bone marrow biopsy

PATHOLOGIC DIAGNOSIS:

BONE MARROW BIOPSY, ASPIRATE SMEAR AND PERIPHERAL: MYELOMA.

MICROSCOPIC DESCRIPTION:

The bone marrow is variably cellular ranging from 50 to 95 % and shows sheets of plasma cells including many immature forms. The residual bone marrow shows trilineage hematopoiesis with an ME ratio of approximately 3:1. Megakaryocytes are present and structurally unremarkable. Bone marrow iron is present and not increased. Reticulin stain shows no increase of fibrosis. Aspirate smears show adequate marrow cellularity. Maturation of both myeloid and erythroid elements is synchronous and progressive. Megakaryocytes are present and structurally unremarkable. Storage iron is present. Multiple aggregates of plasma cells including immature forms and binuclear cells are present. Peripheral smear shows Rouleaux phenomenon. Red cells are normochromic. There is anisocytosis and poikilocytosis with tear drop cells.

Recent hematologic and chemical data show white blood count 6.0, red blood count 4.66, hemoglobin 12.3, hematocrit 26.4, MCV 78.1, MCH 26.3, RDW 15.6, platelets 367,000, granulocytes 80. 3 %, lymphocytes 8.9 %, monocytes 10.1 %, eosinophil 0.4 %, and basophil 0.3 %. Immunoglobulin from February 3, 2004: IgG total 596 mg/dl, IgA 3,664 mg/dl and IgM 9 mg/dl.

COMMENT: Bone marrow morphology and immunochemistry are diagnostic of myeloma.

GROSS DESCRIPTION:

The specimen labeled "BONE MARROW BIOPSY" consists of bone marrow core biopsy measuring 2 cm in length, and is submitted after decalcification. The clot portion measures 2 x 2 x 0.8 cm in aggregate is bisected and the entire specimen is submitted in one cassette. 4 slides of aspirate smears and one peripheral smear are received.

MEH:jak

Pathologist
Electronically signed 02/06/2004

Figure 2.5   Sample bone marrow report.

2004), most physicians reported that the most preferred information was the Hgb, Hct, platelet count, and WBC. The MCV was generally viewed as important by primary care physicians. The RDW and automated reticulocyte count were used primarily by "newer" clinicians.

THE MORPHOLOGICAL CLASSIFICATION OF THE ANEMIAS

Generally, anemias are classified either morphologically or according to pathophysiological cause. The pathophysiological approach refers to the cause of anemias—whether the anemia is caused by excessive destruction or diminished production of red cells. Although this is certainly a respected approach, more clinicians are familiar with the morphological classification of anemias that relies on the red blood cell indices. This classification is readily available using CBC data and can be acted on fairly quickly as a means to start an investigation into cause. There are three morphological classifications of anemia:

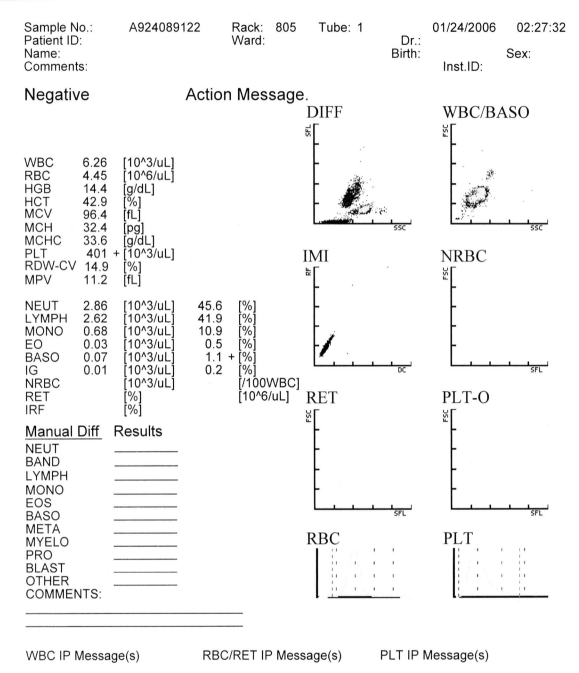

Figure 2.6   Sample CBC.

- Normochromic normocytic anemia
- Microcytic hypochromic anemia
- Macrocytic normochromic anemia

A *normocytic normochromic anemia* implies a normal red cell MCV (80 to 100 fL) and normal Hgb content of red cells (MCHC of 32% to 36%). Although the red cell and Hgb values may be reduced in this anemia, the size and Hgb content per cell are in the normal range. Red cells are normal size with a normal Hgb content. A *microcytic hypochromic anemia* implies an MCV of less than 80 fL with an MCHC of less than 32%. In this blood picture, the red cells are microcytic and smaller and lack Hgb, having an area of central pallor much greater than the usual 3-μm area. A *macrocytic normochromic anemia* implies an MCV of greater than 100 fL. Red cells are larger than 8 μm with an Hgb content in the normal range. If an anemia is suspected and confirmed by a CBC, the peripheral smear picture should reflect the morphological classification generated by automated results. For example, a patient sample with an MCV of 67 fL and an MCHC of 30% should have red cells that are small and pale. If the peripheral smear results do not correlate with the auto-

Table 2.3 ◯ Normal Values Using SI Units	
WBC	4.8 to 10.8 × 10^9/L
RBC	Males 4.7 to 6.1 × 10^{12}/L
	Females 4.2 to 5.4 × 10^{12}/L
Hgb	Males 14 to 18 g/dL
	Females 12 to 16 g/dL
Hct	Males 42% to 52%
	Females 37% to 47%
MCV	80 to 100 fL
MCH	27 to 31 pg
MCHC	32% to 36%
RDW	11.5% to 14.5%
Platelet count	150,000 to 350,000 × 10^9/L

mated results, an investigation should be initiated to determine the cause of the discrepancy. A detailed explanation of anemias under each morphological classification follows in the subsequent chapters.

CALCULATING RED CELL INDICES AND THEIR ROLE IN SAMPLE INTEGRITY

The red cell indices provide information concerning the size and Hgb content of red cells by providing the MCV, MCH, and MCHC. The MCV is one of the most stable parameters in the CBC, with little variability over a period of time: less than 1%.[13] For this reason, the MCV plays an extremely valuable role in monitoring the pre-analytic and analytic qualities of the sample. The MCV is either directly read by the instrumentation method, or it is a calculated value. If it is calculated, the formula is as follows:

$$MCV = (hematocrit/red\ cell\ count) \times 100$$

The normal value is between 80 and 100 fL and implies a red cell that has a size of 6 to 8 μm. Legitimate explanations for a shift in MCV include the presence of cold agglutinins (red cells coated with cold antibody, causing a false increase in size), transfusion therapy (newly transfused cells are larger), and reticulocytosis (presence of polychromatophilic macrocytes). Specimen or preanalytic factors that may account for a shifting MCV include the following[14,15]:

1. Contamination by drawing through the intravenous lines or in-dwelling catheters
2. Specimens from hyperglycemic patients
3. Patients on some chemotherapy drugs or zidovudine (AZT) therapy

Any shift in MCV that cannot be explained as a result of the circumstances listed should prompt the laboratory to investigate a possible sample mismatch or misidentification. As a delta check parameter, the MCV has a high value when determining sample integrity. See Table 2.5 for causes of MCV shifts.

The MCH and MCHC provide information concerning red cell hemoglobinization. The MCH can be calculated by the following formula:

$$MCH = (hemoglobin/red\ cell\ count) \times 100$$

The normal value is 27 to 31 pg, which implies that the average weight of Hgb in a given amount of red cells is in the appropriate range. The MCHC content can be calculated using the following formula (expressed in percentage):

$$MCHC = (hemoglobin/hematocrit) \times 10$$

The normal value is 32% to 36%, which implies that the amount of Hgb per red cell is in the appropriate concentration.

THE VALUE OF THE RED CELL DISTRIBUTION WIDTH

The eighth parameter of the CBC is the RDW, a mathematical calculation that gives insight into the amount of anisocytosis (variation in size) and, to some degree,

Table 2.4 ◯ Selected Red Cell Values for the Newborn
RBC 4.4 to 5.8 × 10^{12}/L
Hgb 17 to 23 g/dL
Hct 53% to 65%
MCV 98 to 108 fL

Table 2.5 ◯ Conditions Relating to Shifts in MCV
• Cold agglutinins
• Transfusions
• Chemotherapy—not all drugs
• AZT therapy
• Hyperglycemia—transient shifts

poikilocytosis (variation in shape) in a peripheral smear. The RDW is derived as follows:

(Standard deviation of RBC volume/mean MCV) × 100

The normal value for RDW is 11.5% to 14.5%. The standard deviation of red cell volume is derived from size histogram data that plot red cell size after a large number of red cells has been analyzed by the instrument. The usefulness of the RDW is that in many cases the RDW will become abnormal earlier in the anemia process than the MCV. Because many anemias (like iron deficiency anemias) develop over a period of time, this parameter may provide a sensitive indicator of red blood size change[16] before the red cell indices become overtly abnormal.

The final item in the CBC is a platelet count. Information regarding platelet estimates and platelet morphology is given in Chapter 20.

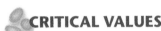CRITICAL VALUES

As mentioned in Chapter 1, critical values are those that are outside the reference range and that demand immediate action by the operator or technologist. A list of critical values is given in Table 2.6. If a patient presents with a critical value on a CBC, the physician or unit must be notified immediately. Records of this communication are essential and are a major part of quality assurance. All technologists should realize the importance and urgency of acting appropriately once a critical value has been obtained.

THE CLINICAL APPROACH TO ANEMIAS

Anemia is defined as a reduction in Hgb, red cell count, and Hct in a given age group and gender where refer-

ence ranges have been established. Many anemias develop secondary to other conditions; yet there are those that are primarily a result of diseased red cells. Establishing a diagnosis of anemia requires a careful history and physical examination, as well as an assessment of the patient's symptoms. A thorough family history can provide information on diet, ethnicity, history of bleeding or anemia, and medical history of relatives. Patients with moderate anemias, having a Hgb of between 7 and 10 g/dL, may show few physical symptoms because of the compensatory nature of the bone marrow. Yet once the Hgb drops below 7 g/dL, symptoms invariably develop. Pallor, fatigue, **tachycardia, syncope,** and hypotension are some of the most common signs of anemia. Pallor and hypotension are associated with decreased blood volume, while fatigue and syncope are associated with decreased oxygen transport, and tachycardia and heart murmur are associated with increased cardiac output (Table 2.7).

THE VALUE OF THE RETICULOCYTE COUNT

The reticulocyte count is the most effective means of assessing red cell generation or response to anemia. Reticulocytes are red cells that are nonnucleated and that contain remnant RNA material, reticulum. Reticulum cannot be visualized by Wright's stain; to be counted and evaluated, reticulocytes must be stained with supravital stains, like new methylene blue or brilliant cresyl blue. On Wright's stain, reticulocytes are seen as polychromatophilic macrocytes, or large, bluish cells. The normal reticulocyte rate is 0.5% to 1.5 % in the adult and 2.0% to 6.0% in the newborn. Because the bone marrow has the capacity to expand its production up to 7 times the normal rate, an elevated reticulocyte count or reticulocytosis is the *appropriate* response in anemic stress. Reticulocytes will be seen in the peripheral smear as polychromatophilic macrocytes; nucle-

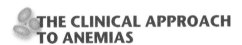

Table 2.6 ◉ Sample Critical Values

WBC
    Low 3.0 × 10⁹/L
    High 25.0 × 10⁹/L
Hgb
    Low 7.0 g/dL
    High 17.0 g/dL
Platelets
    Low 20.0 × 10⁹/L
    High 1000 × 10⁹/L

Table 2.7 ◉ Symptoms of Anemia Linked to Pathophysiology

- Decreased oxygen transport leads to fatigue, **dyspnea, angina pectoris,** and syncope
- Decreased blood volume leads to pallor, **postural hypotension,** and shock
- Increased cardiac output leads to **palpitation,** strong pulse, and heart murmurs

ated red blood cells may also be visualized in the peripheral smear as the bone marrow races to deliver cells prematurely at a rapid rate. EPO production is increased in response to hypoxia (anemia), and erythroid hyperplasia in the bone marrow (the condition in which there are more red cell precursors than white cell precursors being produced) is clear evidence of rapid generation. Failure to produce the expected reticulocyte increase may occur in ineffective erythropoiesis, a condition where red cell precursors are destroyed before they are delivered to the peripheral circulation, or if the bone marrow is infiltrated with tumor or abnormal cells, etc. A decreased reticulocyte count may also be seen in aplastic conditions, where the production of either white or red cells or both is seriously impaired. In any event, the level of reticulocyte response or lack of reticulocyte response is an important indicator of bone marrow function.

CONDENSED CASE 1

It was a busy day in the pediatric ambulatory clinic. At the change of shifts, a nurse discovered a labeled purple top tube sitting on the countertop with doctor's orders attached. The nurse had no idea when the sample was drawn, and neither did any of the other personnel. A CBC and differential were ordered. What is the next course of action?

Answer
This sample needs to be redrawn if in fact the physician is still interested in the results. CBC testing is best done within a 4-hour time period, and within 24 hours if the sample is refrigerated. Red cell morphology will be significantly affected within 2 to 3 hours at room temperature. Peripheral smears made within 12 hours on a refrigerated sample will still be viable. Testing personnel need to be aware of time limits and their effect on sample integrity.

CONDENSED CASE 2

A 47-year-old man on a surgical floor was having daily CBCs ordered. A sample was received at 8 a.m. in the morning with the morning draw specimen. The results were delta checked and reported to the floor. Later in the day, the technologist received another sample for the same patient at 2 p.m. The results on this sample were vastly different and failed the delta check. On a hunch, the technologist retrieved the sample from the a.m. draw and took both samples to the blood bank for an ABO type. The ABO on the morning sample was type O; the ABO on the 2 p.m. sample was type A. The patient has a history of receiving O blood from the blood bank. What is the next course of action?

Answer
Proper patient identification is essential for accurate test results in the clinical laboratory. Extreme care must be taken by everyone involved in drawing and labeling a specimen to be analyzed. Samples may be drawn by the nursing staff, the physician, the infusion team, and the phlebotomist. Each of these individuals must never allow distractions or interruptions to interfere with the essential job of patient identification. In this case, the technologist called up to the surgical floor, explained the situation, and determined that the 2 p.m. sample had been mislabeled. The results on the afternoon sample were voided.

Summary Points

- Hematopoiesis is defined as the production, development, and maturation of all blood cells.

- Erythropoiesis in the fetus takes place in the yolk sac, spleen, and liver.

- Erythropoiesis in the adult takes place primarily in the bone marrow.

- Hematopoiesis within the bone marrow is termed *intramedullary hematopoiesis;* outside the bone marrow, it is termed *extramedullary hematopoiesis.*

- The bone marrow is one of the largest nonsolid organs of the body.

- The M:E ratio (3 to 4:1) reflects the amount of myeloid elements in the bone marrow compared with the erythroid elements in the bone marrow.

- Multipotential stem cells are capable of differentiating into nonlymphoid or lymphoid precursor committed cells.

- EPO is a hormone produced by the kidneys that regulates erythroid production.
- A bone marrow aspirate and biopsy are invasive procedures usually performed at the location of the iliac crest in adults.
- The CBC consists of nine parameters: WBC, RBC, Hgb, Hct, MCV, MCH, MCHC, RDW, and platelet count.
- The MCV is one of the most stable CBC parameters over time.
- Increases in MCV can occur as a result of transfusion, reticulocytosis, hyperglycemia, and methotrexate.
- The RDW may be an early indicator of an anemic process.
- Critical values are those that are outside the reference range and that need to be immediately reported and acted on.
- The reticulocyte count is the most effective means of assessing red cell regeneration in response to anemic stress.

- Red cell production is effective when the bone marrow responds to anemic stress by producing an increased number of reticulocytes and nucleated red cells.
- Ineffective red cell production is described as death of red cell precursors in the bone marrow before they can be delivered to the peripheral circulation.
- Morphological classification of anemias is determined by the red cell indices.
- Microcytic, hypochromic anemias are characterized by an MCV of less than 80 fL and an MCHC of less than 32%.
- Macrocytic, normochromic anemias are characterized by an MCV of greater than 100 fL.
- Normocytic, normochromic anemias are characterized by an MCV between 80 and 100 fL and an MCHC of 32% to 36%.
- Normal red cells are disk-shaped flexible sacs filled with Hgb and having a size of 6 to 8 μm.

CASE STUDY

A 50-year-old woman was referred to a hematologist for recurring pancytopenia. At present, her WBC was 2.5×10^9/L; RBC, 3.0×10^{12}/L; Hct, 30%; platelet count, 40×10^9/L; MCV, 68 fL; MCH, 26 pg; and MCHC, 36.5%. In addition to pancytopenia, she has been experiencing shortness of breath and fatigue for the past 3 weeks, and lately these symptoms had gotten worse. Her family history was unremarkable, but she explained that she has had excessive menstrual bleeding for the past 4 months. A CBC and differential were ordered, as well as a bone marrow examination. *What is the likely cause for this patient's pancytopenia?*

Insights to the Case Study
This patient has a microcytic, hypochromic anemia characterized by small cells lacking Hgb. The MCV and MCHC are both outside of the normal range and are decreased. Additional studies such as serum iron, total iron binding capacity, and serum ferritin need to be initiated to determine the cause of her anemia, but with a history of menorrhagia for approximately 3 weeks, iron deficiency anemia is the most likely diagnosis. Other diagnostic possibilities include hereditary hemochromatosis, thalassemia minor, or the anemia of inflammation, all of which present with hypochromic microcytic indices. Additionally, the patient's bone marrow showed 60% myeloid elements and 20% erythroid elements. A normal level of megakaryocytes was noted. The M:E ratio was designated as 3:1. No atypical cellular formations or abnormal changes to the bone marrow architecture were noted. No specific diagnostic cause for the pancytopenia was determined, and the patient will be followed with a CBC every 3 months.

Review Questions

1. What are the organs of hematopoiesis in fetal life?
   a. Bone marrow
   b. Thymus and thyroid gland
   c. Spleen and liver
   d. Pancreas and kidneys

2. How does the bone marrow respond to anemic stress?
   a. Production is expanded, and red cells are released to the circulation prematurely.
   b. Production is expanded, and platelets are rushed into circulation.

c. Production is diminished, and the M:E ratio is increased.

d. Production is diminished, and the M:E ratio is unaffected.

3. Which chemical substances are responsible for differentiation and replication of the pluripotent stem cell?
   a. Cytokines
   b. Insulin
   c. Thyroxin
   d. Oxygen

4. A hormone released from the kidney that is unique for the erythroid regeneration is
   a. estrogen.
   b. erythropoietin.
   c. progestin.
   d. testosterone.

5. In the adult, the usual location for obtaining a bone marrow aspirate is the
   a. sternum.
   b. iliac crest.
   c. long bones.
   d. lower lumbar spine.

6. What is the most stable parameter of the complete blood count?
   a. White blood cell count
   b. Mean corpuscular volume
   c. Red cell distribution width
   d. Platelet count

7. Which one of the red cell indices reflects the amount of hemoglobin per individual red cell?
   a. Hgb
   b. MCV
   c. MCHC
   d. MCH

8. Given the formulas below, which formula indicates the correlation check between hemoglobin and hematocrit?
   a. (Hgb/Hct) × 100
   b. Hgb × 3 = Hct
   c. Hct = MCV × RBC
   d. (Hgb/RBC) × 100

9. Which of the following CBC parameters may provide an indication of anemia before the MCV indicates an overt size change?
   a. RDW
   b. MCH
   c. WBC
   d. MCHC

10. Which of the following tests is the most effective means of assessing red cell generation in response to anemia?
    a. RDW
    b. Reticulocyte count
    c. Platelet count
    d. CBC

⦿ TROUBLESHOOTING

What Do I Do When the Red Cell Indices Are Extremely Elevated?

A specimen from a 36-year-old man with a history of HIV infection was received in the clinical laboratory. The patient had a history of multiple admissions and was being admitted this time for hyponatremia and severe anemia. The initial results are as follows:

WBC	2.3 × 10⁹/L
RBC	2.02 × 10¹²/L
Hgb	7.8 g/dL
Hct	19.0%
MCV	102.5 fL*
MCH	38.8 pg*
MCHC	41.1%*
RDW	14.5%
Platelets	85 × 10⁶/L

In this sample, the Hgb and Hct have failed the correlation check, and the red cell indices in this individual are astronomically high and have been flagged by the automated instrument. The most likely explanation for these results is the development of a strong cold agglutinin in the patient's sample. Cold agglutinins or cold antibodies were first described by Landsteiner in 1903 and are usually IgM in origin. These agglutinins may occur as a primary anemia or a secondary development to a primary disorder. Individuals who have cold agglutinin disease are usually elderly and have a

(continued on following page)

● TROUBLESHOOTING *(continued)*

chronic hemolytic anemia combined with extreme sensitivity to cold temperatures leading to Raynaud's syndrome. These individuals may bind complement at colder temperature and hemolyze, causing a decreased Hgb and Hct. Agglutination in the digits and extremities may cause vascular obstruction and lead to **acrocyanosis**. In many cases, relocation to a warmer climate results in far fewer hemolytic episodes. Secondary cold agglutinins are observed in individuals with infectious mononucleosis, anti-mycoplasma antibodies, cytomegalovirus antibodies, malaria, anti-hepatitis antibodies, and HIV antibodies. In each of these cases, the immune system is compromised and sets the conditions for the development of an autoantibody against the patient's cells. The resolution of the CBC is to warm the sample in a 37°C water bath for a prescribed amount of time according to laboratory proto-

col. The sample is then recycled through the automated instrument, and the results are compared and then reported. If the cold agglutinin persists, the sample may need to be warmed for a second time to allow the results to equilibrate within reportable range. The CBC results show the patient's results after a 30-minute warming:

WBC	2.2×10^9/L
RBC	2.69×10^{12}/L
Hgb	7.8 g/dL
Hct	22.9%
MCV	85.1 fL
MCH	29.0 pg
MCHC	34.1%
RDW	20.4%
Platelets	87×10^6/L

(*Refer to reference values on front inside cover of this text.)

WORD KEY

Acrocyanosis • Blue or purple mottled discoloration of the fingers, toes, and/or nose

Angina pectoris • Oppressive pain or pressure in the chest

Chemotherapy • Drug therapy used to treat infections, cancers, and other diseases

Dyspnea • Shortness of breath

Hepatosplenomegaly • Enlargement of liver and spleen

Hypoxia • Decreased oxygen

Myelotoxic • Chemicals that destroy white cells

Palpitation • Sensation of rapid or irregular beating of the heart

Postural hypotension • Change in blood pressure from sitting to standing

RES system • Reticuloendothelial system, the mononuclear phagocytic system

Syncope • Fainting

Tachycardia • Fast and hard heartbeat

References

1. Wallace MS. Hematopoietic theory. In: Rodak B, ed. Hematology: Clinical Procedure and Applications, 2nd ed. Philadelphia: WB Saunders, 2002; 73.
2. Tablin F, Chamberlain JK, Weiss L. The microanatomy of the mammalian spleen. In: Bowdler AJ, eds. The Complete Spleen: Structure, Function and Clinical Disorder, 2nd ed. Totowa, NJ: Humana Press, 2002; 18–20.
3. Dailey MO. The immune function of the spleen. In: Bowdler AF, ed. The Complete Spleen: Structure, Function and Clinical Disorders, 2nd ed. Totowa, NJ: Humana Press, 2001; 54–56.
4. Singer SJ, Nicholson L. The fluid mosaic of the structure of cell membranes. Annu Rev Biochem 43:805, 1974.
5. Eshan A. Bone marrow. In: Harmening D. Clinical Hematology and Fundamentals of Hemostasis, 4th ed. Philadelphia: FA Davis, 2002.
6. Crosby WH, Akeroyd JH. The limit of hemoglobin synthesis in hereditary hemolytic anemia. Am J Med 13:273–283, 1952.
7. Herzog EL, Chai L, Krause DS. Plasticity of marrow derived stem cells. Blood 102:3483–3493, 2003.
8. Roath S, Laver J, Lawman JP, et al. Biologic control mechanism. In: Gross S, Roath S, eds. Hematology: A Problem-Oriented Approach. Baltimore: Williams & Wilkins, 1996; 7.
9. Bell A. Morphology of human blood and marrow cells. In: Harmening D, ed. Clinical Hematology and Fundamentals of Hemostasis, 4th ed. Philadelphia: FA Davis, 2002; 30–32.
10. Lappin TRJ, Rich IN. Erythropoietin: The first 90 years. Clin Lab Hematol 18:137, 1996.
11. Jamshidi K, Swaim WR. Bone marrow biopsy with unaltered architecture: A new biopsy device. J Lab Clin Med 77:335, 1971.

12. Krause J. Bone marrow overview. In: Rodak B, ed. Hematology: Clinical Procedures and Applications, 2nd ed. Philadelphia: WB Saunders, 2002; 188–195.

13. Lombarts AJPF, Leijsne B. Outdated blood and redundant buffy-coats as sources for the preparation of multiparameter controls for Coulter-type (resistive-particle) hemocytometry. Clin Chim Acta 143:7–15, 1984.

14. Savage RA, Hoffman GC. Clinical significance of osmotic matrix errors in automated hematology: The frequency of hyperglycemic osmotic matrix errors producing spurious macrocytosis. Am J Clin Pathol 80:861–865, 1983.

15. Pauler DK, Laird NM. Non-linear hierarchical models for monitoring compliance. Stat Med 21:219–229, 2002.

16. Adams-Graves P. Approach to anemia. In: Ling F, Duff P, eds. Obstetrics and Gynecology: Principles for Practice. New York: McGraw-Hill, 2001.

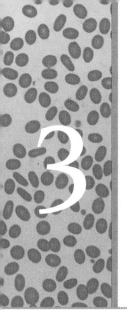
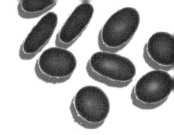

3 Red Blood Cell Production, Function, and Relevant Red Cell Morphology

Betty Ciesla

Basic Red Cell Production

Red Cell Maturation

Red Cell Terminology

Maturation Stages of the Red Cell
  Pronormoblast
  Basophilic Normoblast
  Polychromatophilic Normoblast
  Orthochromic Normoblast-Nucleated (nRBC)
  Reticulocyte
  Mature Red Cell

Red Blood Cell Membrane Development and Function
  Composition of Lipids in the Interior and Exterior Layers
  Composition of Proteins in the Lipid Bilayers
  The Cytoskeleton

Red Cell Metabolism

Abnormal Red Cell Morphology
  Variations in Red Cell Size
  Variations in Red Cell Color
  Variations in Red Cell Shape

Red Cell Inclusions

Objectives

After completing this chapter, the student will be able to:

1. Outline erythropoietic production from origin to maturation with emphasis on stages of red cell development.

2. Describe immature red cells with regard to nucleus:cytoplasm ratio, cytoplasm, nuclear structure, and size.

3. Clarify the role of erythropoietin in health and disease.

4. Differentiate between American Society of Clinical Pathology and College of American Pathologists terminology for the red cell series.

5. Review red cell metabolism with regard to energy needs.

6. Describe the composition of the red cell membrane with regard to key proteins and lipids.

7. Describe the components necessary for maintaining a normal red cell life span.

8. Outline the plasma factors that affect red cell life span.

9. Define *anisocytosis* and *poikilocytosis*.

10. Differentiate between microcyte and macrocyte.

11. Indicate the clinical conditions in which variations in size are seen.

12. Indicate the clinical conditions in which the variations in hemoglobin content are seen.

13. Describe the clinical conditions that show polychromatophilic cells.

14. Identify the pathophysiology and the clinical conditions that may lead to target cells, spherocytes, ovalocytes/elliptocytes, sickle cells, and the fragmented cells.

15. List the most common red cell inclusions and the disease states in which they are observed.

BASIC RED CELL PRODUCTION

Red blood cell production is a dynamic process that originates from pluripotent stem cells, a phenomenal structure whose cells can give rise to many tissues, including skin, bone, and nerve cells. Next to the mapping of the human genome, the use of stem cells as agents of therapy is one of the paramount discoveries of the 20th century. What makes stem cells so appealing is their versatility. They will respond to a programmed chemical environment in bone marrow or in cell culture, replicating and eventually producing the tissue that corresponds to their chemical menu. Red cells derive from the committed stem cells, the CFU-GEMM described in Chapter 2. This cell, derived from the pluripotential stem cell, is under the influence of chemical signals, the cytokines that orchestrate the differentiation and maturation of the cell to a committed pathway. Red cells are under the control of erythropoietin (EPO), a low-molecular-weight hormone produced by the kidneys, which is dedicated to red cell regeneration. EPO makes its way through the circulation and locks onto a receptor on the pronormoblast, the youngest red cell precursor, stimulating the production of 16 mature red cells from every pronormoblast precursor cell (pluripotent stem cell) (Fig. 3.1) .[1]

RED CELL MATURATION

Mature red cells are one of the few cellular structures in the human body that begin as nucleated cells and become anucleate. This remarkable development takes place in the bone marrow over a period of 5 days as each precursor cell goes through three successive divisions, yielding smaller and more compact red cells.[1] Several features of the red cell change dramatically: the cell size reduces, the nucleus:cytoplasm (N:C) ratio reduces, nuclear chromatin becomes more condensed, and the cytoplasm color is altered as hemoglobinization becomes more prominent (Table 3.1). In the bone marrow, erythrocytes at various stages of maturation seem to cluster in specific areas, the so-called erythroblastic island, easily identified in the bone marrow aspirate by the tell-tale morphological clues of erythropoiesis—extremely round nuclear material, combined with basophilic cytoplasm. The main site of adult erythropoiesis is the bone marrow located in the sternum and iliac crest, whereas erythropoiesis in children takes place in the long bones and sternum.

RED CELL TERMINOLOGY

Several nomenclatures are used to describe the maturation stages of the red cell. Both are presented here because many textbooks use them interchangeably. There seems to be little advantage in using one terminology over the other; however, the original intent of creating the terminologies was to clarify the terms created in the 1800s to describe red cell maturation and make the stages of maturation easier to remember and master. The College of American Pathologists (CAP) uses the word "blast" in the description of maturation

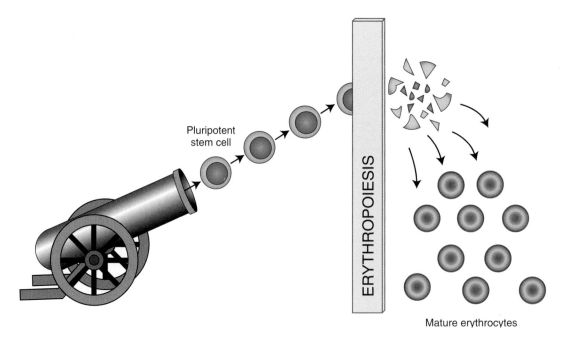

Pluripotent
stem cell

ERYTHROPOIESIS

Mature erythrocytes

Figure 3.1   Through the erythropoietic process, a single pluripotent stem cell will yield 16 mature erythrocytes.

Table 3.1 ⊙ Key Features of Red Cell Development

- Nuclei are always "baseball" round.
- Basophila of cytoplasm is an indicator of immaturity.
- Cell size reduces with maturity.
- As hemoglobin develops, the cytoplasm becomes more magenta.
- The N:C ratio decreases as the cell matures.
- The cytoplasm of the red cell does not contain specific granulation.
- Nuclear chromatin becomes more condensed with age.
- Nucleated red cells (orthochromic normoblasts) are not a physiological component of the normal peripheral smear.

stages, whereas the American Society of Clinical Pathologists (ASCP) incorporates "rubri" into the first four maturation stages (Table 3.2). Throughout this textbook, CAP terminology is used.[2]

MATURATION STAGES OF THE RED CELL

There are six stages of maturation in the red cell series: pronormoblast, basophilic normoblast, polychromatophilic normoblast, orthochromic normoblast, reticulocyte, and mature red cell. In general, several morphological clues mark the red cell maturation series:

- When the red cell is nucleated, the nucleus is "baseball" round.

Table 3.2 ⊙ College of American Pathologists (CAP) vs. American Society for Clinical Pathology (ASCP) Terminology for Red Cells

CAP	ASCP
Pronormoblast	Rubriblast
Basophilic normoblast	Prorubricyte
Polychromatophilic normoblast	Rubricyte
Orthochromic normoblast	Metarubricyte
Reticulocyte	Reticulocyte
Erythrocyte	Erythrocyte

- There are no granules in the cytoplasm of red cells.
- The cytoplasm in younger cells is extremely basophilic and becomes more lavender tinged as hemoglobin is synthesized.
- Size decreases as the cell matures.
- Nuclear chromatin material becomes more condensed in preparation for extrusion from the nucleus.
- The N:C ratio decreases as the nuclear material becomes more condensed and smaller in relationship to the entire red cell.

In the bone marrow and in the peripheral smear, each of these clues is helpful in enabling the technologist to stage a particular red cell. Identification of immature red cells should be systematic and based on reliable morphological criteria. Each red cell maturation stage will be described using size, N:C ratio, nuclear chromatin characteristics, and cytoplasm descriptions. N:C ratio implies the amount of nucleus to the amount of cytoplasm present; the higher the N:C ratio, the more immature is the cell. Nuclear chromatin will be described with respect to chromatin distribution, chromatin texture, and color.

Pronormoblast (Fig. 3.2)

Size: 18 to 20 μm, the largest and most immature, the "mother cell"
N:C ratio: 4:1
Nuclear chromatin: Round nucleus with a densely packed chromatin, evenly distributed, fine texture with deep violet color, nucleoli may be present but are hard to visualize
Cytoplasm: Dark marine blue definitive areas of clearing

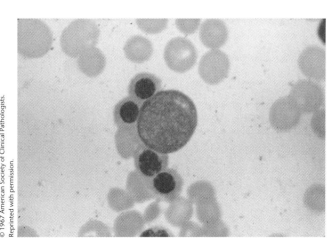

Figure 3.2   Pronormoblast.

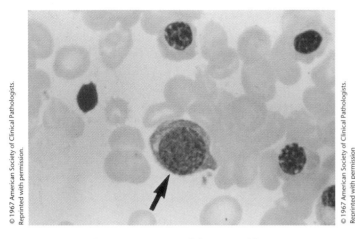

Figure 3.3 Basophilic normoblast.

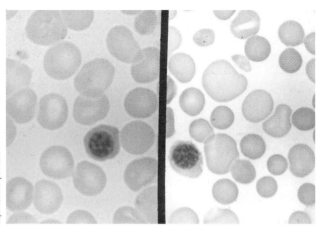

Figure 3.5 Orthochromic normoblast.

Basophilic Normoblast (Fig. 3.3)

Size: 16 µm

N:C ratio: 4:1

Nuclear chromatin: Round nucleus with crystalline chromatin appearance, parachromatin underlayer may be visible, red-purple color to chromatin

Cytoplasm: Cornflower blue with indistinct areas of clearing

Polychromatophilic Normoblast (Fig. 3.4)

Size: 13 µm

N:C ratio: 2:1

Nuclear chromatin: Chromatin is condensed, moderately compacted

Cytoplasm: A color mixture, blue layered with tinges of orange red, "the dawn of hemoglobinization" as hemoglobin begins to be synthesized

Orthochromic Normoblast-Nucleated (nRBC) (Fig. 3.5)

Size: 8 µms

N:C ratio: 1:1

Nuclear chromatin: Dense, velvet-appearing homogenous chromatin

Cytoplasm: Increased volume, with orange-red color tinges with slight blue tone

Reticulocyte (Fig. 3.6)

Size: 8 µm

Appearance: Remnant of RNA visualized as reticulum, filamentous structure in chains or as a single dotted structure in new methylene blue stain: seen in Wright's stain as large bluish-red cells, polychromatophilic macrocytes

Mature Red Cell (Fig. 3.7)

Size: 6 to 8 µm

Appearance: Disk-shaped cell filled with hemoglobin, having an area of central pallor of 1 to 3 µm

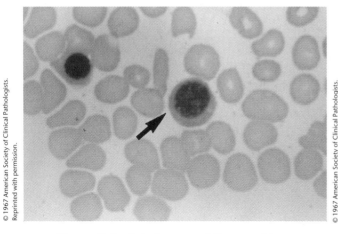

Figure 3.4 Polychromatophilic normoblast.

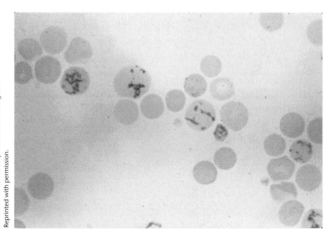

Figure 3.6 Reticulocyte.

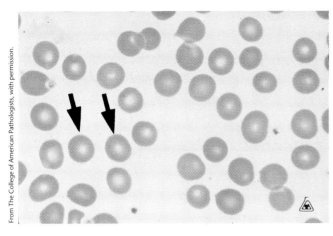

Figure 3.7   Normal red blood cell. Note discocyte shape and small area of central pallor.

RED BLOOD CELL MEMBRANE DEVELOPMENT AND FUNCTION

The mature red blood cell is a magnificently designed instrument for hemoglobin delivery. As a hemoglobin-filled sac, the red cell travels more than 300 miles through the peripheral circulation, submitting itself to the swift waters of the circulatory system, squeezing itself through the threadlike splenic sinuses, and bathing itself in the plasma microenvironment. Cellular and environmental factors contribute to red cell survival. In order for the red cell to survive for its 120-day life cycle, these conditions are necessary:

- The red cell membrane must be deformable.
- Hemoglobin structure and function must be adequate.
- The red cell must maintain osmotic balance and permeability.

The mature red blood cell is an anucleate structure with no capacity to synthesize protein, yet it is capable of a limited metabolism, which enables it to survive 120 days.[3] An intact, competent, and fully functioning red cell membrane is an essential ingredient to a successful red cell life span. The membrane of the red cell is a trilaminar and three-dimensional structure containing glycolipids and glycoproteins on the outermost layer directly beneath the red cell membrane surface. Cholesterol and phospholipids form the central layer, and the inner layer, the **cytoskeleton**, contains the specific membrane protein, spectrin, and ankyrin (Fig. 3.8).

Composition of Lipids in the Interior and Exterior Layers

Fifty percent of the red cell membrane is protein, while 40% is lipid and the remaining 10% is cholesterol. The lipid fraction is a two-dimensional interactive fluid that serves as a barrier to most water-soluble molecules. Cholesterol is equally distributed through the red cell membrane and comprises 25% of the membrane lipid; however, plasma cholesterol and membrane cholesterol are in constant exchange. Cholesterol may accumulate

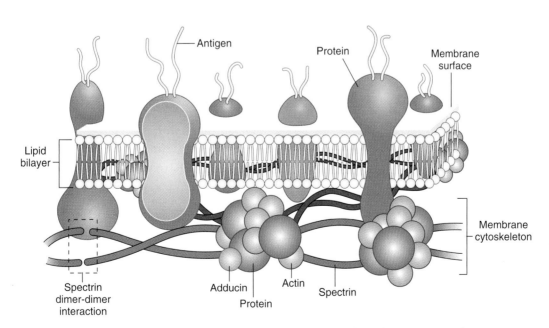

Figure 3.8   Red blood cell membrane. Note placement of integral proteins (glycophorins—in purple) versus peripheral proteins (spectrin, ankyrin).

on the surface of the red cell membrane in response to excessive accumulation in the plasma. Increased plasma cholesterol causes increased deposition of cholesterol on the red cell surface. The red cell becomes heavier and thicker, causing rearrangement of hemoglobin. This may be one pathway to the formation of target cells and acanthocytes, red cell morphologies that exhibit decreased red cell survival. Acanthocytes may also develop subsequent to cholesterol depositions in patients with liver disease and lecithin cholesterol acetyltransferase (LCAT) deficiency.

Composition of Proteins in the Lipid Bilayers

The protein matrix of the red cell membrane is supported by two types of protein. The integral proteins start from the cytoskeleton and expand through the membrane to penetrate the other edge of the red cell surface. Peripheral proteins are confined to the red cell cytoskeleton. The integral proteins provide the backbone for the active and passive transport of the red cell as well as provide supporting structure for more than 30 red cell antigens.[3] Ions and gases move across the red cell membrane in an organized and harmonious fashion. Water (H_2O), chloride (Cl), and bicarbonate (HCO_3) diffuse freely across the red cell membrane as a result of specialized channels, like aquaphorins. Other ions like sodium (Na^+), potassium (K^+), and calcium (Ca^{2+}) are more highly regulated by a careful intracellular-to-extracellular balance. For sodium, the ratio is 1:12, and for potassium, 25:1,[4] the ratio that represents the amount of sodium and potassium transport in and out of the cell. This ratio is the optimum ratio for red cell survival and is controlled by cationic energy pumps requiring ATP for Na^+ and K^+ and by calmodulin, which regulates calcium migration through the calcium-ATPase pumps. If the membrane becomes more permeable to Na^+, rigid red cells may develop leading to spherocytes, which have a decreased life span. Red cells, which are more water permeable, may hemolyze and burst prematurely, again leading to reduced life span. Glycophorins A, B, and C are additional integral membrane proteins, containing 60% carbohydrates and most of the membrane sialic acid, which imparts a net negative charge to the red cell surface. Many red cell antigens are located on this portion of the membrane. Red cell antigens M and N are located on glycophorin A, while red cell antigens S and s are located on glycophorin B. Glycophorin C provides a point of attachment to the cytoskeleton or inner layer of the red cell membrane.

The Cytoskeleton

The cytoskeleton is an interlocking network of proteins that play a significant role in the deformability and elasticity of the red cell membrane. The third layer of the red cell membrane supports the lipid bilayer and also supplies the peripheral proteins. Spectrin and ankyrin are peripheral proteins that are responsible for the deformability properties of the red cell. Deformability and elasticity are crucial properties to the red cell, because the red cell with an average diameter of 6 to 8 μm must maneuver through vascular apertures like the splenic cords and capillary arterioles, which have diameters of 1 to 3 μm. Indeed, the intact and deformable red cell can stretch 117% of its surface area as it weathers the turmoil of circulation, squeezing through small spaces. Inherited abnormalities of spectrin can lead to the production of spherocytes, a more compact red cell with a reduced life span. Spectrin-deficient red cells are normal size and shaped once they exit the bone marrow. It is only when they are pushed into the systemic circulation and are subjected to the rigors of the spleen that the outer layer of the red cell membrane is shaved, leading to the more compact and damaged cell, the spherocyte. This particular spherocyte mechanism, which occurs in hereditary spherocytosis, best illustrates the progressive loss of membrane that occurs in hereditary spherocytosis. Once the spherocyte is reviewed by the spleen, the membrane is removed, leaving a remodeled red cell. Other mechanisms for the formation of spherocytes may occur, but these are discussed later.

RED CELL METABOLISM

Because the mature red cell is an anucleate structure, it has no nuclear or mitochondrial architecture for metabolizing fatty or amino acids. Consequently, it derives all of its energy from the breakdown of glucose. Within this framework, the red cell must maintain its shape, keep hemoglobin in the reduced (Fe^{2+}) state, and move electrolytes across the membrane. There are three metabolic pathways that are essential for red cell function, as follows:

1. The Embden-Meyerhof pathway provides 90% of the cellular ATP because red cell metabolism is essentially **anaerobic.** The functions of ATP are multifactorial and include maintenance of membrane integrity, regulation of the intracellular and extracellular pumps, maintenance of hemoglobin function, and replacement of membrane lipids.[5] This pathway also generates NAD^+ from NADH, an important structure in

the formation of 2,3-diphosphoglycerate, a key element to oxygen loading and unloading.

2. The hexose monophosphate shunt provides 5% to 10% of the ATP necessary so that NADPH is produced and globin chains will not be degraded when subjected to oxidative stress and the accumulation of hydrogen peroxide. If this pathway is deficient, globin chains may precipitate, forming Heinz body inclusions in the red cell. Heinz body inclusions will lead to the formation of bite cells in the peripheral blood as Heinz bodies are pitted from the cell by the spleen.

3. The methemoglobin reductase pathway, which maintains hemoglobin iron in the reduced ferrous state, Fe^{2+}, so that oxygen can be delivered to the tissues, is dependent on the reduction of NAD to NADPH (Fig. 3.9). If this enzyme is absent, methemoglobin accumulates in the red cells. Oxygen transport capabilities are seriously impaired because methemoglobin cannot combine with oxygen.

ABNORMAL RED CELL MORPHOLOGY

Automated instrumentation in hematology has redefined the level of practice in most hematology laboratories. Along with the complete blood count (CBC), most instruments offer an automated differential count. When values from the differential or CBC are out of the reference range, results are flagged. If a result is flagged, the operator or technologist must make a decision to perform reflex testing or pull a peripheral smear for review or complete differential in order to resolve the abnormal result. Therefore, far fewer peripheral smears are being reviewed or given a complete differential count. Those smears that are scanned or reviewed, however, are from patients who are more seriously ill and may have illness with multiple **pathologies.** For this reason, proficiency in normal and abnormal identification of red cells is a desirable skill and one that must be practiced as a student or an employee. This section concentrates on defining abnormal red cell morphology and the pathologies that are causative to that morphology. Automated cell counting and differential counters have not yet replaced the well-trained eye with respect to the subtleties of red cell morphology.

There is no substitute for a well-distributed, well-stained peripheral smear when assessing red cell morphology. Once this is established, there are two principal questions that must be asked when an abnormal morphology is observed:

1. Is the morphology in every field?
2. Is the morphology artificial or pathological?

Technologists review approximately 10 well-stained and well-distributed fields in a peripheral smear and then make a judgment as to whether anisocytosis (variation in size) and poikilocytosis (variation in shape) are present. If these are present, technologists proceed to record and quantitate those shape and size changes that are responsible for anisocytosis and poikilocytosis observation. A numerical scale or qualitative remarks are used to grade the specific morphology. Numeric procedures for assessing red cell morphology can be reviewed in Chapter 20 "Hematology Procedures." What is most important in the assessment of red cell morphology is the discovery of the physiological cause for the creation of that morphology so that the patient can be treated and his or her hematological health restored.

Variations in Red Cell Size

The normal red cell is a disk-shaped structure that is approximately 6 to 8 µm and has an MCV of between 80 and 100 fL and an MCHC of between 32% and 36%. Variations in size are seen as microcytes (less than 6 µm) or macrocytes (greater than 9 µm). Microcytic cells result from four main clinical conditions: iron deficiency anemia, thalassemic syndromes, iron overload conditions, and the anemia of chronic disorders. Microcytic cells are part of the clinical picture in iron deficiency anemia and result from impaired iron metabolism as a result of either deficient iron intake or defective iron absorption.[6] Iron is an essential element to the formation of the hemoglobin molecule. The heme portion of hemoglobin is formed from having four iron atoms surrounded by the protoporphyrin ring. Two pairs of globin chains are then assembled onto the molecule with the heme structure lodged in the pockets of the globin chains. Iron needs to be incorporated into the four heme structures of each hemoglobin molecule, and also needs to be absorbed from the bloodstream and transferred, via transferrin, to the pronormoblasts of the bone marrow for incorporation in the heme structure. Iron-starved red cells divide more rapidly than normal red cells, searching for iron, and are smaller because of these rapid divisions. The thalassemic conditions give rise to microcytes owing to decreased or absent globin synthesis. When either alpha or beta chains are missing or diminished, normal adult hemoglobin is not synthesized and hemoglobin configuration is impaired, leading to microcytic cells that have an increased central pallor, known as hypochromia. The

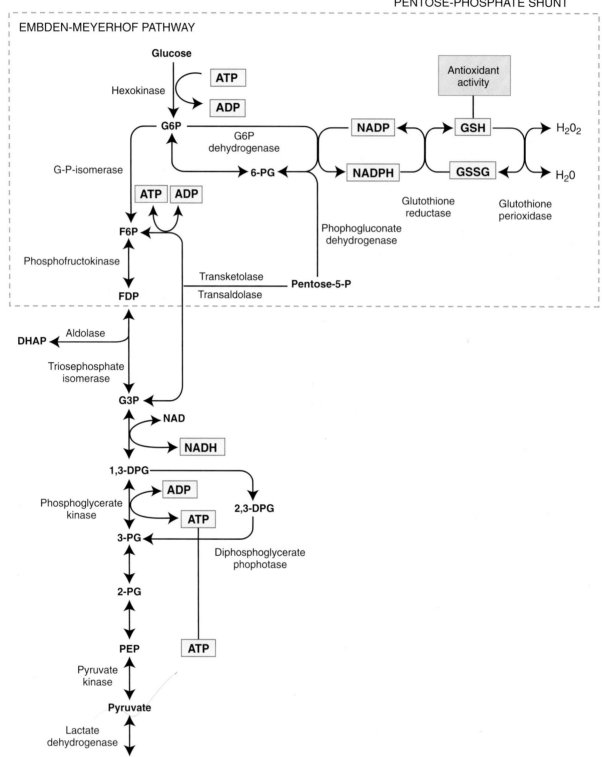

Figure 3.9   Anaerobic breakdown of glucose in red cell metabolism.

third microcytic mechanism occurs in red cells from individuals who have iron overload disorders like hereditary hemochromatosis. These individuals will show a dimorphic blood smear, some microcytes mixed with macrocytes, some red cells exhibiting normal hemoglobin levels, and some showing hypochromia. The final microcytic mechanism is from those individuals who have the anemia of inflammation. Approximately 10% of these individuals who have the anemia of inflammation arising from renal failure or thyroid dysfunction also show microcytic red cells in their peripheral smear as iron delivery to the reticuloendothelial system is impaired.

All immature red blood cells are nucleated structures, and nuclear synthesis depends on vitamin B_{12} and folic acid. If either of these vitamins is unavailable or cannot be absorbed through the gastrointestinal system, a macrocytic cell evolves. More information concerning vitamin B_{12} and folic acid is available in Chapter 6. Macrocytic red blood cells have a diminished life span, and a megaloblastic anemia develops with an MCV in excess of 110 fL. In the bone marrow, the erythropoiesis is ineffective as the red cell precursors are prematurely destroyed before they are released into the peripheral circulation.[7] Additionally, an **asynchrony** develops between the nuclear structure and the cytoplasm, as nuclear development and hemoglobin development become unbalanced. The nuclear age appears to be out of sync with the cytoplasm development. A pancytopenia develops in the CBC and hypersegmented neutrophils, and macro-ovalocytes are also part of the megaloblastic picture. In individuals who have borderline increased MCV, large cells may be generated subsequent to alcoholism and liver disease, or the increase in MCV may be as a result of high reticulocyte counts where polychromatophilic macrocytes are seen in the peripheral smear (Fig. 3.10).

Variations in Red Cell Color

Color variations in the red cells are observed as polychromasia or hypochromia. Polychromasia occurs subsequent to excessive production of red cell precursors in response to anemic stress. When the bone marrow responds to anemic stress, it releases reticulocytes and, at times, orthochromic normoblasts (nucleated red blood cells [nRBCs]) prematurely. What is seen in the peripheral smear is increased polychromasia, red cells that are gray-blue and larger than normal. Polychromatophilic macrocytes are actually reticulocytes; however, the reticulum can be visualized only when these cells are stained with supravital stain. The presence of polychromasia is an excellent indicator of bone marrow health. Polychromasia will be observed

- When the bone marrow is responding to anemia.
- When therapy is instituted for iron deficiency anemia or megaloblastic anemia.
- When the bone marrow is being stimulated as a result of a chronic hematological condition, such as thalassemia or sickle cell disorders.

Hypochromic red cells exhibit a larger than normal area of central pallor, greater than 3 μm, and are usually seen in conditions in which hemoglobin synthesis is impaired. Most hypochromic cells will have an MCHC of less than 32%. The development of hypochromia is usually a gradual process and can be seen on the peripheral smear as a delicately shaded area of hemoglobin within the red cell structure. Any starkly defined area of red cell pallor is usually artifactual and not true hypochromia. Not all hypochromic cells are microcytic, but all microcytic cells are hypochromic. Hypochromia of varying degrees can be seen in iron deficiency anemia, in the thalassemic conditions, and in the sideroblastic, iron-loading processes (Fig. 3.11).

Variations in Red Cell Shape

Shape variations in the red cell are always linked to a defined red cell pathophysiology. Abnormal red cell morphology presents the morphologist with visual

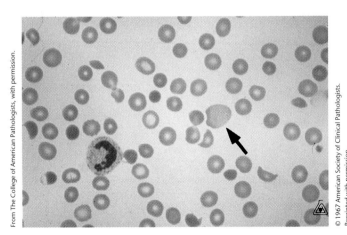

Figure 3.10   Polychromatophilic macrocyte.

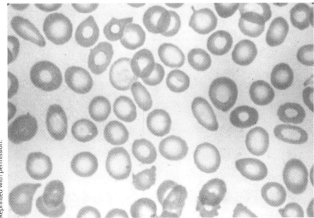

Figure 3.11   Hypochromia.

clues as to what might be the source of the patient's hematological problems, whether they are hemolysis, anemia, or defective splenic function. Five distinct morphologies will be discussed. While these are not all inclusive, they represent the majority of abnormalities seen in a metropolitan population.

Spherocytes

Spherocytes are compact red cells with a near normal MCV and an elevated MCHC, usually above 36%. They are easily recognized from the rest of the red cell background on the peripheral smear because they are dense, dark, and small (Fig. 3.12). Spherocytes arrive in the peripheral circulation via three distinct mechanisms. Individuals who have inherited abnormalities in spectrin will have the condition hereditary spherocytosis (HS). Mature red cells in HS individuals arrive in the peripheral circulation with a normal appearance, but as they try to negotiate the splenic sinuses, the spleen, sensing the membrane imperfections, shears the exterior membrane, leaving a more compact structure, the spherocyte, which is osmotically fragile. The restructured red cell has a reduced life span, and the patient has a lifelong moderate anemia. As red cells age, pieces of membrane are lost in the senescent, or aging, process. Because red cells pass through the spleen hundreds of times in their 120-day life cycle, older and less perfect red cells are trapped by this organ and rendered as spherocytes, where they are eventually removed by the reticuloendothelial system. The final pathophysiology producing a spherocyte is antibody-coated red cells formed subsequent to an autoimmune or immune process. As antibody-coated cells percolate through the spleen, the antibody coating is removed and small amounts of red cell membrane are lost. The cell, the

spherocyte, that is left to traverse the circulation is smaller, denser, and more fragile in its microenvironment.

Sickle Cells

Sickle cells are a highly recognizable red cell morphology, with their crescent shape and pointed projections at one of the terminal ends of the red cells (Fig. 3.13). Individuals who possess sickle cells have sickle hemoglobin as one component of their adult hemoglobin complement. Sickle hemoglobin, hemoglobin S, is an abnormal hemoglobin. Red cells containing this hemoglobin homozygously have a dramatically reduced life span owing to the fact that sickle hemoglobin is intractable and forms tactoids under conditions of hypoxic stress. When red cells containing hemoglobin S try to maneuver through the spleen and the kidney, the hemoglobin lines up in stiff bundles. This makes the red cell less elastic and unable to squeeze through the microcirculation of the spleen. The cell deforms, takes the sickle shape, and is permanently harmed. Many sickle cells may revert to normal disk shape upon oxygenation, but approximately 10% are unable to revert and these are labeled as irreversible sickle cells. Reversible sickle cells, on the other hand, appear in the peripheral smear as thicker, more rounded, half moon–shaped cells with no pointed projections. When properly oxygenated, they resume the normal disk-shaped structure of the red cells. Sickle cells may appear in combination with other hemoglobinopathies like hemoglobin SC and hemoglobin S-thalassemia.

Ovalocytes and Elliptocytes

Ovalocytes and elliptocytes are red cell morphologies that are often used interchangeably, yet these two dis-

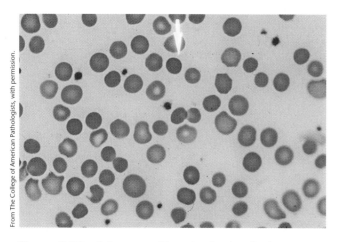

From The College of American Pathologists, with permission.

Figure 3.12   Spherocyte. Note the density of spherocytes in comparison to the red cell background.

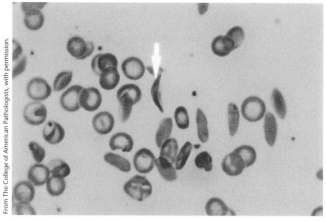

From The College of American Pathologists, with permission.

Figure 3.13   Sickle cell. Note pointed projection.

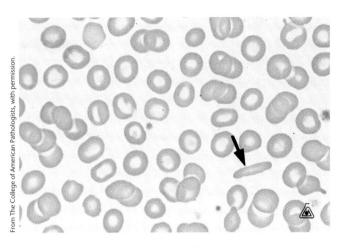

Figure 3.14   Elliptocyte.

tinct morphologies have several recognizable differences (Fig. 3.14). Ovalocytes are egg shaped and capable of many variations of hemoglobin distribution. These cells may appear macrocytic, hypochromic, or normochromic. Ovalocytes—more specifically, macroovalocytes—may be observed in the megaloblastic process. Normochromic ovalocytes are typically seen in thalassemic syndromes. Elliptocytes, on the other hand, are a distinct morphology derived from abnormal spectrin and protein 4.1 component, both red cell membrane proteins. In the primary condition, hereditary elliptocytosis, elliptocytes are the predominant morphology, yet this condition is fairly benign with little consequence to the red cell. The other two genotypes of this disorder, hereditary pyropoikilocytosis and spherocytic hereditary elliptocytosis, are a much more serious morphology with severe anemia and are discussed in a subsequent chapter. Elliptocytes may also be present in the peripheral smear of iron-deficient individuals as well as in patients with idiopathic myelofibrosis.

Target Cells

Target cells appear in the peripheral smear as a bull's eye–shaped cell. They are seen in the peripheral blood due to three mechanisms: (a) as an artifact, (b) due to decreased volume because of loss of hemoglobin, and (c) due to increased red cell surface membrane (Fig. 3.15). As cholesterol increases in the plasma, the red cell surface expands, resulting in increased surface area. Target cells appear as hypochromic with a volume of hemoglobin rimming the cells and a thin layer of hemoglobin located centrally, eccentrically, or as a thick band. As a morphology, target cells appear in iron deficiency anemia, hemoglobin C disease and associated conditions, liver disease, and post splenectomy. When hemo-

globin is affected qualitatively, target cells will appear (Fig. 3.16).

Fragmented Cells

The fragmented cells represent a group of variant morphologies ranging from the schistocytes to the helmet cell. Regardless of the pathophysiology, these cells appear fragmented; indeed, pieces of the red cell membranes have been sheared and hemoglobin leaks through the membranes, causing anemia. Physiological events that may cause this situation are the formation of large inclusions (Heinz bodies) or the predispositions of **thrombi**. Heinz bodies are large inclusions formed in the red cell as a result of oxidative stress, usually in patients with glucose-6-phosphate dehydrogenase deficiency (see Chapter 7). As the inclusion-rich red cells try to negotiate the spleen, the inclusion-rich cell is pitted, leaving a helmet cell (Fig. 3.17). Schistocytes may be encountered as a result of shear stress from systemic thrombin disposition resulting from **disseminated intravascular coagulation** or thrombotic thrombocytopenic purpura.[8] They may also occur in burn patients or in individuals with heart valve surgery. Burr cells, on the other hand, are usually seen in conditions of uremia or dehydration, both conditions that result from a change in tonicity of circulating fluids (Fig. 3.18). Additionally, burr cells may occur as artifacts in blood smears that have forced to dry through repeated shaking.

RED CELL INCLUSIONS

The cytoplasm of all red cells is free of debris, granules, or other structures. Inclusions that find their way into the cytoplasm are the result of distinctive conditions. This section summarizes four of the most common red cell inclusions (Table 3.3): Howell-Jolly bodies, siderotic granules/Pappenheimer bodies, basophilic stippling, and Heinz bodies.

Howell-Jolly bodies are remnants of DNA that appear in the red cell as round, deep purple, nondeformable structures 1 to 2 µm in size. They are eccentrically located in the cytoplasm and are seen when erythropoiesis is rushed. It is thought that the Howell-Jolly bodies represent remnants of the orthochromic normoblast nucleus as it is extruded from the cytoplasm. The spleen usually pits these inclusions from the cytoplasm, yet when the bone marrow is responding to anemic conditions, the spleen cannot keep pace with Howell-Jolly body formation. In post **splenectomy** individuals, however, large numbers of Howell-Jolly bodies may be observed, because the spleen is not avail-

How Target Cells Are Formed

As a result of artifacts, air-drying and hemoglobin precipitation:

Examples: High humidity, slow drying, and hemoglobin C

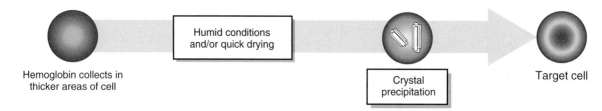

Hemoglobin collects in thicker areas of cell

Humid conditions and/or quick drying

Crystal precipitation

Target cell

As a result of decreased volume:

Examples: Iron deficiency, thalassemia, and hemoglobinopathies (Hb S,E)

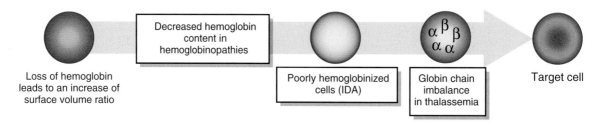

Loss of hemoglobin leads to an increase of surface volume ratio

Decreased hemoglobin content in hemoglobinopathies

Poorly hemoglobinized cells (IDA)

Globin chain imbalance in thalassemia

Target cell

As a result of increased surface membrane:

Examples: Liver disease (obstructive jaundice), LCAT deficiency, and asplenism

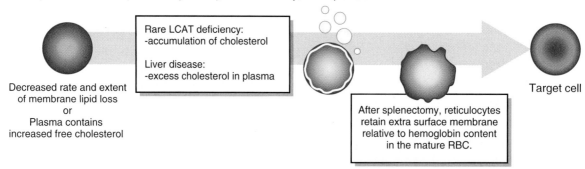

Decreased rate and extent of membrane lipid loss
or
Plasma contains increased free cholesterol

Rare LCAT deficiency:
-accumulation of cholesterol

Liver disease:
-excess cholesterol in plasma

After splenectomy, reticulocytes retain extra surface membrane relative to hemoglobin content in the mature RBC.

Target cell

Figure 3.15   Three possibilities for target cell formation.

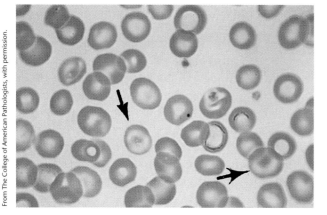

Figure 3.16   Target cell.

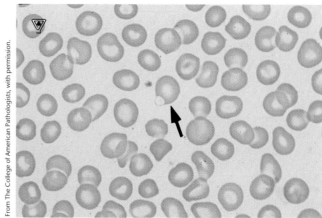

Figure 3.17   Bite cells (helmet cells).

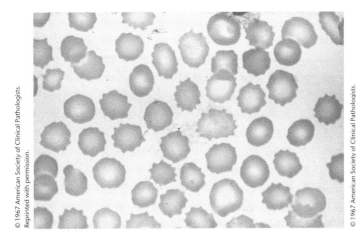

Figure 3.18   Burr cells.

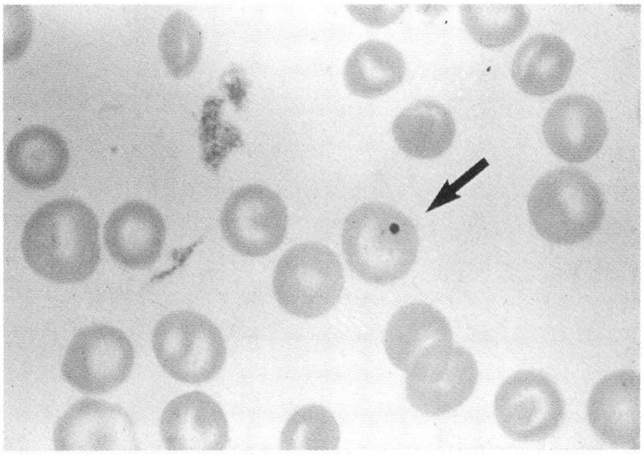

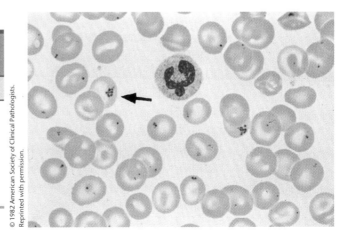

Figure 3.19   Howell-Jolly bodies.

able to inspect and remove them from the cell cytoplasm (Fig. 3.19).

Siderotic granules/Pappenheimer bodies are seen in the iron loading processes such as hereditary hemochromatosis and iron loading anemias subsequent to transfusion therapy. They appear as small beaded inclusions, light purple and located along the periphery of the red cells. Prussian blue staining is the confirmatory staining in determining whether these inclusions are iron in origin; consequently, these inclusions are termed siderotic granules in Prussian blue staining and Pappenheimer bodies in Wright's stain. Siderotic granules may also be viewed in thalassemic conditions and in patients post splenectomy (Fig. 3.20).

Basophilic stippling is a result of RNA and mitochondrial remnants. These remnants appear as diffusely basophilic granules located throughout the cytoplasm and are either dustlike or coarse in appearance. They are difficult to visualize in the peripheral smear without

fine focusing, but red cell–containing basophilic stippling will often be polychromatophilic. Whenever erythropoiesis is accelerated, basophilic stippling is likely to be found as well in individuals with lead poisoning (Fig. 3.21).

Heinz bodies result from denatured hemoglobin and are defined as large structures approximately 1 to 3 μm in diameter located toward the periphery of the red cell membrane (Fig. 3.21). Although they cannot be visualized by Wright's stain, bite cells in the peripheral smear are evidence that a Heinz body has been formed and removed by the spleen. To visualize the actual Heinz body inclusion, staining with a supravital stain such as brilliant cresyl blue or crystal violet may be necessary. Heinz bodies are seen in glucose-6-phosphate dehydrogenase deficiency or in any unstable hemoglobinopathy such as hemoglobin Zurich (Fig. 3.22). See Figure 3.23 for a schematic representation of Heinz body formation.

Table 3.3 ⊙ Summary of Inclusions	
Inclusion	**Composition**
Howell-Jolly body	DNA in origin
Basophilic stippling	RNA remnants
Siderotic granules/ Pappenheimer bodies	Iron
Heinz bodies	Denatured hemoglobin

Figure 3.20   Siderotic granules.

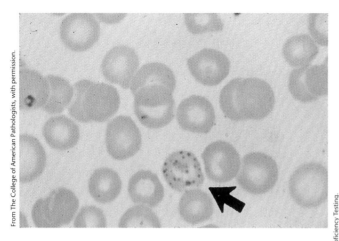

From The College of American Pathologists, with permission.

Figure 3.21   Basophilic stippling.

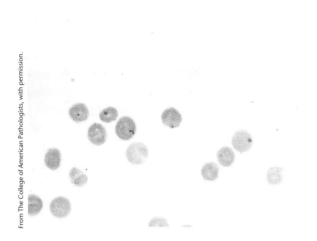

From The College of American Pathologists, with permission.

Figure 3.22   Heinz bodies.

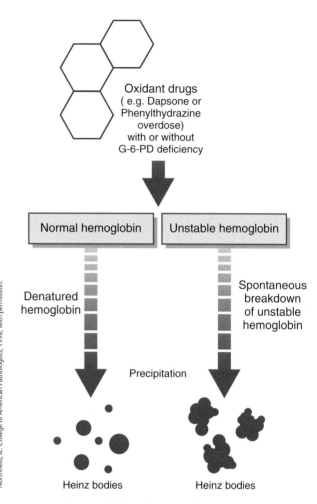

Adapted from Glassy E. Color Atlas of Hematology: An Illustrated Guide Based on Proficiency Testing. Northfield, IL: College of American Pathologists, 1998, with permission.

Oxidant drugs (e.g. Dapsone or Phenylthydrazine overdose) with or without G-6-PD deficiency

Normal hemoglobin   Unstable hemoglobin

Denatured hemoglobin   Spontaneous breakdown of unstable hemoglobin

Precipitation

Heinz bodies   Heinz bodies

Figure 3.23   Heinz body formation.

CONDENSED CASE

At a local physician office lab (POL), one technologist was assigned to do complete differentials or to review smears depending on the automated count. She noticed that in every smear she reviewed, burr cells were a prominent part of the red cell morphology. She began to get suspicious and consider the possibility that the burr cells were artifactual. **What are the potential causes for artifactually induced burr cells?**

Answer

Burr cells can be artifactual if (1) the blood smears that are made are forced to air dry through repeated shaking or (2) the buffer used in staining is not at the proper pH.

Summary Points

- Red cell production is under the control of erythropoietin (EPO), a hormone released from the kidney
- The main sites of adult erythropoiesis are the sternum and iliac crest.
- Each pronormoblast produces 16 mature red cells.
- As they mature, red cells decrease in size, become less basophilic in their cytoplasm, develop the orange tinge of hemoglobin, and lose their nucleus.
- Another name for an orthochromic normoblast is a nucleated red blood cell (nRBC).
- The red cell membrane is a trilaminar structure containing glycolipids, glycoproteins, cholesterol, and proteins that anchor the cell and provide deformability such as spectrin and ankyrin.
- Integral proteins start from the cytoskeleton and expand through the entire red cell membrane.

- Peripheral proteins are confined to the red cell cytoskeleton.
- Sodium and potassium migrate from the plasma across the red cell membranes in an organized fashion controlled by cationic pumps.
- Deformability and elasticity are crucial properties of the red cell membrane, which must be able to extend is surface area up to 117% to accommodate its passage through arterioles and capillary space.
- The Embden-Meyerhof pathway provides 90% of cellular ATP necessary for anaerobic red cell metabolism.
- Microcytes and macrocytes represent size changes in the red cells determined by abnormal pathologies.
- Microcytes are seen in iron deficiency anemia, thalassemic conditions, iron loading processes, and, in some individuals, with the anemia of inflammation.
- Macrocytes are associated with megaloblastic processes, liver disease, and high reticulocyte counts.
- Polychromasia is the peripheral cell response to accelerated erythropoiesis.
- Hypochromia is a color variation in the red cell determined by lack of hemoglobin synthesis.
- Sickle cells are observed when hemoglobin S is part of the hemoglobin component; there are two types of sickle cells: irreversible or reversible or oat-shaped sickle cells.
- Spherocytes are seen in hereditary spherocytosis, in autoimmune hemolytic anemias, or as a part of red cell senescence.
- Target cells are seen in any condition affecting hemoglobin function and also in liver disease or other processes where cholesterol is loaded in the circulation.
- Fragmented cells occur as a result of membrane loss and may be seen in heart valve disease, in burns, or in conditions where there is a predisposition of thrombi.
- Ovalocytes can be seen in thalassemic processes and in the megaloblastic anemias where macro-ovalocytes are seen.
- Elliptocytes are seen in iron deficiency anemia, hereditary elliptocytosis, and idiopathic myelofibrosis.
- Howell-Jolly bodies are DNA in origin and seen in conditions of accelerated erythropoiesis: basophilic stippling is RNA in origin and is seen in lead poisoning and accelerated erythropoiesis.
- Heinz bodies are formed from denatured hemoglobin, usually from individuals with glucose-6-phosphate dehydrogenase deficiency.
- Pappenheimer bodies/siderotic granules are iron in origin and seen in iron loading process or in patients who are hypertransfused.

CASE STUDY

A 55-year-old woman complained to her physician that her finger and toes became blue during cold weather. When she warmed them up, her digits became painful. She also noted that she has been feeling extremely fatigued, with tachycardia and dyspnea. There was no family history of anemia or any other inherited hematological condition, but there has been a history of vascular disease in her paternal side. A CBC and differential were ordered with the following results: WBC 8.0×10^9/L, RBC 3.04×10^{12}/L, Hgb 9.0 g/dL, Hct 28.0%, MCV 82 fL, MCH 28 pg, and MCHC 30.2%. A reticulocyte count was ordered once the CBC was performed. **Which anemic condition can lead to this patient's unusual symptoms?**

Insights to the Case Study

This patient is showing signs of anemia with a low RBC, Hgb, and Hct. Additionally, she is showing the physical symptoms of anemia, which include shortness of breath (dyspnea), heart palpitations (tachycardia), and fatigue.

Her symptoms related to her fingers and toes suggest Raynaud's syndrome, and her physician proceeded to order a direct antiglobulin test battery using all three anti-human globulin reagents. This test was positive with agglutination in the complement anti-human globulin reagent, indicating complement coating of the red cells. Her physician diagnosed cold agglutinin syndrome in the early stages. Cold agglutinin syndrome is a hemolytic anemia most often associated with cold reactive autoantibodies, which are complement binding. This syndrome accounts for approximately 16% to 23% of all cases of immune hemolytic processes. Patients experience hemolysis and hemoglobinuria at cold temperatures as well as the physical symptoms indicated in this case. Many individuals move to warmer climates to prevent hemolytic episodes or if symptoms exacerbate. In addition, our patient's peripheral blood smear showed occasional spherocytes and moderate polychromasia, and her reticulocyte count was 3.0% (normal value, 0.5% to 1.5%).

Review Questions

1. What is a significant morphological difference between irreversibly sickled cells and reversible sickled cells?
   a. Puddled hemoglobin
   b. Crystal formation central to the sickle cells
   c. Pointed projections to the sickle cell
   d. Fragmentation of the red cell membrane

2. What are two integral proteins in the red cell structure that house red cell antigens?
   a. Glycoproteins and glycolipids
   b. Glycophorin A and glycophorin B
   c. Cholesterol and spectrin
   d. Sodium and potassium

3. All of the following are characteristic of the red cell in stages of development *except*
   a. nuclei are "baseball" round.
   b. immature cells are larger.
   c. N:C ratio decreases as the cell matures.
   d. distinct granulation in the cytoplasm.

4. Which red cell inclusions originate as a result of denatured hemoglobin?
   a. Howell-Jolly bodies
   b. Heinz bodies

   c. Pappenheimer bodies
   d. Malarial parasites

5. In which conditions can you see elliptocytes?
   a. Iron loading processes
   b. Sickle cell anemia
   c. Iron deficiency anemia
   d. Thalassemia

6. Which red cell morphology may form as a result of excess cholesterol taken upon the red cell membrane?
   a. Macrocytes
   b. Target cells
   c. Schistocytes
   d. Ovalocytes

7. Hypochromia is used to define
   a. color change in the red cell.
   b. variation in shape of the red cell.
   c. variation in size of the red cell.
   d. decrease in hemoglobin content of the red cell.

○ TROUBLESHOOTING

What Do I Do When There Is a Drastic Change in a Patient's Differential Results During the Same Shift?

A 47-year-old male patient recovering from bacterial meningitis was having his blood drawn on a daily basis for CBCs. His sample was received in the morning with the morning draw at 8 a.m. (see the chart). Later in the day, the technologist received another request for a CBC on the same patient and noticed quite a difference in the automated differential. The RBC, Hgb, Hct, MCV, and RDW all resembled the first sample from the a.m. draw. The technologist suspected that the second sample has been mislabeled. She retrieved both samples and asked the blood bank to perform ABO grouping on the samples. Results are as follows.

8 a.m. Draw		2 p.m. Draw	
CBC	**Differential**	**CBC**	**Differential**
WBC 11.1	Neutrophils 86%	12.4	Neutrophils 66%
RBC 3.97	Lymphocytes 8%	3.82	Lymphocytes 20%
Hgb 12.7	Monocytes 5%	12.5	Monocytes 12%
Hct 38.0	Eosinophils 1	36.0	Eosinophils 2%
MCV 95.6	Basophils 0	94.3	Basophils 0%
MCH 32.0		32.7	
MCHC 33.5		34.7	
RDW 13.9		12.6	
Platelets 224		313	

Blood Banking Report

8 a.m. sample: O pos

2 p.m. sample: A pos

The CBCs of both samples were fairly equal with no cause for alarm, however, there were some disparities in the differential of the two samples. Even though both sets of results were acceptable and no result was flagged, the technologist had a nagging suspicion that the second sample was mislabeled. She took both samples, the a.m. and p.m. samples, to the blood bank to be ABO typed. The blood types on these samples did not match, but the patient has a history of type O blood from blood bank files. The floor was notified that the sample was mislabeled, the sample was discarded, and the afternoon results on that patient were negated. Putting all of the pieces of this puzzle together led to a confirmation of the patient's original suspicions of the p.m. sample. Rather than verify the p.m. results, the technologist chose to investigate the possibility of a mislabeled sample. Discovering an error in patient sample collection provides an opportunity for the laboratory to remind the hospital units that accurate patient collection and identification procedures are tantamount to accurate patient results.

WORD KEY

Anaerobic • Able to live without oxygen

Asynchrony • Failure of event to occur at the same time

Cytoskeleton • Internal structural framework of the cell

Disseminated intravascular coagulation • Pathological condition in which the coagulation pathways are hyperstimulated, either excessive fibrin disposition or excess fibrinolysis

Pathology • Study of the nature and cause of disease which involved changes in structure and function

Splenectomy • Removal of the spleen

Thrombi • Plural of thrombus; a blood clot that obstructs a blood vessel or a cavity of the heart

References

1. Bell A. Morphology of human blood and marrow cells. In: Harmening D, ed. Clinical Hematology and Fundamentals of Hemostasis, 4th ed. Philadelphia: FA Davis, 2002; 10.

2. Schwabbauer M. Normal erythrocyte production, physiology and destruction. In: Steine-Martin E, Lotspeich-Steininger C, Koeple JA, eds. Clinical Hematology: Principles, Procedures and Correlations, 2nd ed. Philadelphia: Lippincott, 1998; 61.

3. Hubbard JD. A concise review of clinical laboratory sciences. Baltimore, MD: Williams & Wilkins, 1997; 139–140.

4. Harmening D, Hughes V, Del Toro C. The red cell: Structure and function. In: Harmening D, ed. Clinical Hematology and Fundamentals of Hemostasis, 4th ed. Philadelphia: FA Davis, 2002; 62.

5. Besa E. Hemolytic anemia in hematology. Besa E, Catalano P, Kant JA, eds. Philadelphia: Harwal Publishing, 1992; 98–99.

6. Hussong JW. Iron metabolism and hypochromic anemias. In Harmening, D: Clinical Hematology and Fundamentals of Hemostasis, 4th ed. Philadelphia: FA Davis, 2002; 105.

7. Ciesla B. Pondering red cell morphology. ADVANCE for Medical Laboratory Professionals 15:10–11, 2003.

8. Womack EP. Treating thrombotic thrombocytopenic purpura with plasma exchange. Lab Med 30:279, 1999.

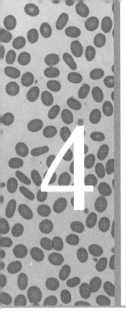
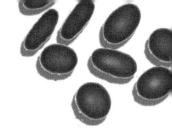

4

Hemoglobin Function and Principles of Hemolysis

Betty Ciesla

Hemoglobin Structure and Synthesis
  Types of Hemoglobin
  Hemoglobin Function
  Abnormal Hemoglobins

The Hemolytic Process
  Types of Hemolysis
  Laboratory Evidence of Hemolysis
  The Physiology of Hemolysis

Terminology Relevant to the Hemolytic Anemias

Objectives

After completing this chapter, the student will be able to:

1. Identify the components of hemoglobin.

2. Define the normal structural elements related to hemoglobin synthesis.

3. Describe hemoglobin function.

4. Describe the origin of hemoglobin synthesis in erythroid precursors.

5. List the normal adult hemoglobins.

6. Describe the chemical configuration and percentages of the normal adult hemoglobins, Hgb A, Hgb A_2, and Hgb F.

7. Relate the shift from fetal hemoglobin to adult hemoglobin in terms of fetal to adult development.

8. Outline the steps involved in oxygen delivery and the elimination of carbon dioxide.

9. Describe the oxygen dissociation curve in general terms.

10. Differentiate the abnormal hemoglobins in terms of toxicity and oxygen capacity.

11. Describe hemolysis in terms of its effect on the bone marrow, blood smear, and blood chemistry.

12. Define *extravascular hemolysis* with respect to organ of origin and laboratory diagnosis.

13. Define *intravascular hemolysis* with respect to organs affected and laboratory diagnosis.

14. Recall the terminologies used to classify the hemolytic anemias.

HEMOGLOBIN STRUCTURE AND SYNTHESIS

Hemoglobin is the life-giving substance of every red cell, the oxygen-carrying component of the red cell. Each red blood cell is nothing more than a fluid-filled sac, with the fluid being hemoglobin. In 4 months, or 120 days, red cells with normal hemoglobin content submit to the rigors of circulation. Red cells are stretched, twisted, pummeled, and squeezed as they make their way through the circulatory watershed. Each major organ in the human body depends on oxygenation for growth and function, and this process is ultimately under the control of hemoglobin. The hemoglobin molecule consists of two primary structures:

- *Heme portion*. This structure involves four iron atoms in the ferrous state (Fe^{2+} because iron in the ferric state, Fe^{3+}, cannot bind oxygen) surrounded by protoporphyrin IX, or the porphyrin ring, a structure formed in the nucleated red cells. Protoporphyrin IX is the final product in the synthesis of the heme molecule. It results from the interaction of succinyl coenzyme A and delta-aminolevulinic acid in the mitochondria of the nucleated red cells. Several intermediate by products are formed: porphobilinogen, uroporphyrinogen, and coproporphyrin. Once iron in incorporated, it combines with protoporphyrin to form the complete heme molecule. Defects in any of the intermediate products can impair hemoglobin function.
- *Globin portion*. These consist of **amino acids** linked together to form a polypeptide chain, a bracelet of amino acids. The most significant chains for adult hemoglobins are the alpha and beta chains. Alpha chains have 141 amino acids in a unique arrangement, and beta chains have 146 amino acids in a unique arrangement. The heme and globin portions of the hemoglobin molecule are linked together by chemical bonds.
- An additional structure that supports the hemoglobin molecule is *2,3-diphosphoglycerate* (2,3-DPG), a substance produced via the Embden-Meyerhof pathway during anaerobic glycolysis.[1] This structure is intimately related to oxygen affinity of hemoglobin and is explained in that section.

Each heme molecule consists of four heme structures with iron at the center and two pairs of globin chains (Fig. 4.1). The heme structure sits lodged in the pocket of the globin chains. Hemoglobin begins to be synthesized at the polychromatic normoblast stage of red cell development. This synthesis is visualized by the change in cytoplasmic color from a deep blue to a lavender-tinged cytoplasmic color. Sixty-five percent of hemoglobin is synthesized before the red cell nucleus is extruded, with an additional 35% synthesized by the reticulocyte stage.[2] Normal mature red cells have a full complement of hemoglobin, which occupies a little less than one half of the surface area of the red cell.

Types of Hemoglobin

There are three types of hemoglobin that are synthesized: embryonic hemoglobins, fetal hemoglobin, and the adult hemoglobins. Each of these types of hemoglobins has a specific arrangement of globin chains and each globin chain is under the influence of a specific chromosome. Chromosome 11 contains the genes for the production of epsilon, beta, gamma, and delta chains. Each parent contributes one gene for the production of each of these chains. Therefore, each individual has two genes for the production of any of these chains. Chromosome 16 is responsible for the alpha and zeta genes. There are two genes on the chromosome for the production of alpha chains and one gene for the production of zeta chains (Fig. 4.2). Thus, each parent contributes two genes for the production of alpha chains and one for the zeta chains. Thus, each individual has four genes for the production of alpha chains and two for zeta chains. Alpha chains are a constant component of adult hemoglobin; therefore, each hemoglobin has two obligatory alpha chains as part of its chemical configuration. The epsilon and zeta chains are

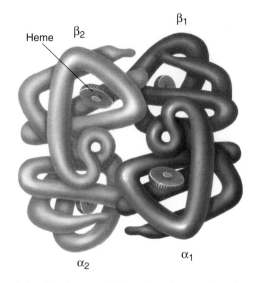

Figure 4.1 The hemoglobin molecule: note four heme molecules tucked inside globin chains.

reserved for the production of embryonic hemoglobins. As the embryo develops, hemoglobins Gower I and II (α_2, ε_2) and hemoglobin Portland ($\gamma_2\delta_2$), are synthesized and remain in the embryo for the 3 months. Hemoglobin F ($\alpha_2\gamma_2$), fetal hemoglobin, begins to be synthesized at approximately 3 months in fetal development and remains as the majority hemoglobin at birth. Between 3 and 6 months post delivery, the amount of gamma chains declines and the amount of beta chains increases, making hemoglobin A ($\alpha_2\beta_2$) the majority adult hemoglobin, 95% to 98%. Hemoglobin A_2 ($\alpha_2\delta_2$), 1% to 3%, and hemoglobin F, less than 1%, are also part of the normal adult hemoglobin **complement**. Amino acids are an essential component of each of the globin chains. The unique position of amino acids in each chain, as well as the specificity of the amino acid itself, is essential to the normal function of the hemoglobin molecule. Synthetic or structural abnormalities of the protein chains may lead to hemoglobin defects.

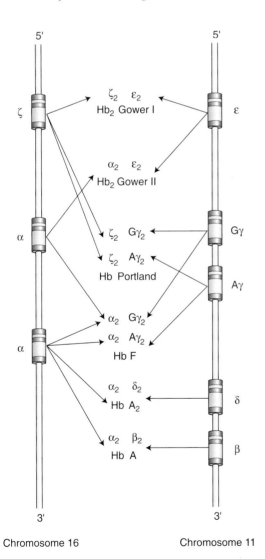

Figure 4.2 Specific chromosomes relative to human hemoglobin formation.

Hemoglobin Function

Oxygen delivery is the principal purpose of the hemoglobin molecule. Additionally, it is a structure capable of pulling CO_2 away from the tissues, as well as keeping the blood in a balanced pH. The hemoglobin molecule loads oxygen on a one-to-one basis, one molecule of hemoglobin to one molecule of oxygen in the oxygen-rich environment of the alveoli of the lungs. Hemoglobin becomes saturated with oxygen, oxyhemoglobin, and has a high affinity for oxygen in this pulmonary environment, because the network of capillaries in the lungs makes the diffusion of oxygen a rapid process. As the molecule transits through the circulation, deoxyhemoglobin is able to transport oxygen and unload to the tissues in areas of low oxygen affinity. As hemoglobin goes through the loading and unloading process, changes appear in the molecule. These changes are termed **allosteric** changes, a term that relates to the way hemoglobin is able to rotate on its axis, determine the action of salt bridges between the globin structures, and dictate the movement of 2,3-DPG. The hemoglobin molecule appears in a tense and a relaxed form.[3] When tense, hemoglobin in not oxygenated, 2,3-DPG is at the center of the molecule, and the salt bridges between the globin chains are in place. When oxygenated, the relaxed form is in place; 2,3-DPG is expelled, salt bridges are broken, and the molecule is capable of fully loading oxygen.

The binding and release of oxygen from the hemoglobin molecule are defined by the oxygen dissociation curve (OD curve) (Fig. 4.3). This curve is represented as a sigmoid shape, an "S" shape, not the straight-line shape familiar to most students. The curve is designed to illustrate the unique qualities of oxygen dissociation and to attempt to graphically demonstrate how the hemoglobin molecule and oxygen respond to normal and abnormal physiologies.[4] What is essential when considering the hemoglobin molecule is that when the molecule is fully saturated, it has all of the oxygen it needs and a high level of oxygen tension. As it travels from the pulmonary circulation to the venous circulation, it has more of an inclination to give up its oxygen in response to the oxygen needs of the tissue it is serving. Figure 4-3 demonstrates the following:[5]

1. There is a progressive increase in the percentage of the hemoglobin that is bound with oxygen as the blood P_{O_2} increases.
2. In the lungs in which the blood P_{O_2} is 100 mm Hg, hemoglobin is 97% saturated with oxygen.
3. In venous circulation, in which the P_{O_2} is 40 mm Hg, 75% of the hemoglobin molecule is saturated with oxygen and 25% of the oxy-

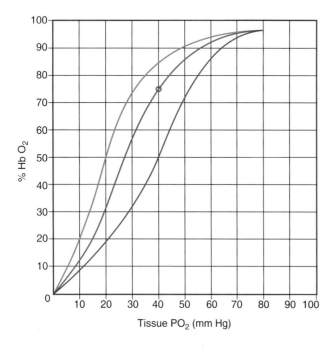

■ = Normal 7.4
■ = Right shift 7.2
■ = Left shift 7.6

Figure 4.3   The oxygen dissociation curve. In the normal curve (blue) at 40 mm Hg, 75% of the hemoglobin molecule is saturated with oxygen, leaving 25% capable of being released to tissue. Note the right-shifted curve (red). At 40 mm Hg, hemoglobin is 50% saturated but willing to give up 50% of its oxygen to the tissues. Note the left-shifted curve (black). At 40 mm Hg, hemoglobin is 75% saturated but willing to release only 12% to the tissues.

gen is capable of being released when the hemoglobin level is normal.

Two things are demonstrated by this relationship: depending on the need of tissues for oxygen, the hemoglobin molecule will either hold onto oxygen, oxygen affinity, or it will release more oxygen as physiological circumstances dictate.

• When referring to the OD curve, we speak about it in terms of having a "shift to the right" or a "shift to the left."
• Shifting the curve means that physiological conditions are present in the body that will impact the relationship of oxygen and hemoglobin. In most cases, the hemoglobin molecule will compensate by holding or delivering oxygen depending on tissue need. This compensatory mechanism can be demonstrated through the OD curve.
• When the curve is right shifted, hemoglobin has less attraction for oxygen and is more will-

ing to release oxygen to the tissues. In a right-shifted OD curve, at 40 mm Hg, hemoglobin is 50% saturated but willing to give up 50% of its oxygen to the tissue because of need.
• When the curve is left shifted, hemoglobin has more of an attraction for oxygen and is less willing to release it to the tissues. In a left-shifted OD curve, at 40 mm Hg, hemoglobin is 75% saturated but willing to release only 12% to the tissues.

Physiological conditions that will shift the curve to the right are

a. Anemia
b. Decreased pH (**acidosis**)
c. Increase in 2,3-DPG

Therefore, in the anemic state, even though there are fewer red cells and less hemoglobin, the cells act more efficiently to deliver oxygen to the tissues. In fact, the compensatory mechanism of the OD curve works quite adequately if the hemoglobin level is between 8 and 12 g/dL. It is only when the hemoglobin level drops below 8 g/dL that symptoms start to develop, for the most part. Conditions that shift the OD curve to the left are

a. Decrease in 2,3-DPG
b. Higher body temperatures
c. Presence of abnormal hemoglobins or high oxygen affinity hemoglobins
d. Multiple transfusions of stored blood where 2,3-DPG is depleted by virtue of the storage process
e. Increased pH (**alkalosis**)

Less oxygen is released to tissues under these conditions when 2,3-DPG is lower. Consider this analogy for the OD curve. The OD curve is like a roller coaster. As you start up the incline, you are holding on tight, and then as you roll down the hill, you are more willing to throw your arms up in the air and release or relax your grip. So it is with the right-shifted OD curve.

Abnormal Hemoglobins

Normal hemoglobin is a highly stable protein, which can be converted to cyanmethemoglobin, a colored pigment. This conversion is the basis for most of the colorimetric procedures used to measure hemoglobin, and it depends on a versatile and viable hemoglobin compound. Hemoglobins that are physiologically abnormal have a higher oxygen affinity and produce conditions that are usually toxic to the human body.

Three abnormal hemoglobins are methemoglobin, sulfhemoglobin, and carboxyhemoglobin. Increasing the amounts of any of these abnormal hemoglobins in the bloodstream can be potentially fatal. Often, the production of abnormal hemoglobins results from accidental or purposeful ingestion or absorption of substances, drugs, and so on that are harmful. At times, abnormal hemoglobins are produced as a result of inherited defects. In the abnormal hemoglobin methemoglobin, iron has been oxidized to the Fe^{3+} state, which is no longer capable of binding oxygen. Methemoglobin builds up in the circulation and if the level is above 10%, individuals appear **cyanotic,** having a blue color, especially in the lips and fingers.[6] Aniline drugs and some antimalarial treatments may induce a methemoglobinemia in individuals who are unable to reduce methemoglobin. Hemoglobin M, an inherited condition arising from an amino acid substitution, may also result in cyanotic conditions. Carboxyhemoglobin levels are increased in smokers and certain industrial workers. As a hemoglobin derivative, carboxyhemoglobin has an affinity for carbon monoxide that is 200 times greater than for oxygen; therefore, no oxygen is delivered to the tissues. For this reason, carbon monoxide poisoning, either deliberate or accidental, is efficient and relatively painless. Sulfhemoglobin can be formed on exposure to agents such as sulfonamides or sulfa-containing drugs. The affinity of sulfhemoglobin for oxygen is 100 times lower than that of normal hemoglobin. It may be toxic at a very low level (Table 4.1).

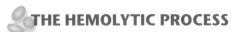 THE HEMOLYTIC PROCESS

Red cell senescence or death is a natural process for red cells at the end of their 120-day life span. As a natural byproduct, the contents of the red cell are released and returned to various parts of the circulation to be recycled in the process of red cell regeneration. When red cell death occurs in an orderly fashion, the hematological balance is maintained. Hemoglobin is kept at normal levels, and the bone marrow maintains a steady production of red cells. If premature red cell death or hemolysis occurs, a series of events begin to cascade, which provide laboratory evidence that red cells are dying faster than their normal 120-day life cycle (Table 4.2). When this happens, the body's peripheral circulation begins its intervention process. There is evidence

Table 4.1 ◉ Abnormal Hemoglobins

- Sulfhemoglobin
- Carboxyhemoglobin
- Methemoglobin

Table 4.2 ◉ Relationship of Hemolysis and Clinical Events

Clinical Events	Physical Symptoms
↓ RBC, Hgb, Hct	Symptoms of anemia: pallor, fatigue, tachycardia
↑ Bilirubin	Jaundice
Hemoglobinemia	Blood-tinged plasma
Hemoglobinuria	Blood-tinged urine

for hemolysis in the bone marrow, in the peripheral circulation, and in the blood plasma. The bone marrow will show erythroid **hyperplasia,** meaning an increase in red blood cell precursors and premature release of reticulocytes and young red cells. The normal M:E ratio of 3 to 4:1 will be shifted toward the red blood cell, giving a ratio of perhaps 1:2. The peripheral smear will provide visual clues of hemolysis by showing an increase in **polychromasia** and the presence of nucleated red cells and possibly spherocytes. Spherocytes may appear in the peripheral circulation if red cells become coated with antibody. As antibody-coated red cells travel through the spleen, the spleen subsequently shears off the antibody as the red cell percolates through this organ.[7] None of these visual indicators are likely to be observed in the *normal* peripheral smear. They are seen in the peripheral smear in *response* to a hemolytic event. Plasma changes are discussed later in the chapter.

Types of Hemolysis

Hemolysis can be an extravascular or an intravascular process. Ninety percent of all hemolysis is extravascular and occurs in the spleen, liver, lymph nodes, and the bone marrow, the organs of the reticuloendothelial system. Red cells are destroyed and their contents are phagocytized with hemoglobin released into the macrophages. Extravascular hemolysis is a well-established pathway in which red cell breakdown leads to the release of the internal products of hemoglobin, primarily heme and globin (Fig. 4.4). The amino acids of the globin chains are recycled into the amino acid pool, while the products of heme are taken through different pathways. Iron is transported via transferrin; the transport protein to the bone marrow or storage sites to be used in erythropoiesis, while the rest of the hemoglobin molecule reacts with hemoxygenase, yielding a byproduct biliverdin, which is reduced to unconjugated bilirubin. This bilirubin product attaches to albumin and is then transported to the liver.

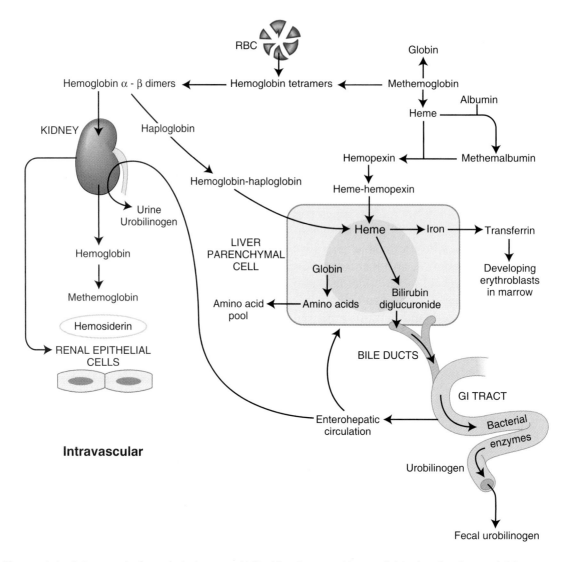

Figure 4.4   Intravascular hemolysis: increased bilirubin, decreased haptoglobin, but free hemoglobin present.

Ten percent of hemolysis is intravascular, and it occurs as hemoglobin is lysed directly in the blood. Intravascular lysis takes place directly inside the vessel, and hemoglobin is released into the plasma (Fig. 4.5). Hemoglobinemia, red-tinged hemoglobin seen directly in the plasma after the blood sample is centrifuged, is an unusual finding seen only in intravascular lysis. Blood in the urine, hemoglobinuria, may also be a byproduct of direct intravascular lysis that may be complement mediated. If complement is activated as in the case of ABO transfusion reaction, a complex of proteins are introduced that cause additional damage to the red cell membrane.[8] Evidence of intravascular lysis indicates a serious condition that must be acted on promptly.

Laboratory Evidence of Hemolysis

Hemolysis can be distinguished in the laboratory by a variety of methods. Most of these measurements are obtained in the hematology and chemistry laboratories by routine laboratory procedures. There is no need to consider expensive reference procedures. The first consideration is to establish whether the patient is hemolyzing. The second consideration is to establish the cause and type of hemolysis. If the patient is experiencing *intravascular* lysis, these conditions are present:

• Hemoglobin, hematocrit, and red cell count are low.
• Serum bilirubin is elevated.
• Serum haptoglobin is low.
• Hemoglobinemia (free hemoglobin in plasma) may be present.
• Hemoglobinuria (hemoglobin in urine) may be present.
• Reticulocyte count is elevated.
• Lactate dehydrogenase (LDH) is elevated.

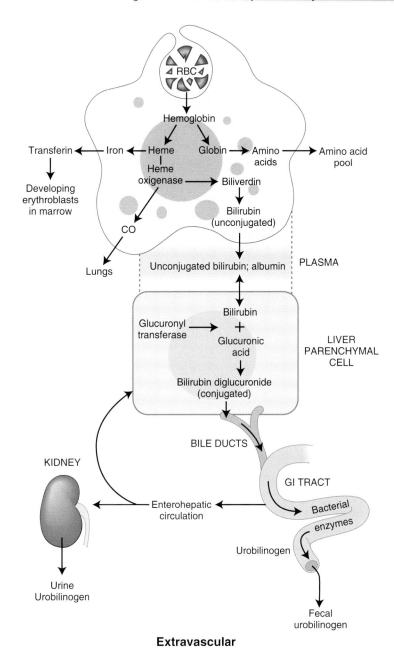

Figure 4.5 Extravascular hemolysis: increased bilirubin and decreased haptoglobin.

Extravascular

Under conditions of *extravascular* lysis, these conditions are present:

- Hemoglobin, hematocrit, and red cell count are low.
- Serum bilirubin is elevated.
- Reticulocyte count is elevated.
- Haptoglobin is low.
- Hepatosplenomegaly may be seen.
- LDH is elevated.

The Physiology of Hemolysis

Distinguishing between intravascular and extravascular hemolysis can be accomplished by paying careful atten-

tion to laboratory data. Yet, it is imperative for a student to understand why each of these events is taking place. When considering intravascular lysis, conditions that may predispose to rapid and volatile lysis within vessels may activate complement, an efficient accessory to the hemolytic process. Red blood cells burst, releasing their contents, and the alpha and beta dimers of hemoglobin are released immediately into the plasma. From the plasma they are bound to haptoglobin. The hemoglobin-haptoglobin complex is too large to be filtered by the kidneys, so it is not excreted but rather transported to the liver, where it is destroyed and broken down. The actual haptoglobin measurement of the plasma is lower in a hemolytic event, indicating that there are no sites left for this molecule to be bound with hemoglobin. The CBC will show reduced hemoglobin, hematocrit, and red cell count in response to excessive red cell destruction, and the reticulocyte count is elevated in response to the erythroid hyperplasia of the bone marrow. Reticulocytes are released prematurely in response to the red cell need in anemic conditions; therefore, the reticulocyte count is almost always elevated. Additionally, LDH is increased. LDH is a red blood cell enzyme that will increase in the plasma as red blood cells are lysed prematurely. Hemoglobinemia may appear as red-tinged plasma, because the red cells have burst directly inside the vessels; consequently, centrifuged blood samples may have a red or pink-tinged plasma component. Hemoglobinuria is a direct representation of free hemoglobin being filtered by the kidney into the urine; therefore, urine samples may be blood tinged. Intravascular events may take as long as 48 hours to manifest through laboratory results. Many of the same processes that occur in intravascular events may occur in extravascular hemolysis, with the exception of hemoglobinuria and hemoglobinemia. Additionally, the spleen may become enlarged in extravascular hemolysis because damaged red cells may become sequestered in this organ.

TERMINOLOGY RELEVANT TO THE HEMOLYTIC ANEMIAS

The hemolytic anemias are classified according to many different schemes. In this chapter, we have classified the hemolytic anemias according to the site of hemolysis by classifying hemolytic events as either extravascular or intravascular. Yet many textbooks discuss the

Table 4.3 ● Hemolytic Anemias Classified by Intrinsic or Extrinsic Defects (Modified List)	
Intrinsic Red Cell Defects Leading to Hemolysis	**Extrinsic Defects Leading to Hemolysis**
Hemoglobinopathies: structural and synthetic	Autoimmune hemolytic anemia
Red cell membrane defects	Parasitic infection
Red cell enzyme defects	Microangiopathic hemolytic anemia
Stem cell defects	Environmental agents, including venoms and chemical agents

hemolytic anemias in terms of those that result from intrinsic defects of the red cell as opposed to those that result from extrinsic events that are not necessarily related to the structure of the red cell but affect its life span. Intrinsic defects of the red cell relate to inherited deficiencies of the red cell membrane, hemoglobin structure or synthesis, or biochemical components. Extrinsic defects relate to those events that are secondary to red cell structure and function but may still result in a hemolytic event. Regardless of the classification, it is paramount that the hemolytic anemias be recognized, evaluated, and managed so that life-threatening sequelae do not arise.[9] See Table 4.3 for a modified list of those anemias classified by intrinsic or extrinsic defects.

CONDENSED CASE

An 80-year-old woman visited the emergency department at 9 p.m. with complaints of dizziness of 3 days' duration and right-sided abdominal pain. Once in the treatment room, three tubes of blood were drawn from the patient: a purple top, a blue top, and a tiger top. The samples were not inverted, and they remained unlabeled in the treatment room for at least 1 hour, sitting in an emesis basin. The patient was subsequently admitted to the hospital at 3 a.m. and all of her blood work was redrawn. **What was the probable cause for the second stick?**

Answer

This scenario represents two important breakdowns of phlebotomy protocol—lack of inversion of anticoagulated tubes and lack of labeling. Tubes that are anticoagulated should be inverted no less than six times for proper mixing of blood and anticoagulant. Failure to do so could easily result in clotted tubes. Proper labeling of tubes should take place at the bedside, immediately after the sample has been drawn. The patient should identify himself or herself verbally, and this identification should be verified through the identification bracelet. Rigorous efforts must be taken for proper patient identification.

Summary Points

- Hemoglobin has two main components: heme and globin.
- Heme consists of iron and the protoporphyrin ring.
- Globin consists of amino acid chains of specific lengths and specific amino acids; alpha and beta chains are the two most significant amino acid chains.
- Alpha chains have 141 amino acids, and beta chains have 146 amino acids.
- Hemoglobins Gower and Portland are embryonic hemoglobins; hemoglobin F is fetal hemoglobin, and the adult hemoglobins are hemoglobins A, A_2, and F.
- Oxygen delivery is the primary purpose of the hemoglobin molecule.
- 2,3-DPG is intimately related to the oxygen affinity of hemoglobin.
- The OD curve schematically represents the saturation of hemoglobin with oxygen and the release of oxygen from the hemoglobin molecule under normal and abnormal physiological conditions.
- Hemolysis is the premature destruction of the red cell before its 120-day life cycle.
- Hemolysis may be classified as intravascular or extravascular, which relates to the site of hemolysis.
- Intravascular hemolysis takes place inside the blood vessels; extravascular hemolysis takes place outside the blood vessels, primarily in the RES system.
- Hemolytic anemias may be classified by intrinsic defects of the red cell or extrinsic defects that affect the red cell.

CASE STUDY

Eight-year-old twin boys were brought into the emergency department with complaints of intermittent fevers and lethargy. The boys had not been feeling well for the last 2 weeks. They had recently returned from a trip to Nigeria with their parents. All members of the family had been treated with antimalarial medication before the trip. Neither parent exhibited any of the symptoms of the children. A CBC with differential was ordered as well as a peripheral smear for malarial parasites. The children were slightly anemic, with hematocrits at 33%, and both boys had elevated white counts of around 15.0×10^9/L.

Insights to the Case Study

Both of these young boys had malaria, and ring forms were observed in the thin preparation on the peripheral smear. *Plasmodium falciparum* was identified. Additionally, they had begun to show slight hemolysis as evidenced by their slightly abnormal hematocrits. Drug-resistant strains of malaria are becoming increasingly common in the world, and cases of malaria are on the rise not only in endemic areas in Africa but also in countries like Peru and Tajikistan, areas where malaria infections were unlikely. When one considers that malaria is still killing 1.1 million individuals a year and still infecting up to a half-billion people a year,[10] this health situation is of major impact and significance. Hardest hit are the most vulnerable populations like young children in remote villages who may not have access to vaccine or treatment. Death or life-changing neurological manifestations are common in this population. Many strains of the malaria parasite have also become resistant to chloroquine, once the panacea for malarial protection. Factors such as noncompliance with drug protocol (not taking the drug as long as is necessary) and the indiscriminant use of this drug have led the malarial parasite to adapt to the drug and become resistant to the more common remedies. Our patients were thought to have a drug-resistant strain of malaria, were placed on Fansidar, and made a good recovery.

Review Questions

1. Which of these hemoglobins is an embryonic hemoglobin?
   a. Hemoglobin A
   b. Hemoglobin Gower
   c. Hemoglobin F
   d. Hemoglobin A 2

2. How many total genes does a person possess for the production of alpha chains?
   a. One
   b. Two
   c. Four
   d. Three

3. Name one condition that may shift the OD curve to the left.
   a. Inheriting a high oxygen affinity hemoglobin
   b. Metabolic acidosis
   c. Anemia
   d. Increased hemoglobin concentration

4. If polychromasia is increased in the peripheral smear, the _____ should be elevated.
   a. white cell count
   b. red cell count
   c. reticulocyte count
   d. basophil count

5. If 2,3-DPG increases, then the hemoglobin molecule will release more oxygen. This is known as a _____OD curve.
   a. left-shifted
   b. normal physiological
   c. right-shifted
   d. neutral

6. Which of the following statements regarding 2,3-DPG is correct?
   a. It catalyzes porphyrin synthesis.
   b. It controls hemoglobin affinity for oxygen.
   c. It prevents oxidative penetration of hemoglobin.
   d. It converts methemoglobin to oxyhemoglobin.

7. When the iron in the hemoglobin molecule is in the ferric (Fe^{3+}) state, hemoglobin is termed
   a. carboxyhemoglobin.
   b. methemoglobin.
   c. ferrihemoglobin.
   d. sulfhemoglobin.

● TROUBLESHOOTING

What Do I Do When There Is a Discrepancy in the Hemoglobin Value?

A 50-year-old man presented to the emergency department with chest pain, shortness of breath, and tightness in the chest area. He was immediately moved to the treatment room, where cardiac enzymes, troponin, CBC, cholesterol, and triglycerides were ordered. For illustrative purposes, only the results of the CBC are given, as follows:

WBC	12.0×10^9/L
RBC	4.83×10^{12}/L
Hgb	15.0 g/dL
Hct	39.0%
MCV	84 fL
MCH	31 pg
MCHC	39%
Platelet	$340,000 \times 10^9$/L

While the other results were pending, the CBC was run on automated instrumentation. The operator noticed that the hemoglobin and hematocrit failed the correlation check by not adhering to the rule of three: hemoglobin $\times$ 3 = hematocrit $\pm$3%. Because the hemoglobin was significantly elevated in comparison to the hematocrit, the hemoglobin value was suspect. The patient sample was spun and observed for lipemia. The plasma was cloudy and grossly lipemic, and when remixed, a milky appearance could be seen in the mixed sample. Lipemia interferes with the optical measurement of hemoglobin, giving a false elevation of hemoglobin, and all subsequent measurements that depend on a hemoglobin value in the calculation, namely MCH and MCHC. It became clear that corrective action needed to be taken to provide valid results. Corrections for lipemia can occur via one of two methods: the plasma blank correction method or the plasma by dilution replacement method. The most frequently encountered method is the plasma blank correction method, in which the sample is spun, a plasma aliquot is removed, and then the spun plasma is recycled through the instrument. This plasma value is used in the following formula to correct the hemoglobin result

Corrected hemoglobin = Initial whole blood hemoglobin–(Plasma hemoglobin blank × [1 − Initial whole blood hematocrit/100])

When our plasma blank was run, we obtained a value of 3.0.

Therefore, our correction would be as follows:

= 15.5 – (3.0 × [1 − 0.39])

= 15.5 − 1.83

= 13.7

This hemoglobin value is now used in the calculation for MCH and MCHC, to yield corrected MCH and MCHC results of 28.3 and 35.1, respectively.

The second corrective method is the diluent replacement method. Once the whole blood has been cycled through the automated instrument, an aliquot of the sample is removed and spun. The plasma from the spun sample is carefully removed and replaced by an equal amount of saline or other diluent. The removal of plasma and replacement with saline are critical in this procedure. If this step has been done accurately, there will be little difference in the red cell count and this will serve as a quality control for the accuracy of pipetting in this method. Too wide a variation in the red cell counts will indicate poor pipetting. Once an accurate replacement has been established, the saline sample is cycled and the hemoglobin can be reported directly from this sample and used to recalculate indices.

Either of these methods involves labor-intensive, yet essential, steps in reporting an accurate CBC. The operator must first recognize the discrepancy between hemoglobin and hematocrit and then be familiar with the corrective steps that need to be taken to provide a reliable CBC.[11]

(Refer to normal values in Chapter 2.)

WORD KEY

Acidosis • Increase in the acidity of blood (as in diabetic acidosis) due to an excessive loss of bicarbonate (as in renal disease)

Alkalosis • Increase in blood alkalinity due to an accumulation of alkaline or reduction in acid

Allosteric • Shape change

Amino acid • One of a large group of organic compounds marked by the presence of both an amino group (NH_2) and a carboxyl group (COOH); the building blocks of protein and the end products of protein digestion

Complement • Group of proteins in the blood that play a vital role in the body's immune defenses through a cascade of interaction

Cyanosis • Blue tinge to the extremities (lips, fingers, toes)

Hyperplasia • Excessive proliferation of normal cells in the normal tissue of an organ

Polychromasia • Blue tinge to the red cells indicating premature release

References

1. Brown BA. Hematology: Principles and Procedures, 6th ed. Philadelphia: Lippincott Williams and Wilkins, 2003; 42–43.
2. Turgeon ML. Normal erythrocyte lifecycle and physiology. In: Turgeon ML, ed. Clinical Hematology: Theory and Procedures, 3rd ed. Philadelphia: Lippincott Williams and Wilkins, 1999; 66.
3. Ludvigsen FB. Hemoglobin synthesis and function. In: Steine-Martin EA, Lotspeich-Steininger CA, Koepke JA, eds. Clinical Hematology: Principles, Procedures and Correlations, 2nd ed. Philadelphia: Lippincott, 1998; 75.
4. Hillman RS, Finch CA. General characteristics of the erythron. In: Hillman R, Finch C, eds. Red Cell Manual, 7th ed. Philadelphia: FA Davis, 1996; 17–19.
5. Harmening DM, Hughes VC, DelToro C. The red blood cell: Structure and function. In: Harmening D, ed. Clinical Hematology and Fundamentals of Hemostasis, 4th ed. Philadelphia: FA Davis, 2002; 66–67.
6. Bunn HF. Human hemoglobins: Normal and abnormal: Methemoglobinemia. In: Nathan SH, Oski A, eds. Hematology of Infancy and Childhood, 4th ed. Philadelphia: WB Saunders, 1993; 720–723.
7. Wright MS, Smith LA. Laboratory investigation of autoimmune hemolytic anemias. Clin Lab Sci 12:119–122, 1999.
8. Nemchik L. Introduction to anemias of increased erythrocyte destruction. In: Steine-Martin EA, Lotspeich-Steininger CA, Koepke JA, eds. Clinical Hematology: Principles, Procedures and Correlations, 2nd ed. Philadelphia: Lippincott, 1998; 245.
9. Ucar K. Clinical presentation and management of hemolytic anemias. Oncology 10:163–170, 2002.
10. Birch D. Malaria: Quest for a Vaccine. *Baltimore Sun*, June 18, 2000.
11. Lemery L, Ciesla B. Why Did this Sample Fail the Correlation Checks? American Society of Clinical Pathologists Tech Sample 1997 G-12. Chicago, Ill.

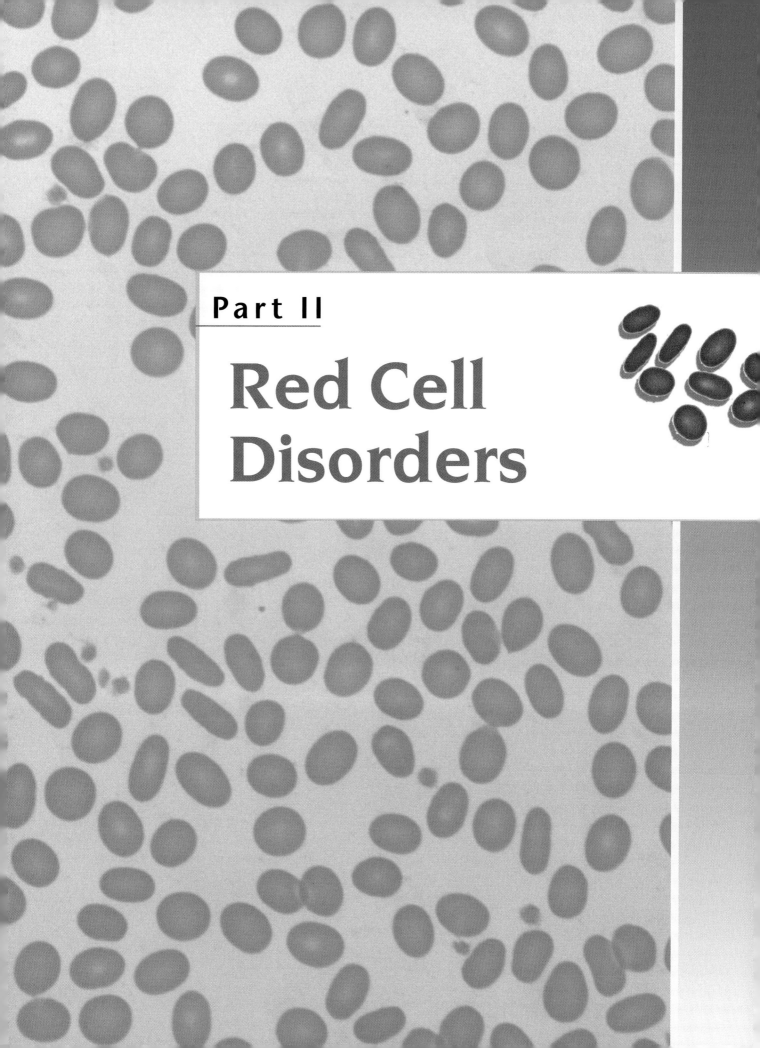

Part II

Red Cell Disorders

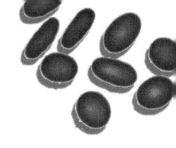

5

The Microcytic Anemias

Betty Ciesla

Iron Intake and Iron Absorption

Iron Storage and Recycled Iron

Iron Deficiency Anemia

Pathophysiology and Symptoms

Tests Used to Diagnose Iron Deficiency

Causes of Iron Deficiency

Treatment for Iron Deficiency

Anemia of Chronic Disease and Inflammation: Pathophysiology, Diagnosis, and Treatment

Anemias Related to Iron Overload Conditions, the Sideroblastic Anemias

Hereditary Hemochromatosis

The Thalassemia Syndromes

Brief History and Demographics

The Pathophysiology of the Thalassemias

The Alpha Thalassemias

Beta Thalassemia Major: Cooley's Anemia, Mediterranean Fever

Thalassemia Intermedia and Beta Thalassemia Trait

Objectives

After completing this chapter, the student will be able to:

1. Describe the red blood cell indices related to the microcytic anemias.
2. List the microcytic anemias considered in a differential diagnosis of microcytic processes.
3. Describe iron transport from ingestion to incorporation in hemoglobin.
4. List the three stages of iron deficiency.
5. Describe the physical symptoms of an individual with iron deficiency anemia.
6. Identify the iron needs of children and adults.
7. Identify the laboratory tests for an individual with iron deficiency anemia.
8. Describe the iron overload conditions.
9. Define the pathophysiology of hereditary hemochromatosis.
10. Outline the symptoms of individuals with hereditary hemochromatosis.
11. Describe the diagnosis and clinical management of individuals with hereditary hemochromatosis.
12. Describe the basic pathophysiological defect in the thalassemia syndromes.
13. Describe the alpha thalassemic conditions with regard to gene deletions and clinical symptoms.
14. List the three types of beta thalassemia.
15. Discuss the clinical manifestations of the beta thalassemias with regard to bone marrow changes, splenic changes, skeletal changes, and hematological changes.
16. Correlate the morphological changes in the red cell with the defect in the alpha and beta thalassemias.
17. Describe the major hemoglobin in each of the thalassemic states.
18. Describe the transfusion protocols of thalassemia major patients and their contraindications.

Anemia is a significant health issue in the world population, affecting every ethnic class and social strata. The clinical laboratory plays a decisive role in supplying the physician with clinical data in defining the cause and determining the treatment of this condition. Broadly defined, when red cells are no longer able to supply oxygen to the body's tissues, the individual becomes *anemic*. Anemias may be classified according to their physiology or their morphology. The morphological classification is based on red blood cell indices, while the physiological classification is determined based on symptoms and bone marrow response. This chapter will stress the morphological classification of anemias. Normal red cell indices are MCV of 80 to 100 fL, MCH of 27 to 31 pg, and MCHC of 32% to 36%. If a microcytic process is present, then hemoglobin synthesis is disrupted and the MCV is less than 80 fL and the MCHC is less than 32%. The red cells are termed microcytic, hypochromic and appear as small red cells, deficient in hemoglobin. The laboratorian can be instrumental in helping the physician to recognize that a microcytic anemic process is occurring, determine the cause, and decide on a management or therapeutic plan. The microcytic anemias are iron deficiency anemia (IDA), sideroblastic anemias (acquired and inherited), the thalassemias, and a percentage of anemia of inflammation that transcend into IDA.

IRON INTAKE AND IRON ABSORPTION

Iron is one of the most abundant metals in the world, yet IDA continues to be one the most prominent nutritional disorders worldwide.[1] Many factors contribute to this situation and they need to be understood to have a fuller appreciation of iron balance. Iron balance is regulated by several conditions: (a) the amount of iron ingested, (b) the amount of iron absorbed, (c) red blood cell formation using recycled and new iron, (d) iron stores, and (e) iron loss through blood loss or other sources (Fig. 5.1).

The amount of iron that needs to be obtained through the diet varies according to age and gender. Males need to absorb about 1 mg/day, premenopausal females about 0.2 to 2.0 mg/day, and children approximately 0.5 mg/day.[2] For perspective, if an adult male eats a 2500-calorie diet, he will ingest about 15 mg of iron of which only 10% will be absorbed, giving him 1.5 mg/day of iron that can be used for red cell production or stored in the reticuloendothelial system (RES).[3] Iron in the diet is available as heme iron through meats or as nonheme/nonmeat iron. For a listing of sources, see Table 5-1. For the infant, iron-fortified formulas and breast milk are major sources of iron. As the infant develops and rapidly gains weight, there is a high demand for iron. Most infants and young children will need some dietary supplementation to maintain iron balance (see Table 5.7).

Once iron is ingested, it is absorbed in the gastrointestinal (GI) tract and then transported into the circulation. The main portion of the GI tract involved is the duodenum and jejunum of the small intestine, where on average only about 10% of ingested iron is absorbed. This absorption rate is not static, however, and it decreases or increases relative to iron stores and the body's needs. Once absorbed, the iron molecule is converted from the Fe^{3+} (ferric) to the Fe^{2+} (ferrous) state by stomach acid, and then the iron molecules are transported through the circulation to the bone marrow via transferrin. Transferrin, the transport vehicle, is a plasma protein formed in the liver that assists iron delivery to the erythroblasts in the bone marrow. Transferrin receptors on the pronormoblast bind iron, so that iron molecules can immediately start being incorporated into the heme molecule during erythropoiesis. The willingness for the transferrin receptor to bind iron is influenced by the iron being delivered, the pH of the body, and, on the molecular level, the influence of an iron regulatory factor, ferritin repressor protein.[4] An essential ingredient to seamless iron absorption and transport is a healthy GI tract. Procedures such a **gastrectomy** or gastric bypass, atrophic gastritis, or celiac disease may compromise iron absorption.[5] There are dietary substances that enhance or diminish the absorption of iron from the diet (Tables 5.2 and 5.3), as well as foods with a high iron value (Table 5.4).

IRON STORAGE AND RECYCLED IRON

Ferritin and hemosiderin are the primary storage forms of iron. These compounds are harbored in the liver, spleen, bone marrow, and skeletal muscle. Ferritin can be measured in plasma, while hemosiderin is more often identified in the urine or stained through the bone marrow. Iron stores in men are generally 1.0 to 1.4 g of body iron, and for women, 0.2 to 0.4 g. Given these figures and with the realization that the iron absorption requirement is on average 1 mg/day, it is easy to understand why in adults with iron-poor diets anemia may take years to develop. Specifically, body stores in men of 1 g would last 3 to 4 years before iron depletion takes place.[6] Indeed, most cases of iron deficiency are directly related to external blood loss, especially **menorrhagia**

The Iron Cycle: Ingestion, Absorption, Storage

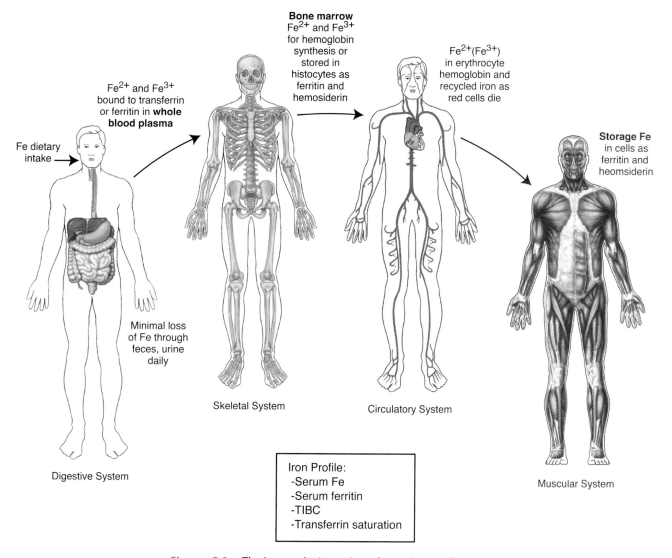

Fe dietary intake →

Fe^{2+} and Fe^{3+} bound to transferrin or ferritin in **whole blood plasma**

Bone marrow
Fe^{2+} and Fe^{3+} for hemoglobin synthesis or stored in histocytes as ferritin and hemosiderin

$Fe^{2+}(Fe^{3+})$ in erythrocyte hemoglobin and recycled iron as red cells die

Storage Fe in cells as ferritin and heomsiderin

Minimal loss of Fe through feces, urine daily

Digestive System

Skeletal System

Circulatory System

Muscular System

Iron Profile:
-Serum Fe
-Serum ferritin
-TIBC
-Transferrin saturation

Figure 5.1   The iron cycle: Ingestion, absorption, and storage.

or slow GI bleed. Blood lost outside the body has no chance of being recycled into the usable byproduct of heme and globin.

The recycling of iron from heme and amino acids from globin following the lysis of aged red cells is a very efficient process. Heme is returned to the bone marrow, and the amino acids of the globin chain are returned to the amino acid pool. Each of these products will later be recruited for hemoglobin formation and red cell production. In the adult, approximately 95% of recycled iron is used for red cell production, whereas in the infant, only 70% is used for this purpose (Fig. 5.2). Because of this relationship, it is easy to understand the significance of adequate iron sources in the early years of development.

Table 5.1 ⊙ The Multiple Forms of Iron in the Body

Iron in Food

Heme sources: Meat

Nonheme sources: Beans, clams, vegetables

Iron in Storage

Ferritin: Found in liver, spleen, skeletal muscle, bone marrow

Hemosiderin: Found in excreted urine

Iron in Circulation

Iron and globin are recycled as a result of red cell senescence

Table 5.2 ○	Enhancers of Iron Absorption

- Orange juice
- Vitamin C
- Pickles
- Soy sauce
- Vinegar
- Alcohol

IRON DEFICIENCY ANEMIA

Pathophysiology and Symptoms

IDA can be a primary condition due to blood loss or inadequate iron intake. It may also be a secondary condition due to a disease process or conditions that deplete iron stores, such as GI bleed or pregnancy. In either case, IDA will manifest itself as a microcytic, hypochromic process, where the red cells are small and deficient in hemoglobin (Table 5.5). The CBC will be characterized by a low red count, hemoglobin, hematocrit, MCV, and MCHC. The development of IDA is a three-stage process:

- Stage I: Continuum of iron depletion from the marrow (Prussian blue stain will show absence of iron)
- Stage II: Iron deficient erythropoiesis
- Stage III: Finally, a frank case of IDA in the peripheral circulation

In most cases, the patient will not present with overt symptoms until anemia develops (stage III); however, serum ferritin will be decreased at every stage. Diagnostic laboratory tests such as serum iron and serum ferritin may be used by the physician to diagnose an individual well before anemia develops. Individuals in high-risk groups should be periodically monitored for iron status (Table 5.6).

Table 5.3 ○	Inhibitors of Iron Absorption

- Tea
- Coffee
- Oregano
- Milk

Table 5.4 ○	Foods With High Iron Value

- Clams
- Soybeans
- Lentils
- Pinto beans
- Liver
- Garbanzo beans
- Tofu
- Packaged oatmeal

There are many symptoms that mark an individual as being iron deficient. Some of these symptoms are unique to iron deficiency and some are general symptoms of anemia. Clinically, a patient with anemia may present with

- Fatigue
- Pallor
- Vertigo
- Dyspnea
- Cold intolerance
- Lethargy

Additionally, these patients may experience cardiac problems such as palpitations and angina (see Table 2.7). Symptoms *unique* to the IDA patient are pica (an abnormal craving for unusual substances such as dirt, ice, or clay), cheilitis (inflammation around the lips), and koilonychias (spooning of the nail beds) (Fig. 5.3). Additionally, evidence suggests that iron deficiency in infants may result in developmental delays and behavioral disturbances.[7] In pregnant women, iron deficiency in the first two trimesters may lead to an increase in preterm delivery and an increase in delivering a low-birth-weight child.[7] Anemia affects 3.5 million individuals in the United States, with approximately 50% of these cases being IDA.[1] Sensitivity to the possibility of iron deficiency backed by good diagnostic data is the best weapon to eliminate IDA in the Western world.

Tests Used to Diagnose Iron Deficiency

From a clinical standpoint, if iron deficiency is suspected, testing for iron deficiency must analyze the patient's *red cell status* and *iron status*. In terms of the CBC, all parameters except the white cell and platelet counts will be below the normal reference range (see Table 2.3). In some cases, if a patient is actively bleeding,

ADULT

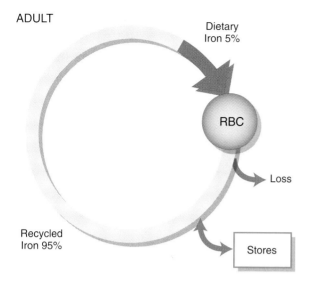

INFANT 1YR

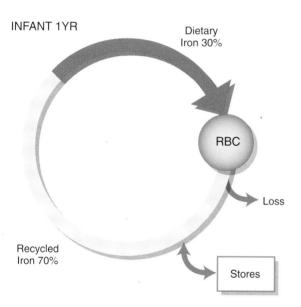

Figure 5.2 Iron need versus amount of recycled iron available.

the platelet count will be elevated. The MCV and MCHC will be markedly lower than normal, the RDW may be mildly elevated, and the peripheral smear will show small red cells, which are deficient in hemoglobin. Target cells and elliptocytes may occasionally be seen (Fig. 5.4). The reticulocyte count will be low in comparison to the level of anemia, indicating a slightly ineffective erythropoiesis.

Tests to assess a patient's iron status include serum iron, serum ferritin, transferrin or total iron binding capacity (TIBC), and transferrin saturation. Serum iron is a measure of the total amount of iron in the serum with a normal value of 50 to 150 µg/L. Serum ferritin is

Table 5.5 ⊙ Stages of Iron Deficiency Anemia Matched to Diagnostic Signals

Stage 1: Iron Stores Depleted. Test for

Absence of stainable bone marrow iron

Decreased serum ferritin level

Increased TIBC

Stage 2: Iron-Deficient Erythropoiesis. Test for

Slight microcytosis

Slight decreased hemoglobin

Decreased transferrin saturation

Stage 3: Iron Deficiency Anemia. Test for

Decreased serum iron

Decreased serum ferritin

Increased TIBC

Decreased transferring saturation

one of the most sensitive indicators of iron stores, with a normal value of 20 to 250 µg/L for men and 10 to 120 µg/L for women. Ferritin is an acute phase reactant, and conditions such as chronic inflammation or chronic infection may falsely elevate the serum ferritin level. In these cases, an accurate assessment of iron stores will be difficult. The TIBC measures the availability of iron binding sites on the transferrin molecule. If an individual is iron deficient, there will be many binding sites available searching for iron and the TIBC

Table 5.6 ⊙ Causes of Iron Deficiency Anemia

Related to Increased Iron Demands

Growth spurts in infants and children

Pregnancy and nursing

Related to Lack of Iron Intake

Poor diet

Conditions that diminish absorption

Related to Blood Loss

Menorrhagia

Gastrointestinal bleeding (GI bleed)

Hemolysis

Other physical causes of bleeding

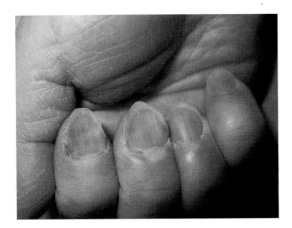

Figure 5.3   Koilonychia.

value will be increased. This value is elevated in iron-deficient patients (reference range, 250 to 450 µg/L) but subject to fluctuations in patients who use oral contraceptives or have liver disease, chronic infections, or nephrotic syndrome. The TIBC is less sensitive to iron deficiency and must be evaluated in terms of the patient's other health issues. Transferrin saturation (% saturation) is derived as the product of the serum iron concentration divided by the TIBC and multiplied by 100. The normal value is 20% to 50%.

There are occasions when a diagnosis of IDA is made too casually and is based on a patient's age group, gender, or vague complaints. Young women who give a history of fatigue or menstrual problems are often simply given a trial of iron therapy with no supporting laboratory workup. A diagnosis of IDA should be made ONLY with the supporting laboratory data that reflect the patient's red cell and iron status. The patient should insist that this work be done before therapy is initiated as unnecessary iron use has the potential for serious consequences.

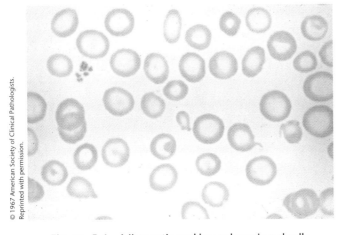

© 1967 American Society of Clinical Pathologists. Reprinted with permission.

Figure 5.4   Microcytic and hypochromic red cells.

Causes of Iron Deficiency

There are many populations that are vulnerable to IDA. Infants and pregnant women may suffer from nutritional deficiency, young children may develop IDA when their growth and development rate outstrip their iron intake, and young women who have increased iron need due to menstruation or pregnancy may develop IDA (see Table 5.6). But the primary cause of iron deficiency in the Western world is GI bleeding for males and excessive menses for females. In both of these cases, blood is lost from the body. External blood loss presents a significant challenge to the body because millions of shed red cells can never be used for recycling new red cells. Slow GI bleeds and dysfunctional uterine bleeding over time will lead to a depletion of iron stores and IDA will commence. Storage iron, represented by ferritin, represents a primary reservoir of iron that can be used as other iron sources are depleted. The average ferritin concentrations in males are 135 µg/L, females, 43 µg/L, and children, 30 µg/L.[7] Barring any other external loss of blood, iron deficiency solely due to lack of dietary sources would develop over a protracted period of time.

Treatment for Iron Deficiency

Treatment for iron deficiency is given orally in the form of drops (good for infants and children) or tablets. Iron preparations are in the form of ferrous sulfate, ferrous gluconate, and ferrous fumerate and are readily available over the counter in most places.[8] Side effects from oral iron therapy may include constipation, stomach discomfort, or diarrhea. Most side effects can be overcome with consultation from the pharmacist for a gentler preparation. What is essential is to remain compliant and to continue on iron therapy despite side effects. Laboratory evaluations such as the CBC and the reticulocyte count should show marked improvement in a few weeks. Additionally, the microcytosis and hypochromia seen in the peripheral smear will eventually be replaced by normocytic and normochromic red cells. Although oral iron will normalize the hematological picture, an investigation should commence as to the source of the anemia and whether there are any underlying causes that are contributory. Table 5.7 provides recommendations to prevent and control iron deficiency in the United States.

ANEMIA OF CHRONIC DISEASE AND INFLAMMATION: PATHOPHYSIOLOGY, DIAGNOSIS, AND TREATMENT

The anemia of chronic disease or the anemia of inflammation is one of the most common anemias in hospital

Table 5.7 ● Recommendations to Prevent and Control Iron Deficiency in the United States

For infants (0 to 12 months) and children (1 to 5 years)
- Encourage breastfeeding or
- Iron-fortified formula
- Serve one serving of fruits, vegetables, juice by 6 months
- Screen children for anemia every 6 months

School-age children (5 to 12 years) and adolescent boys (12 to 18 years)
- Screen only those with history of IDA or low iron intake groups

Adolescent girls (12 to 18 years) and nonpregnant women of childbearing age
- Encourage intake of iron-rich food and foods that increase iron absorption
- Screen nonpregnant women every 5 to 10 years through childbearing years

Pregnant women
- Start oral doses of iron at first prenatal visit
- Screen for anemia at first prenatal visit
- If hemoglobin is <9 g/dL, provide further medical attention

Postpartum women
- Risk factors include continued anemia, excessive blood loss, and multiple births

Males older than 18 years/postmenopausal women
- No routine screening is recommended

Modified from Centers for Disease Control and Prevention. Recommendations to Prevent and Control Iron Deficiency in the United States. April 1998. Available at http://www.cdc.gov/mmnr/preview/mmwrhtml/100051880.htm. Accessed September 24, 2006.

Table 5.8 ● Conditions Leading to Anemia of Inflammation or Anemia of Chronic Disease

- Rheumatoid arthritis
- Chronic renal disease
- Thyroid disorders
- Malignancies
- Inflammatory bowel disease

populations and second only to iron deficiency in terms of frequency.

Many individuals with chronic disorders such **collagen vascular disease,** chronic kidney disease, thyroid disorders, malignancies, and so on may show an anemia that will eventually develop into a microcytic anemia (Table 5.8). When this occurs, most physicians will order laboratory testing to establish whether there is also an iron deficiency process. This is termed *differential diagnosis.* Differential diagnosis is a process by which a physician examines a group of laboratory values and symptoms and tries to correlate them to a particular physiology. Patients with the anemia of chronic disease will show a borderline low red cell count, hemoglobin, and hematocrit, a slightly low MCV, and a normal MCHC. The peripheral smear will be essentially normal with slight variation in size and chroma. Serum iron will be low, serum ferritin will be normal or increased, and serum TIBC will be decreased. Although this is NOT the profile for a patient with IDA, in both conditions the patient will have a low serum iron. There are several theories to account for these data. In the anemias of inflammation, iron is blocked from reaching erythroid precursors because of impaired release from macrophages; there is impaired EPO production; and the pronormoblasts are not as responsive to EPO from patients with chronic disease.[9] Few individuals require a blood transfusion for treatment of their anemia. On most occasions, once the underlying disease is successfully managed, symptoms of anemia seem to resolve. Recently, a new hormone, hepcidin, was discovered. Hepcidin is linked to the immune response and has been identified as a regulator of iron transit. As more information unfolds, undoubtedly this discovery will have major implications for iron use and the inflammatory process.[10]

ANEMIAS RELATED TO IRON OVERLOAD CONDITIONS, THE SIDEROBLASTIC ANEMIAS

The disorders in this category are either inherited or acquired. There is an excessive accumulation of iron in the mitochondria. This leads to the presence of iron deposits in the red cell precursors in the marrow called ringed sideroblasts (Fig. 5.5), a dimorphic blood picture, as well as increased serum ferritin. If the iron loading is an acquired process, it may result from diseases such as thalassemia major or sickle cell anemia that require a high transfusion protocol. Additionally, acquired iron loading may occur from alcoholism, lead poisoning, or chloramphenicol use. Inherited sideroblastic anemias will be the result of inherited abnormal genes, which is discussed later in the chapter.

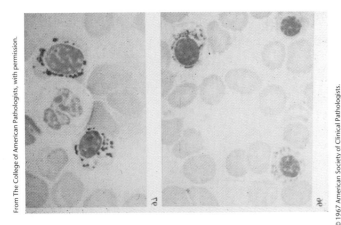

Figure 5.5   Ringed sideroblast in the bone marrow.

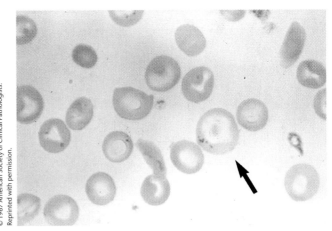

Figure 5.7   Pappenheimer bodies.

In any case, the patient's peripheral smear will show a microcytic process, with dimorphism (some microcytes and some normal cells, some hypochromic and some normochromic) (Fig. 5.6) and the presence of Pappenheimer bodies (Fig. 5.7), red cells with precipitated iron inclusions that look like grape clusters in the periphery of the red cell. An iron profile will reveal an increased serum ferritin and an increased serum iron. As can be expected, once the underlying condition is successfully managed, the iron overload conditions will be resolved.

Hereditary Hemochromatosis

Hereditary hemochromatosis (HH) is one of the most common genetic disorder in persons with European ancestry and a major *inherited* sideroblastic anemia. More than a million persons are affected in the United States.[11] Caucasians, African Americans, and Hispanics are particularly at risk. Yet this disorder has a low profile, relative to other blood disorders, partially because it is almost always a diagnosis of exclusion. HH is an autosomal recessive disorder carried on chromosome 6 that is closely linked to HLA-A3. It may be inherited homozygously or heterozygously with homozygotes more prone to iron overload. However, 10% of heterozygotes will also show signs of excessive iron loading.[12] Because of this inheritance, individuals with HH begin to load iron excessively from a young age and continue iron loading with every decade. Most are diagnosed accidentally, as a result of blood screening for a totally unrelated issue. In these individuals, the customary process of iron absorption and storage become unbalanced due to the inheritance of an abnormal gene, *HFE,* the gene that regulates the amount of iron absorbed from the diet. Two mutations, C282Y and H63D, have been described.[12] The complete role of these mutant variations in the *HFE* gene is not fully understood, yet it is known that the normal product of these genes does not bind to the transferrin receptor in the normal iron delivery process. As a result of this faulty mechanism, iron is constantly loaded into the storage sites and leads to multiorgan damage and symptoms over the decades.[13]

Symptoms and Laboratory Diagnosis of Hereditary Hemochromatosis

HH is a great impersonator with a myriad of symptoms that usually serve to confuse rather than lead to a direct diagnosis. A few of the more common symptoms are

- Chronic fatigue and weakness
- Cirrhosis of the liver
- Hyperpigmentation
- Diabetes
- Impotence

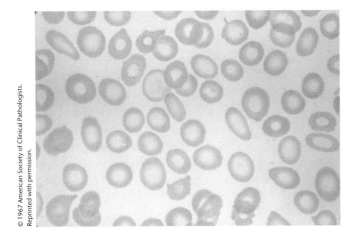

Figure 5.6   Dimorphism in the red cells: Two cell populations and different levels of hypochromia.

- Sterility
- Cardiac arrhythmias
- Tender swollen joints
- Hair loss
- Abdominal symptoms (Table 5.9)

As can be imagined, each of these symptoms alone could point a physician in a direction other than HH, yet when these symptoms are combined with a microcytic process, a screening for iron status will provide relevant information. As has already been indicated, screening for iron status would include

- Serum iron
- Serum transferrin level
- TIBC
- Possibly transferrin saturation

In patients with HH, serum iron, serum ferritin, and transferrin saturation will be elevated, while TIBC and transferrin will fall in the normal reference range. It should be noted that symptoms may not be seen and blood values may not be elevated in younger individuals. Serum ferritin levels above 150 μg/L and transferrin saturation levels of greater than 45% are indicative of HH. Genetic testing would be appropriate for these individuals to establish if they possess the G282Y and the H63D mutation present in 80% to 95% of patients with HH, yet this testing is expensive and should be ordered judiciously. The laboratory is critical in the diagnosis of HH and its value cannot be underestimated in providing definitive data for this crucial diagnosis.

Treatment for Hereditary Hemochromatosis

Untreated HH can be fatal, and advanced iron overload frequently leads to liver cancer (Fig. 5.8). The treatment of choice for individuals newly diagnosed with HH is aggressive therapeutic phlebotomy, or bloodletting, as it used to be termed. The goal of this procedure is to reduce the serum ferritin level to less than 10 μg/dL and to keep the patient's hematocrit at around 35%. For most patients, there will be one or two phlebotomies performed per week as long as the patient can tolerate the procedure. Once the patient serum ferritin has returned to near normal, phlebotomies will occur three

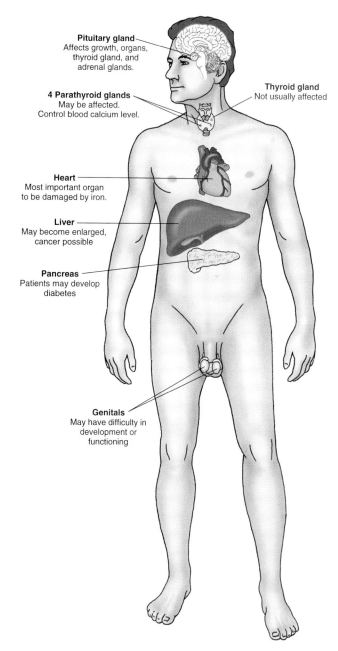

Figure 5.8   Organs of the body damaged by iron overload.

Table 5.9 ◉ The Confusing Symptoms of Hereditary Hemochromatosis	
Symptom	**Possible Other Cause**
Chronic fatigue weakness	Could be seen in IDA
Cirrhosis of the liver	Could be seen in alcoholism
Cardiac arrhythmias	Could be seen in valve problems, congestive heart failure
Tender swollen joints	Could be seen in collagen vascular diseases
Hair loss, hyperpigmentation	Could be seen in endocrine disorders

or four times a year to keep the serum ferritin in range. Symptoms will lessen and in some cases disappear completely once the iron level is reduced. Excess iron lowers the immune system, and it has been suggested that iron overload causes a significant amount of diabetes. For patients who cannot tolerate phlebotomies or are unwilling to go through the procedure, desferrioxamine (Desferal), an iron-**chelating** agent, can be used. In this procedure, the dose of Desferal matched to body weight is delivered through a continuous 12- to 16-hour infusion pump. Patients usually use a subcutaneous injection site for infusion and infuse during the nighttime hours. Excess iron is chelated and then excreted in the urine. Infusion sites need to be rotated often to avoid infections and irritation (Fig. 5.9). Patients who are noncompliant in ridding themselves of iron through either phlebotomy or Desferal will significantly shorten their life span. Early diagnosis of HH disorder can easily be accomplished by adding blood tests such as serum ferritin and transferrin saturation to the menu of tests offered during yearly physical examinations. Slowly, the medical community is becoming aware of this "silent killer" as individual consumers become more knowledgeable of this disease and as organizations like the Iron Overload Disease Association (www.ironoverload.org) become more aggressive in outreach and education. HH is *preventable*, but it will take the efforts of many individuals—nutritionists, physicians, laboratory personnel, and patients—to raise awareness and expand educational outreach.

THE THALASSEMIA SYNDROMES

Brief History and Demographics

Over 2 million Americans carry the gene for thalassemia,[14] yet most have never heard of the word *thalassemia*, which comes from the Greek word *thalassa*, meaning "from the sea." Relatively few individuals develop severe forms of thalassemia, but for those who do, there is a lifetime of transfusions and medical management of multiorgan problems. The thalassemic gene is ubiquitous, yet it has a particular penetration in Mediterranean areas and in Middle Eastern, Northern African, Indian, Asian, and Caribbean populations. More cases are being seen and treated in the United States as more diverse populations enter the country. Fortunately, laboratory professionals seem to be more aware of the possibility of thalassemic conditions when faced with a patient who presents with microcytic process and normal iron status. Physicians and medical students, interns, and residents often fail to consider the thalassemias as reasons for a microcytic process, most likely due to lack of in-depth training or exposure. A respectful relationship between the laboratory and medical staff can be tremendously beneficial in diagnosing and treating new cases of thalassemia.

Dr. Thomas Cooley and Dr. Pearl Lee described the first cases of thalassemia disease in North America in 1925. Clustering together five cases, these clinicians described four children who had anemia, hepatosplenomegaly, skin discoloration, jaundice, and peculiar facial features and bone changes. Their bone marrows showed erythroid hyperplasia (Fig. 5.10), and their peripheral smear showed many nucleated red cells, target cells, and microcytes (Fig. 5.11). Not much has changed in the initial presentation of an individual with thalassemia disease or thalassemia major. The mode of

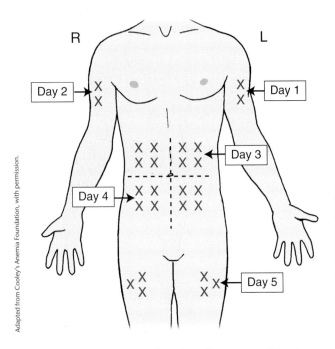

Adapted from Cooley's Anemia Foundation, with permission.

Figure 5.9 Rotation chart for subcutaneous injections.

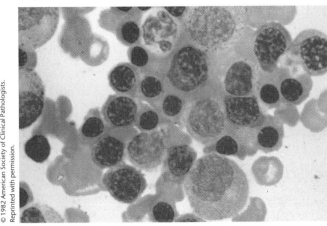

© 1982 American Society of Clinical Pathologists. Reprinted with permission.

Figure 5.10 Erythroid hyperplasia: the bone marrow's response to anemic stress.

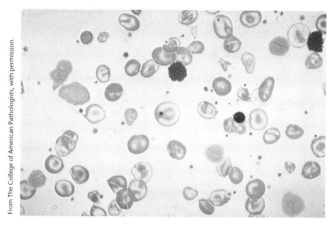

From The College of American Pathologists, with permission.

Figure 5.11 Thalassemia major, showing a high degree of poikilocytosis and nRBCs.

inheritance for this disorder was described by Dr. W. N. Valentine in 1944, and since 1960, the genetic interactions and the cloning of the thalassemic genes have been accomplished. Yet there has been no cure.

The Pathophysiology of the Thalassemias

Unlike the other microcytic processes discussed, the thalassemias have *nothing* to do with iron. The thalassemias are globin chain disorders that are concerned with the lack of production of alpha or beta globin chains. The thalassemias are hemoglobin synthesis defects. Failure to synthesize either the alpha or the beta chain impairs the production of the normal physiological adult hemoglobin, hemoglobin A ($\alpha_2\beta_2$), hemoglobin A2 ($\alpha_2\delta_2$), and hemoglobin F ($\alpha_2\delta_2$). The construction of each of these normal hemoglobins depends on alpha and beta chains being synthesized as part of their normal tetramer. When this synthesis is impaired, the hemoglobins are formed as a result of the unbalanced chain production that negatively affects red cell life span. Additionally, there are multiorgan complications, the development of a microcytic anemia, and a peripheral smear with many red cell morphological abnormalities. There are two major types of thalassemias: alpha thalassemia and beta thalassemian. Put simply, the alpha thalassemias result from gene deletions. Each individual inherits four alpha genes, two maternal and two paternal. Each of the four clinical presentations of alpha thalassemia results from one or more of the alpha genes being deleted. The beta thalassemias revolve around the inheritance of a defective beta gene, either from one parent (heterozygously) or from both parents (homozygously). To date, 200 mutations of the beta gene have been described, and these mutations have been broadly divided into the B^0 or the B^+ gene. In the B^0 individuals, there is a complete lack of synthesis of the beta chain, and in B^+ individuals, a limited amount of the beta chain is synthesized. Both of these mutations affect specific populations (Table 5.10). On the molecular level, beta chain defects result from faulty transcription of messenger RNA.

The Alpha Thalassemias

Symptomatology

The alpha thalassemias have a high incidence in the Asian populations (e.g., Thailand, Vietnam, Cambodia, Indonesia, and Laos).[15] They are also seen in Saudi Arabian and Filipino populations. As you may recall, the alpha chain is the critical building block for construction of all normal adult physiological hemoglobins, because each adult hemoglobin depends on the production of the alpha chain. The alpha chain is also critical in the development of hemoglobin in the fetus; without alpha chain development, there is no Hgb F formed. There are four clinical states of alpha thalassemia that are related to the number of alpha genes deleted (Fig. 5.12).

Gene States of Alpha Hemoglobin

The most severe state is Barts hydrops fetalis, in which there is a total absence of alpha chain synthesis: no hemoglobin A is formed, only hemoglobin Barts ($\gamma4$), a high oxygen affinity hemoglobin. Because this hemoglobin is an abnormal tetramer and oxygen loving (hemoglobin Barts holds onto oxygen and resists delivering oxygen to the tissues), the anemia that develops is severe and usually leads to stillbirth or spontaneous abortion. Hemoglobin H disease is the next most severe condition. Here, there is only one functional alpha gene, and the other three genes are deleted. Little hemoglobin A is produced; instead, a new hemoglobin H is formed, which is also a fairly unstable tetramer ($\beta4$) and repre-

Table 5.10 ◎ Gene Expression in Population	
B^0	B^+
Northern Italy	Mediterranean region
Greece	Southeast Asia
Algeria	Middle East
Saudi Arabia	Indian subcontinent
	West Africa

Normal chromosome 16

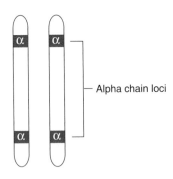

Alpha chain loci

Clinical Conditions of Alpha Thalassemia

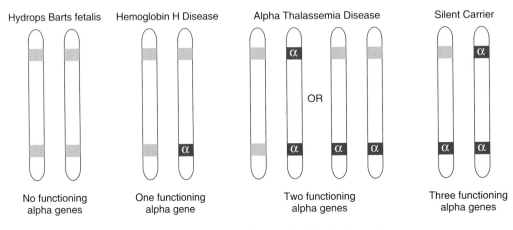

Hydrops Barts fetalis	Hemoglobin H Disease	Alpha Thalassemia Disease	Silent Carrier
No functioning alpha genes	One functioning alpha gene	Two functioning alpha genes	Three functioning alpha genes

OR

Figure 5.12   Clinical states of alpha thalassemia.

sents 5% to 40% on alkaline electrophoresis (see Chapter 8). Hemoglobin levels are less than 10 g/dL (average, 6 to 8 g/dL), and reticulocyte counts are in the range of 5% to 10%. There is a microcytosis and hypochromia observed in the peripheral smear with red cell fragments (Fig. 5.13). An unusual inclusion, hemoglobin H inclusion, is formed. On supravital staining, with brilliant cresyl blue or crystal violet, it looks like a pitted golf ball (Fig. 5.14). In peripheral circulation, this inclusion is usually pitted from the red cell, leaving the cell more fragile and less elastic with a shortened life span. Individuals with hemoglobin H disease have a lifelong anemia with variable splenomegaly and bone changes.

The final two clinical conditions are less severe: the two-gene deletion state, alpha thalassemia trait, and the one-gene deletion state, the silent carrier. The individual with the alpha thalassemia trait possesses only two viable hemoglobin A genes and may only have a mild anemia with many microcytic, hypochromic cells. Some hemoglobin Barts will be formed. The silent carrier will be hematologically normal or slightly micro-

cytic, and therefore the patient may be unaware of his or her alpha gene status. Since diagnosing patients from both of these alpha thalassemia subsets (alpha thal-

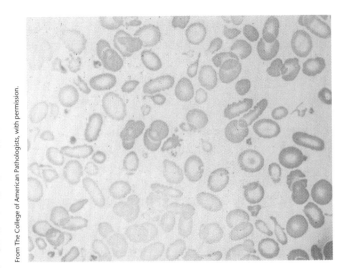

From The College of American Pathologists, with permission.

Figure 5.13   Peripheral smear from an individual with hemoglobin H.

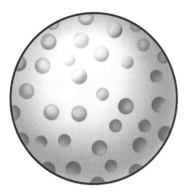

H Bodies in mature red cell

Figure 5.14 Hemoglobin H inclusions as seen after brilliant cresyl blue staining.

assemia trait/silent carrier) may be difficult, it is important to note that the presence of elliptocytes and target cells in their peripheral smears can present a high predictive value, if smears are carefully reviewed for these findings.[16]

Diagnosis and Treatment

If the most severe alpha thalassemic condition is suspected, especially in pregnancy, amniocentesis fluid or chronic villi sampling may be obtained and examined for the presence of alpha genes through molecular diagnostic procedures. In the case of hydrops Barts fetalis, most of these pregnancies are terminated or individuals are delivered of severely edematous fetuses that are not viable. Cord blood is usually tested for hemoglobin electrophoresis, which usually shows a high percentage of hemoglobin Barts. For these individuals and individuals in high-risk ethnic groups, genetic counseling is strongly advised. Hemoglobin H may be suspected if CBCs show slightly elevated red blood cell counts combined with extremely low MCVs, less than 60 fL, and RDW results that are extremely elevated (normal value, 11% to 15%) owing to the misshapened red cells and fragments in comparison to the more homogeneous microcytic hypochromic population as seen in IDA. Although hemoglobin H may be present at 5% to 40%, failure to demonstrate an abnormal hemoglobin band by electrophoresis should not eliminate the patient as suspect.[17] Hemoglobin H, a fast-moving hemoglobin on alkaline electrophoresis, may be missed by traditional methods. The final two conditions—alpha thalassemia trait and the silent carrier condition—may not be recognized on peripheral smear analysis because their hematological pictures are not that abnormal.

Treatment for hemoglobin H disease is supportive, with transfusions given only if necessary. Iron deficiency must be eliminated as a reason for the microcytic indices so that the patient will not be given iron unnecessarily.

Beta Thalassemia Major: Cooley's Anemia, Mediterranean Fever

This inherited blood disorder affects million of individuals worldwide. In the United States alone, over 2 million individuals are carriers of the thalassemic gene, resulting in significant penetrance of this gene, which often results in disease. In beta thalassemia major, there is little or no beta chain being synthesized; consequently, there is no (or a very minor amount of) hemoglobin A being synthesized. This condition results from a union between two carriers, and according to Mendelian genetics, there is a one-in-four chance for a severely affected individual to be born (Fig. 5.15). The other offspring may be carriers. Beta thalassemia major is a serious genetic blood disorder, affecting multiple organs, quality of life, and longevity. Most infants born with thalassemia major will not be ill for the first 6 months. Because fetal hemoglobin is the majority hemoglobin at birth, infants do quite well. But, in the normal sequence of events, gamma chains are silenced and beta chains increase, forming hemoglobin A somewhere between 3 and 6 months. As there are no beta chains to combine with the alpha chains, hemoglobin F continues to be made; but there is an imbalance of alpha chains. When alpha chains cannot combine, they are unpaired and precipitate inside the red cell, causing a markedly decreased life span (7 to 22 days). Between 2 and 4 years old, most young children with beta thalassemia major begin to show a failure to thrive, irritability, enlarged spleens, symptoms of anemia, **jaundice,** and transfusion requirement.

Living With Thalassemia Major

Patients and families with thalassemia major balance multiple health issues on a daily basis as they struggle to maintain a normal life. Medical management of this disease is continuous, frustrating, and disruptive for children who have the disease and parents who are caregivers and carriers. Severe anemia underlies most of the other complications, with hemoglobin values, although variable, often in the range of 6 to 9 g/dL, about one-half the normal level. The patient's peripheral smear shows a severe microcytic hypochromic process with a high number of nucleated red blood cells, marked polychro-

IF.....   Both parents carry the beta thalassemia trait ⊖

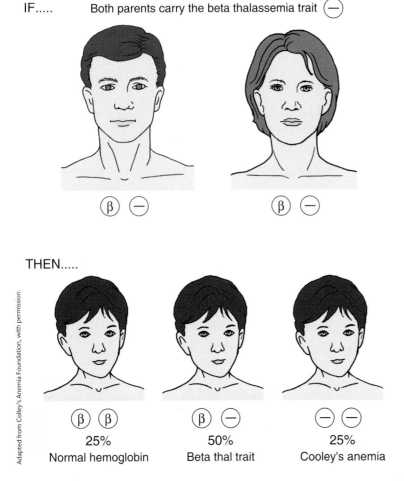

β ⊖   β ⊖

THEN.....

β β   β ⊖   ⊖ ⊖
25%   50%   25%
Normal hemoglobin   Beta thal trait   Cooley's anemia

Figure 5.15   Genetics of beta thalassemia.

masia, and a high degree of red cell morphology. (See Fig. 5.11.) Because this chronic anemic state has led to chronic overexpansion of the capable bone marrow, (the bone marrow increases its output up to 20 times), the quality of bone that is laid down is thin and fragile. Pathological fractures and bony changes in the facial structure (thalassemic facies) and skull are normally seen and give the thalassemic individual a strange look. Bossing or protrusion of the skull is prominent, as is orthodontic misalignment. The spleen reaches enormous proportions because abnormal red cells have been harbored and sequestered on a daily basis. Enlarged spleens cause excessive hemolysis and discomfort. Many patients have splenectomies and this *does* ameliorate some of the anemia issues, but it presents the patient with other challenges, because splenectomy is not a benign procedure (see Chapter 2). Yet one of the gravest problems is iron overload. Patients with beta thalassemia major absorb more iron through diet because of increased erythropoiesis, and they accumulate iron as a result of taking in 200 mg additional iron with each transfusion of packed cells.[18] Thalassemia major patients in the United States have an average transfusion regimen of

blood once every 2 to 5 weeks, so iron accumulation is expected and needs to be medically monitored and managed. The author refers the reader to the Cooley's Anemia Foundation Website for more information (www. cooleysanemia.org).

Treating and Managing Thalassemia Major

Thalassemia major patients will be on either a low-transfusion or a high-transfusion protocol. A low-transfusion protocol treats the patient symptomatically, administering transfusion when symptoms warrant. A high-transfusion protocol aims to keep the patient's hemoglobin level close to 10 g/dL; the patient is transfused every 2 to 5 weeks. There are good arguments for both, bearing in mind that transfusion exposes the individual not only to excess iron but also to foreign red cell antigens and other blood-borne diseases. A high-transfusion protocol gives the patient the best hope for a normal quality of life, by increasing his or her hemoglobin and providing better bone quality, better growth, less iron, and near-normal spleen size. Yet, iron overload looms as a major outcome of the high-transfusion protocol and is the major focus of clinical management.

Patients need to be assessed for liver, pancreatic, endocrine, and cardiac iron. Although noninvasive procedures are available, they are specialized and not available at every clinical facility. Iron overload poses significant risk to cardiac function and leads to hepatic and endocrinological complications. Iron chelation is recommended once the serum ferritin level has reached about 1000 µg/L, and this usually correlates with about 10 to 20 transfusions from the onset of diagnosis.[19] The procedure for chelation with Desferal has been explained earlier in this chapter. Compliance is critical in thalassemia major patients, yet difficult to maintain, as the patient moves from childhood to adolescence and becomes less willing to be hooked up to the infusion pump. In late 2005, an oral chelating agent, Exjade or ICL670 (Novartis), became available to this patient population. Despite compliance with chelating therapy, cardiac complications continue to be the leading cause of death in patients with thalassemia major.

Bone marrow transplantation and stem cell transplantation are therapeutic modalities that are also available for the severe thalassemic patient. For patients considering bone marrow transplant, finding a compatible donor is the necessary first step. If this can be accomplished, then bone marrow transplant should be considered early before the patient develops too many complications of thalassemia. The transplant procedure itself is rigorous and not without risks. Stem cell transplantation, although a viable alternative, takes much forethought and is often limited by the fact that stem cells have not been collected from the umbilical cord post delivery.

Thalassemia Intermedia and Beta Thalassemia Trait

Individuals with thalassemia intermedia are not a well-defined subset of thalassemia major patients. As a clinical group, they develop problems later in life than do thalassemia major individuals and they may *not* need transfusions. They do develop larger spleens, but their transfusion requirements, if present, are less frequent. Bone changes may be present, but they are mild. Individuals with thalassemia intermedia may need to be iron depleted with Desferal therapy, but this is much less frequent than their thalassemia major counterparts.

Beta thalassemia trait is the heterozygous condition, in which only one abnormal beta gene is inherited from the parent. This condition mimics IDA with individuals presenting with microcytic hypochromic indices and moderately low hemoglobin and hematocrit values.[20] Hemoglobin A_2 will be increased to approximately 5% to 10%. Beta thalassemia minor has

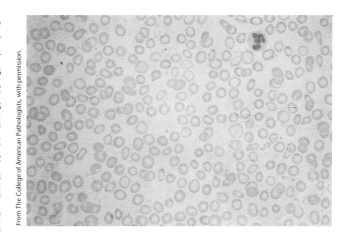

Figure 5.16 Microcytic hypochromic blood smear in thalassemia minor.

often been confused with IDA (Fig. 5.16), but a close examination of the CBC will show an individual with an increased red count. Above all other values, the increased RBC is significant in this condition because it represents that the bone marrow is compensating for having only one half the complement of beta chains. This change, although subtle, is often unrecognized by clinicians, and for this reason, many beta thalassemia minor patients have been put on iron protocols that offer no therapeutic value. Iron is *not* the problem in beta thalassemia minor (Table 5.11). Although a therapeutic trial of iron may not harm the patient in the long run, it is not good medical management. Patients who have microcytic indices may easily represent the largest number of anemia patients. A careful diagnosis that considers broader possibilities for a microcytic presentation is in the best interest of the patient and the health care system as a whole (Table 5.12).

Table 5.11 ● Differential Diagnosis of Microcytic Disorders

Diagnosis	Serum Iron	TIBC	% Saturation	Ferritin
AOI/ACD	↓	↓	↓	↑
HH	↑	↓	↑	↑
IDA	↓	↑	↓	↓
SA	↑	↓	↑	↑
Thalassemia minor	↑/N	N	↑	↑

HH, hereditary hemochromatosis; IDA, iron deficiency anemia; SA, sideroblastic anemia; AOI, anemia of inflammation; ACD, anemia of chronic disease.

Table 5.12 ⦿ Diagnostic Clues for the Thalassemic Conditions

If you are suspecting the two- or three-gene deletion alpha thalassemic state
- The MCVs are much lower than in IDA
- RDW is much more severe in alpha thalassemias

If you suspect the silent carrier alpha thalassemic state
- MCV is in normal or low-normal range
- Presence of elliptocytes on the smear is an indicator

If you suspect beta thalassemia major state
- MCVs are low
- High numbers of nRBCs on smear

- Presence of targets, fragments on smear
- Microcytosis and hypochromia
- Hgb F is major hemoglobin on electrophoresis

If you suspect beta thalassemia minor state
- MCV is lower than in IDA
- RBC count is elevated
- Microcytosis and hypochromia
- May see basophilic stippling, targets on smear
- Hgb A$_2$ is elevated

CONDENSED CASE

A South Vietnamese adolescent girl is seen in the student health clinic for complaints of shortness of breath. Her laboratory results reveal WBC = 9.0×10^9/L, Hgb = 9.0 g/dL, Hct = 27%, MCV = 62 fL, and MCHC = 30.2. The peripheral smear revealed moderate target cells, microcytes, hypochromic, and some fragments. Hemoglobin electrophoresis at pH 8.6 indicates three bands: a heavy band in the A position, a lighter band in the F position, and a moderate band that is faster than Hgb A. **What is your clinical impression?**

Answer

This patient most likely has hemoglobin H disease and is showing signs of anemia. She has done a good job of compensating and probably never needed transfusion. Her peripheral smear abnormalities combined and her electrophoresis results are fairly conclusive for this alpha thalassemia.

Summary Points

- An anemia classified as microcytic, hypochromic means that there is a decreased MCV and decreased MCHC.

- The most common microcytic anemias are IDA, sideroblastic anemias, hereditary hemochromatosis, and anemia of chronic disease.

- Iron is ingested, absorbed from the duodenum and jejunum, and then moved to the bone marrow by transferrin, the transport protein.

- Individuals with IDA will experience symptoms of anemia and perhaps cheilitis, koilonychia, or pica.

- Individuals with iron deficiency will have a decreased serum iron and serum ferritin and increased TIBC.

- The anemia of chronic disease or the anemia of inflammation is one of the most common anemias in the hospital population.

- Hereditary hemochromatosis (HH) is an inherited iron loading anemia.

- Multiple organs are affected in HH, because individuals with HH have been iron loading for decades.

- The serum iron and serum ferritin are high in HH.

- Therapeutic phlebotomy is the therapy of choice for HH.

- The thalassemia syndromes are globin chain synthetic defects.

- There are four clinical conditions of alpha thalassemia, each caused by gene deletions.

- Beta thalassemia major is the most severe of the beta thalassemic conditions.

- Individuals with beta thalassemia major will have a severe anemia, splenomegaly, and thalassemic facies.

- The majority hemoglobin in beta thalassemic major is hemoglobin F.

- Beta thalassemia minor is similar to IDA with the exception of an elevated RBC and an elevated hemoglobin A$_2$.

CASE STUDY

A physician came into the clinical laboratory during the evening shift requesting to review the peripheral smear on one of his patients. This particular 40-year-old patient had been particularly confusing for him because she came into the clinic with a CBC that indicated IDA, with MCV of 76 fL, Hgb 11.3 g/dL, Hct 34%, and RBC 5.8×10^{12}/L. She had complaints of fatigue and lethargy. The physician had put her on a trial therapy with iron supplementation, but 3 weeks later her laboratory results were virtually the same. **What inherited hematological condition shows a clinical picture similar to IDA?**

Insights to the Case Study

This case illustrates a frequent problem in the diagnosis and management of a patient with microcytic indices. This patient was diagnosed with IDA with no clear indication of her iron status and begun on a therapeutic trial of iron. She did not respond, since her CBC remained virtually the same. When a hemoglobin A_2 was ordered, the results were found to be 8.5% (normal value, 2% to 3%), and these results are indicative of beta thalassemia trait. This condition is an inherited disorder in which only one normal beta gene is present. An abnormal beta gene is inherited from one parent; consequently a full complement of hemoglobin A is not formed and hemoglobin A_2 is elevated. The patient has a lifelong moderate microcytic anemia, with an elevated red count. Patients lead a normal life, but conditions such as pregnancy or illness may cause the anemia to worsen, and transfusion in these cases may be warranted. If the information is available, individuals who carry the beta thalassemic trait should identify themselves to their supervising physician.

Review Questions

1. The morphological classification of anemias is based on the
   a. red cell count.
   b. cause of the anemia.
   c. red cell indices.
   d. reticulocyte count.

2. Which of these symptoms is specific for IDA?
   a. Fatigue
   b. Koilonychia
   c. Palpitations
   d. Dizziness

3. Which of the following laboratory tests will be abnormal through each stage of iron deficiency?
   a. Serum iron
   b. Hemoglobin and hematocrit
   c. Red cell count
   d. Serum ferritin

4. A patient presents with a microcytic hypochromia anemia with ragged-looking red cells in the peripheral smear and a high reticulocyte count. A brilliant cresyl blue preparation reveals inclusions that appear like pitted golf balls. These inclusions are suggestive of
   a. hemoglobin H disease.
   b. beta thalassemia major.

   c. hereditary hemochromatosis.
   d. beta thalassemic trait.

5. The most cost-effective therapy for a patient with hereditary hemochromatosis is
   a. Desferal chelation.
   b. bone marrow transplant.
   c. therapeutic phlebotomy.
   d. stem cell transplant.

6. List two sets of laboratory data that can distinguish IDA from beta thalassemia trait.
   a. Serum iron and red count
   b. Hemoglobin and hematocrit
   c. White count and RDW
   d. Red cell indices and platelets

7. What is the majority hemoglobin in thalassemia major?
   a. Hemoglobin A
   b. Hemoglobin A_2
   c. Hemoglobin F
   d. Hemoglobin H

8. Of the four clinical states of alpha thalassemia, which is incompatible with life?
   a. Alpha thalassemia silent carrier
   b. Alpha thalassemia trait
   c. Hemoglobin H disease
   d. Hydrops Barts fetalis

9. Which of the following hemoglobins has the chemical confirmation β_4?
    a. Hemoglobin Barts
    b. Hemoglobin Gower
    c. Hemoglobin H
    d. Hemoglobin Portland

10. Although there are many complications in thalassemia major individuals, which of the following is the leading cause of death?
    a. Splenomegaly
    b. Cardiac complications
    c. Hepatitis C infection
    d. Pathological fractures

● TROUBLESHOOTING

What Do I Do When Red Cell Inclusions Have Been Misidentified?

A 36-year-old chronic alcoholic with liver disease and pneumonia was admitted to the hospital. Her admission was for treatment of the pneumonia. Routine CBCs including differential were ordered daily to monitor her white count during the treatment process. During evaluation of her peripheral smear, a shift to the left was observed. This is a term used to describe the presence of younger white cells from the bone marrow in response to infection and inflammation. On the second day after admission, the patient's smear was being examined on the evening shift by a new laboratory graduate: She noted red cell inclusions and identified them as Howell-Jolly bodies, but she felt insecure about the identity of the inclusion and no one was available to observe the inclusion. After consulting with the lead technologist, they reviewed the smear together to try to identify which inclusion was present. The student preliminarily identified the inclusions as Howell-Jolly bodies, which are single inclusion, DNA in origin, and usually located in the periphery of the red cell. Basophilic stippling was another possibility, but stippling is RNA in origin and seen throughout the red cells; the new employee noted that the inclusion was located toward the periphery of the cell. The next possibility was Pappenheimer bodies, small inclusions that look like grape clusters. Pappenheimer bodies are usually iron deposits either in the form of ferritin or hemosiderin. If they are suspected, an iron stain (Prussian blue) will confirm the presence of iron. A Prussian blue stain was performed, and the inclusions were confirmed to be siderocytes, iron-containing inclusions. These inclusions can be found in hemochromatosis, alcoholism, hemolytic anemia, and post splenectomy.

WORD KEY

Chelation • To remove a heavy compound, like a heavy metal

Collagen vascular disease • Disorder that affects primarily the joints and mobility

Dyspnea • Shortness of breath

Gastrectomy • Removal of a portion of the stomach

Jaundice • Increase in bilirubin leading to a yellow discoloration in the mucous membranes of the eyes and a yellow tone to the skin

Menorrhagia • Excessive menstrual bleeding

Vertigo • Dizziness

References

1. Ogedegbe HO, Csury L, Simmons BH. Anemias: A clinical laboratory perspective. Lab Med 35:177, 2004.
2. Hillman RS, Finch CA. Differential diagnosis of anemia. In: Hillman RS, Finch CA, eds. Red Cell Manual, 7th ed. Philadelphia: FA Davis, 1996; 71.
3. Hussong JW. Iron metabolism and hypochromic anemias. In: Harmening D, ed. Clinical Hematology and Fundamentals of Hemostasis. Philadelphia: FA Davis, 2002; 100.
4. Coleman M. Iron metabolism. In: Rodak B, ed. Hematology: Clinical Principles and Applications, 2nd ed. Philadelphia: WB Saunders, 2002; 118–119.
5. Annibale B, Caparso F, Delle Fave G. The stomach and iron deficiency anemia: A forgotten link. Liver Dis 35:288–295, 2003.
6. Gross S. Disorders of iron metabolism. In: Gross S, Roath S, eds. Routine Hematology: A Problem-Oriented Approach. Baltimore: Williams and Wilkins, 1996; 118.
7. Centers for Disease Control and Prevention. Recommendations to Prevent and Control Iron Deficiency in the United States. April 1998. Available at http://www.cdc.gov/mmnr/preview/mmwrhtml/100051880.htm. Accessed September 24, 2006.

8. Gross S. Disorders of iron metabolism. In: Gross S, Roath S, eds. Routine Hematology: A Problem-Oriented Approach. Baltimore: Williams and Wilkins; 1996; 125.

9. Spivak JL. Iron and the anemia of chronic disease. Oncology 9(Suppl 10):25–33, 2002.

10. Roy CN, Weinstein DA, Andrews NC. The molecular biology of the anemia of chronic disease: A hypothesis. Pediatr Res 53:507–512, 2003.

11. Kaplan LA, Pesce AJ. Iron, porphyrin and bilirubin metabolism. In: Kaplan LA, Pesce AJ, eds. Clinical Chemistry Theory, Analysis, Correlations, 3rd ed. St. Louis: Mosby, 1996; 700–701.

12. Weinberg ED. Laboratory contributions to the diagnosis of common iron loading disorders and anemias. Lab Med 32:507–508, 2002.

13. Galhenge SP, Viiala CH, Olynyk JK. Screening for hemochromatosis: Patients with liver disease, families and populations. Curr Gastroenterol Rep 6:44–51, 2004.

14. Cooley's Anemia Foundation. Leading the Fight Against Thalassemia. Available at www.cooleysanemia.org.

15. Panich V, Pornpatku M, Sriroohgrueng W. The problem of the thalassemias in Thailand. Southeast Asian J Trop Med Public Health Suppl:23, 1992.

16. Teshima D, Hall J, Darniati E, et al. Microscopic erythrocyte morphologic changes associated with alpha thalassemia. Clin Lab Sci 6:236–240, 1993.

17. Hall RB, Haga JA, Guerra CG, et al. Optimizing the detection of hemoglobin H disease. Lab Med 26:736–741, 1995.

18. Vullo R, Moddel B, Georganda E. What Is Cooley's Anemia? 2nd ed. Nicosia, Cyprus/Geneva: Thalassaemia International Federation/World Health Organization, 1995; 17.

19. Eleftheriou A. Compliance to Iron Chelation Therapy with Desferrioxamine. Nicosia, Cyprus: Thalassaemia International Federation, 2000; 15.

20. Nuchprayoon I, Sukthawee B, Nuchprayoon T. Red cell indices and therapeutic trial of iron in diagnostic workup for anemic Thai females. J Med Assoc Thai 86(Suppl 2):S160–S169, 2003.

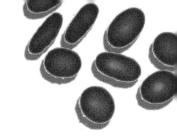

6 The Macrocytic Anemias

Betty Ciesla

The Macrocytic Anemias and the Megaloblastic Process

The Red Cell Precursors in Megaloblastic Anemia

Ineffective Erythropoiesis in Megaloblastic Anemia

Vitamin B$_{12}$ and Folic Acid: Their Role in DNA Synthesis

Nutritional Requirements, Transport, and Metabolism of Vitamin B$_{12}$ and Folic Acid

Incorporating Vitamin B$_{12}$ Into the Bone Marrow

Clinical Features of Patients With Megaloblastic Anemia

Hematological Features of Megaloblastic Anemias

Pernicious Anemia as a Subset of Megaloblastic Anemias

Vitamin B$_{12}$ and Folic Acid Deficiency

Laboratory Diagnosis of Megaloblastic Anemias

Treatment and Response of Individuals With Megaloblastic Anemia

Macrocytic Anemias That Are Not Megaloblastic

Objectives

After completing this chapter, the student will be able to:

1. Define *megaloblastic anemia* as a macrocytic anemia.

2. Compare and contrast the morphological characteristics of megaloblasts and normoblasts in the bone marrow.

3. Differentiate red cell and white cell changes in the peripheral smear that are seen in the megaloblastic anemias.

4. Describe ineffective hematopoiesis as it relates to the megaloblastic process.

5. Describe the pathway of vitamin B$_{12}$ and folic acid from ingestion through incorporation into the red cell.

6. Describe the clinical symptoms of a patient with megaloblastic anemia.

7. List the causes of vitamin B$_{12}$ and folic acid deficiency.

8. Define *pernicious anemia* and its clinical and laboratory findings.

9. Describe the Schilling test and its use in diagnosing megaloblastic anemia.

10. Describe the treatments for the megaloblastic anemias.

11. Differentiate the anemias that are macrocytic but are not megaloblastic.

THE MACROCYTIC ANEMIAS AND THE MEGALOBLASTIC PROCESS

The macrocytic anemias are a morphological classification of anemias that have an MCV of greater than 100 fL. The MCH is also elevated but the MCHC is within normal range, and these anemias are termed macrocytic/normochromic. Broadly defined, the macrocytic anemias are divided into two categories: megaloblastic and nonmegaloblastic processes. If the source of the anemia is a vitamin B_{12} or folic acid deficiency, the anemia is termed megaloblastic. If the source of the anemia is unrelated to a nutritional deficiency, the anemia is macrocytic but *not* megaloblastic. Vitamin B_{12} or folic acid deficiency leads to impaired DNA synthesis, a serious condition, and will affect all readily dividing cells, skin cells, hematopoietic cells, and epithelial cells. The effects on the bone marrow, peripheral smear, and the patient's quality of life are dramatic and substantive.

THE RED CELL PRECURSORS IN MEGALOBLASTIC ANEMIA

Because megaloblastic processes damage DNA synthesis, nucleated cells will be the most affected. There are multiple white cell and red cell changes in the bone marrow structure that should be recognized and appreciated. The megaloblastic red cell precursors are larger, the nuclear structure is less condensed, and the cytoplasm is extremely basophilic or much bluer. There is asynchrony between the age of the nuclear material and the age of the cytoplasm, but this can best be appreciated by making a serious comparison of the nuclear and cytoplasmic material in megaloblastic precursor cells versus normoblastic precursor cells (Fig. 6.1). When a cell stage is asynchronous, the nuclear age and the cytoplasmic age do not correspond. Recall that the normal red cell series is programmed for two specific functions: hemoglobin synthesis and nuclear expulsion. In order for the nucleus to be expelled, certain changes must occur in the size of the nucleus and the consistency of the nucleus structure. Therefore, the chromatin that begins as fine, reticular, and smooth must take on a different texture and conformation before it is expelled from the orthochromic normoblast. In megaloblastic erythropoiesis, the texture and condensation of the nuclear material are disrupted. Megaloblastic chromatin in the megaloblastic pronormoblast and megaloblastic basophilic normoblast is open-weaved with a clockface arrangement of chromatin, easily imagined if you closely look at the chromatin pattern. The nuclear (or chromatin) material is fragile and lacks the composi-

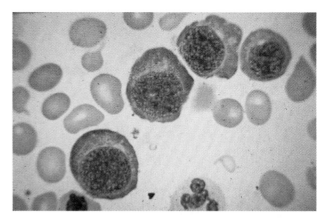

Figure 6.1   Megaloblastic precursors, showing the asynchrony between the nucleus and the chromatin; the cytoplasm of most cells is extremely basophilic.

tion and condensation of a nucleus ready to be delivered from the cell. Likewise, the cytoplasmic material in the early megaloblastic precursors is extremely basophilic, much bluer than normal precursors (Fig. 6.2). Students usually have a difficult time observing the difference between the normal red cell precursors and the megaloblastic precursors. A careful study of the nucleus/cytoplasm (N:C) ratio, size of the cell, nuclear material, and cytoplasm color in each stage of each cell will help to differentiate one from the other.

INEFFECTIVE ERYTHROPOIESIS IN MEGALOBLASTIC ANEMIA

The bone marrow is hypercellular in the megaloblastic conditions and the white cell precursor cells are large, especially the metamyelocytes. The myeloid-to-erythroid (M:E) ratio is 1:1 or 1:3, reflecting erythroid hyperplasia as you would see in the bone marrow

From The College of American Pathologists, with permission.

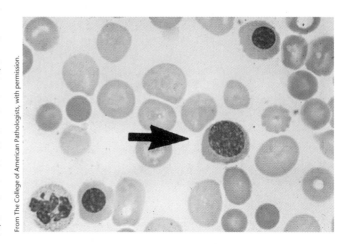

Figure 6.2   Normoblastic erythropoiesis with a polychromatophilic normoblast (*arrow*).

Table 6.1 ○ Consequences of Ineffective Erythropoiesis

- Bone marrow destruction of erythroid precursors
- Lack of regeneration of bone marrow elements during anemic stress
- Lack of nRBCs in peripheral smear
- Lack of polychromasia in peripheral smear
- Reticulocytopenia
- Intramedullary hemolysis
- Increased bilirubin and LDH

responding to anemia. However, in the megaloblastic processes, there is an ineffective erythropoiesis, which means destruction in the bone marrow of red cell precursors before they even reach the peripheral circulation (Table 6.1). Megaloblastic precursor cells, especially at the polychromatophilic and basophilic states, hemolyze before their maturation cycle is completed. Orthochromic normoblasts and/or reticulocytes do not have the opportunity to be delivered from the bone marrow as they NORMALLY would in response to anemic stress. Consequently, the reticulocyte count is inappropriately low. The peripheral smear does not show polychromasia or nucleated red cells, and bilirubin and LDH are elevated. The last two clinical developments signal **intramedullary hemolysis.** If the erythropoiesis was effective and the bone marrow was responding to anemic stress, the peripheral smear would show evidence of a regenerative marrow process. Polychromasia and the presence of nucleated red cells would be self-evident (Table 6.2).

Table 6.2 ○ Bone Marrow Response to Anemic Stress

- The production of red cell precursor cells is accelerated.
- The M:E ratio is adjusted to reflect erythroid hyperplasia.
- Precursor cells, orthochromic normoblasts, are prematurely released from the marrow.
- Reticulocytes are prematurely released from the marrow.
- Polychromasia is seen in the peripheral smear.
- nRBCs are present in the peripheral smear.
- If the reticulocyte count is high, then a slight macrocytosis might develop.

VITAMIN B_{12} AND FOLIC ACID: THEIR ROLE IN DNA SYNTHESIS

DNA synthesis is dependent on a key structure, thymidine triphosphate (TTP). This structure cannot be formed unless it receives a methyl group from methyl tetrahydrofolate or folic acid. Vitamin B_{12} is the cofactor responsible for transferring the methyl group to methyl tetrahydrofolate.[1] Sufficient quantities of vitamin B_{12} and folic acid are key to the formation of TTP. If TTP cannot be synthesized, then it is replaced by deoxyuridine triphosphate (DTP). The synthesis of this component leads to nuclear fragmentation and destruction of cells and impaired cell division. For this reason, vitamin B_{12} and folic acid are essential elements in the DNA pathway.

NUTRITIONAL REQUIREMENTS, TRANSPORT, AND METABOLISM OF VITAMIN B_{12} AND FOLIC ACID

Microorganisms and fungi are the main producers of vitamin B_{12}, a group of vitamins known as cobalamins. This vitamin may also be embedded in liver, meat, fish, eggs, and dairy products. The recommended daily allowance of vitamin B_{12} is 2.0 μg/day with the daily diet providing approximately 5 to 30 μg/day and storage of 1 to 2 mg, in the liver. Dietary requirements will increase during pregnancy and lactation. Depletion of vitamin B_{12} stores takes years to develop. Folic acid, on the other hand, is readily available in green leafy vegetables, fruit, broccoli, and dairy products. The minimum daily requirement is 200 μg/day, a much higher requirement than that of vitamin B_{12}, with body stores of 5 to 10 mg. in the liver. Folic acid is quickly depleted in a matter of months because the daily requirement is so much higher (Table 6.3). Pregnant women are encour-

Table 6.3 ○ Sources of Vitamin B_{12} and Folic Acid

Vitamin B_{12}
- Meat, liver, kidney, oysters, clams, fish
- Eggs, cheese, and other dairy products

Folic Acid
- Green leafy vegetables
- Broccoli
- Fruit
- Whole grains
- Dairy products

aged to increase their folic acid intake because decreased folate may lead to neural tube defects.

INCORPORATING VITAMIN B₁₂ INTO THE BONE MARROW

The incorporation of vitamin B_{12} into bone marrow and other tissues is a multistep process. Initially, the vitamin is taken in from the diet and separated from food by hydrochloric acid, synthesized by gastric cells. Next B_{12} is transported to the stomach and combines with intrinsic factor, a substance secreted by the parietal cells of the stomach. Intrinsic factor and B_{12} form a complex that proceeds to the ileum. Vitamin B_{12} is absorbed through the brush borders of the ileum, and intrinsic factor is neutralized. Once the vitamin leaves the ileum, it is carried across the stomach wall and into the plasma to form a complex with transcobalamin II (TCII), which transports it to the circulation.[2] From the circulation, vitamin B_{12} is transferred to the liver, the bone marrow, and other tissues (Fig. 6.3).

Moving folic acid into the circulation and tissues occurs with a little more ease. Once folic acid is ingested and absorbed through the small intestine, it is reduced to methyl tetrahydrofolate through dihydrofolate reductase, an enzyme available in mucosal cells. It is the reduced form that is delivered to the tissues. Once

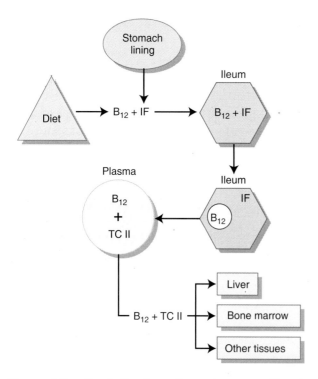

Figure 6.3 Vitamin B_{12} absorption and transport. Vitamin B_{12} must be combined with intrinsic factor (IF) before it enters the blood circulation: transcobalamin II (TC II) is the transport protein that carries vitamin B_{12} to the tissues.

inside the tissues, the methyl group is released to combine with homocysteine, an early precursor to DNA synthesis. Homocysteine is converted to methionine, an amino acid. If folate or vitamin B_{12} metabolism is flawed, homocysteine will accumulate and can potentially lead to thrombosis,[3] a potential consequence to the hemostatic system that is just being realized.

CLINICAL FEATURES OF PATIENTS WITH MEGALOBLASTIC ANEMIA

Megaloblastic anemia is usually a disease of middle-aged to older age with a high predilection for women. Severe anemia, in which the hemoglobin drops to 7 to 8 g/dL, is accompanied by symptoms of anemias such as shortness of breath, light-headedness, extreme weakness, and pallor. Patients may experience glossitis (sore or enlarged tongue), dyspepsia, or diarrhea. Evidence of neurological involvement may be seen with patients experiencing numbness, vibratory loss (**paresthesias**), difficulties in balance and walking, and personality changes. Vitamin B_{12} deficiency causes a **demyelination** of the peripheral nerves, the spinal column, and the brain, which can cause many of the more severe neurological symptoms such as **spasticity** or **paranoia.** Jaundice may be seen, because the average red cell life span in megaloblastic anemia is 75 days, a little more than one half of the average red cell life span of 120 days. The bilirubin level is elevated, and the lactate dehydrogenase (LDH) level is high, signifying hemolysis.

HEMATOLOGICAL FEATURES OF MEGALOBLASTIC ANEMIAS

The CBC shows a pancytopenia (low white count, low red count, and low platelet count), although the platelet count may be only borderline low (see normal values on the front cover of this textbook). Pancytopenia in the CBC combined with macrocytosis should raise the index of suspicion toward a megaloblastic process because few other conditions (aplastic anemia, hypersplenism) show this pattern.[4] Red cell inclusions such as basophilic stippling and Howell-Jolly bodies may be observed. Howell-Jolly bodies formed from megaloblastic erythropoiesis are larger and more fragmented in appearance than normal Howell-Jolly bodies. There is a low reticulocyte count (less than 1%) and the RDW is increased, owing to schistocytes, targets, and teardrop cells. The blood smear in megaloblastic anemia is extremely relevant in the diagnosis and shows macrocytes, macro-ovalocytes, hypersegmented multilobed neutrophils, and little polychromasia with respect to the anemia (Fig. 6.4). The presence of hyper-

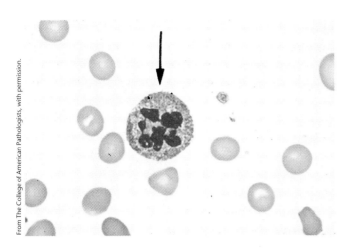

Figure 6.4 Peripheral smear from a patient with mega-loblastic anemia. Note the hypersegmented neutrophils and the macro-ovalocytes.

segmented neutrophils (lobe count of more than five lobes) in combination with macrocytic anemia is a morphological marker for megaloblastic anemias. This qualitative white cell abnormality appears early in the disease and survives through treatment. It is usually the last morphology to disappear. The MCV initially is extremely high and may be in the range of 100 to 140 fL. A bone marrow examination is not necessary for the diagnosis of megaloblastic anemia, because the diagnosis of this disorder can be adequately made without this time-consuming, costly, and invasive procedure.

PERNICIOUS ANEMIA AS A SUBSET OF MEGALOBLASTIC ANEMIAS

Intrinsic factor is the single most important ingredient to the absorption of vitamin B_{12} and subsequent delivery of vitamin B_{12} to the circulation. When problems with intrinsic factor develop, the condition is called pernicious anemia. Drs. George Minot and William Murphy of Boston were awarded the Nobel Prize in 1934 for their discovery that ingestion of liver successfully treated patients with pernicious anemia. Several factors may account for the lack of intrinsic factor in the stomach, including physical factors such as partial or whole gastrectomy, or genetic and immune factors. Whatever the cause, either intrinsic factor is not being secreted or it is being blocked or neutralized in some fashion. Atrophic gastritis may occur in which gastric secretions are diminished and therefore intrinsic factor fails to be secreted. The reasons for this remain unclear but age may play a role.[5] Immune factors may arise that cause antibodies to be produced against intrinsic factor, thyroid tissue, and parietal cells, all of which will decrease the production of intrinsic factor. Antibodies

to intrinsic factor are present in 56% of patients with pernicious anemia, with 90% of patients showing parietal cell antibodies, and this suggests a strong autoimmune component to this disorder. Additionally, there is a higher frequency of pernicious anemias in individuals with diabetes, thyroid conditions, and other autoimmune processes.[6] Pernicious anemia may occur genetically as an autosomal recessive trait in children before the age of 2. Cubilin, a receptor for vitamin B_{12} and intrinsic factor, has been identified since 1998, but its role in juvenile-onset pernicious anemia is still being researched.[7] Adult forms of congenital pernicious anemia do occur and are associated with **achlorhydria** or malabsorption in relatives.

Pernicious anemia is more common in individuals with Irish and Scandinavian ethnicity. Pernicious anemia patients will experience all of the symptoms of a patient with megaloblastic anemia, but they have a higher tendency for neurological involvement including those already mentioned as well as degeneration of peripheral nerves and the spinal column. Neurological symptoms may be slow to develop but include a vast array of symptomatology. Patients may experience paresthesias in the limbs, an abnormal or clumsy walking pattern or stiffness in the limbs. Treatment will usually reverse these symptoms.

VITAMIN B_{12} AND FOLIC ACID DEFICIENCY

Dietary deficiencies are rarely the cause of vitamin B_{12} deficiency, except for individuals who are strictly vegetarians or infants nursed by vegetarian mothers who are not supplementing their diets. Other potential sources of a deficiency in vitamin B_{12} are the malabsorption syndromes, which include any condition that affects B_{12} absorption. Lack of intrinsic factor may occur if a gastrectomy or partial gastrectomy has occurred, and the parietal cells that secrete IF would invariably be affected, thereby affecting vitamin B_{12} absorption. Added to this is a condition called blind loop syndrome, in which there is an overgrowth of bacteria in a small pocket of malformed intestine. The microorganisms take up the vitamin B_{12}, and it is not available to be absorbed. Although unusual, the fish tapeworm *Diphyllobothrium latum* may compete for vitamin B_{12} when it attaches to the intestine. Individuals who have this parasite exhibit signs of megaloblastic anemia, which can be corrected once the parasite is discovered and destroyed.

Dietary deficiency is a serious consideration in folic acid deficiency and may occur in pregnancy or infancy because of increased requirement or in the elderly or alcoholic persons because of lack of availability. Folic acid is depleted from body stores within 3 to 6 months, and in vulnerable populations, folic acid deficiency continues to be one of the most common vitamin deficiencies in the United States. Tropical spue is one of the most common malabsorption syndromes that contributes to folic acid deficiency. This syndrome is usually seen in individuals from tropical or subtropical climates like Haiti, Cuba, and Puerto Rico. Although rare, this condition affects overall digestion and is thought to be a result of infection, overgrowth of bacteria, or poor nutrition. Normally, the villi that line the digestive tract are fingerlike projections whose job is to promote absorption from ingested food. The villi from individuals with tropical sprue are flattened, leading to poor absorption activity. Individuals with sprue will manifest this disease with diarrhea, indigestion, and weight loss. Last, folic acid deficiency may be expected in individuals taking methotrexate or other chemotherapy drugs, because many of these directly affect DNA synthesis of dividing cells, normal and abnormal.

LABORATORY DIAGNOSIS OF MEGALOBLASTIC ANEMIAS

The megaloblastic anemias show striking similarities in their clinical and hematological presentations. Common features of the megaloblastic anemias include

- Pancytopenia
- Increased MCV and MCHC
- Hypersegmented neutrophils (five lobes or more in segmented neutrophils)
- Increased bilirubin
- Increased LDH
- Hyperplasia in the bone marrow
- Decreased M:E ratio
- Reticulocytopenia

The differential diagnosis of these disorders depends on a more sophisticated battery of laboratory tests that can help determine if the patient is lacking vitamin B_{12}, folic acid, or intrinsic factor. Several tests are used to distinguish between these possibilities; they include serum B_{12}, folic acid, or red cell folate determination by radioimmunoassay, gastric analysis to determine achlorhydria or lack of hydrochloric acid in the stomach, or tests to denote intrinsic factor or parietal cell antibodies performed by enzyme-linked immunosorbent assay (ELISA). Parietal cell antibodies are seen in 90% of individuals at the time of initial diagnosis,[8] although the presence of these antibodies is not specific for a diagnosis of pernicious anemia, because parietal cell antibodies are seen in some individuals with endocrine disorders. Intrinsic factor antibody evaluations are cost effective, reliable, and highly specific for a diagnosis of pernicious anemia.[9] There are two classifications of intrinsic antibody: blocking antibodies and binding antibodies. Blocking antibodies inhibit the binding of vitamin B_{12} to intrinsic factor, while binding antibodies prevent the attachment of the intrinsic factor–B_{12} complex to receptors in the small intestine. Radioimmunoassay testing can delineate the nature of the intrinsic factor antibody. The reference procedure for the determination of pernicious anemia, however, continues to be the Schilling test, which measures the intestinal absorption of vitamin B_{12}. This test is performed in two parts, and although it is costly and labor intensive, it provides valuable information on the cause of pernicious anemia. The procedure in part 1 is to give the patient an oral dose of vitamin B_{12} and then, within 2 hours, a flushing dose of vitamin B_{12} via intramuscular injection. The flushing dose saturates all of the liver B_{12} binding sites. The urine is collected in a 24-hour period and the amount of vitamin B_{12} is measured. If intrinsic factor was present and vitamin B_{12} was absorbed, then 5% to 30% of the initial radiolabeled B_{12} will be excreted. If less than this amount is excreted, some type of malabsorption has taken place. In part 2 of the test, intrinsic factor is added to the oral vitamin B_{12} dose and the test proceeds as in part 1, including the flushing dose of B_{12}. If the excretion of B_{12} is in the proper amount, then intrinsic factor is determined as the deficiency. If the excretion of B_{12} is less than expected, then the patient is diagnosed with a malabsorption syndrome. Normal kidney function and conscientious urine collection are essential for the correct interpretation of this test. Once the results are analyzed, the physician will have a clear picture as to whether the lack of vitamin B_{12} absorption is due to intrinsic factor deficiency or malabsorption syndrome (Fig. 6.5).

TREATMENT AND RESPONSE OF INDIVIDUALS WITH MEGALOBLASTIC ANEMIA

Therapeutic vitamin B_{12} is available in the cyanocobalamin or hydroxycobalamin form. The vitamin can be administered orally, intramuscularly, or subcutaneously. If a patient is simply lacking in vitamin B_{12}, this vitamin can be taken orally at a daily dose of 1000 µg.

Oral cyanocobalamin offers a substantial cost savings to the patients compared with intramuscular vitamin B_{12} injections, which need to administered by a health professional.[10] Therapy is lifelong. For a patient with pernicious anemia, about 6000 µg of vitamin B_{12} over a 6-day period is used as an initial dose. At this

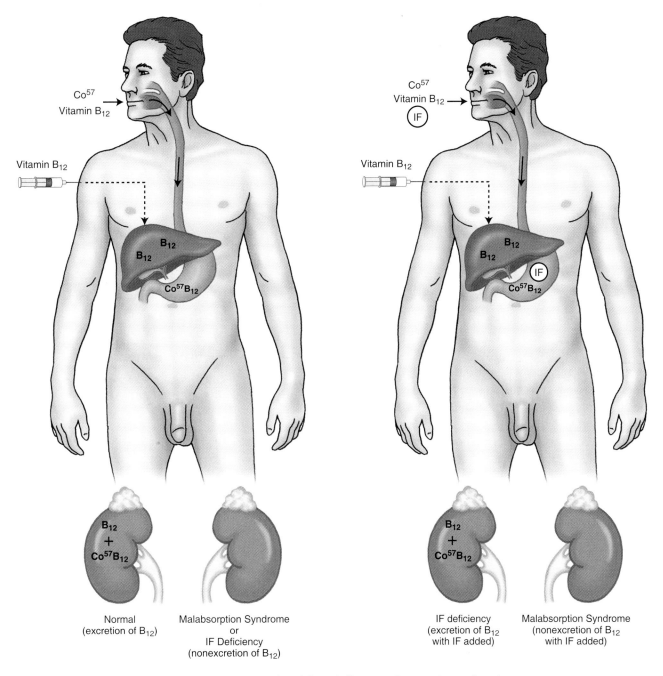

Figure 6.5   Parts 1 and 2 of the Schilling test. See text for explanation.

dosage, all of the body stores are saturated. If the therapy is successful, the patient's symptoms will begin to diminish, and a rapid reticulocyte response will commence in 2 to 3 days. Maintenance therapy of vitamin B_{12} will need to be given every 1 to 2 months for life, and the patient should be monitored by hematological assays.

Folic acid deficiency is fairly easy to treat with oral folate at 1 to 5 mg/day for 2 to 3 weeks. Short-term therapy is usually all that is required, and patients are counseled to increase their dietary intake of folic acid. Changes in the peripheral circulation will be noticed fairly quickly as the MCV comes back into the reference range, the anemia is resolved, and some of the clinical symptoms abate. Dual therapy may be started in those individuals who have a combined deficiency; however, the folic acid will resolve the hematological abnormalities long before the neurological abnormalities are resolved.

MACROCYTIC ANEMIAS THAT ARE NOT MEGALOBLASTIC

When macrocytes appear in the peripheral smear, it is important to observe them carefully for shape, color, or hypochromia, because these morphological clues can aid in determining if the macrocytosis is megaloblastic or nonmegaloblastic. Megaloblastic macrocytes are large and oval, with a thicker exterior membrane and lacking hypochromia. Macrocytes in the peripheral smear that lack any of these characteristics are usually not of megaloblastic origins. Several conditions can contribute to a macrocytic blood picture without a deficiency in vitamin B_{12} and folic acid. The most frequently seen conditions are a compensatory bone marrow response to hemolytic anemia, in which case a reticulocytosis will be seen. Because reticulocytes are polychromatophilic macrocytes and because reticulocytes will be prematurely delivered from the bone marrow in response to hemolysis, it is easy to understand how a macrocytic blood picture would develop. Usually, in these cases, the MCV is only slightly elevated, up to 105 fL. Macrocytosis may also be seen in conditions such as hypothyroidism, chronic liver disease, alcoholism, chemotherapy treatment, or a myelodysplastic disorder. Often, in patients with chronic liver disease and alcoholism, the macrocytes are targeted or hypochromic. Additionally, a macrocytic blood picture is noted in newborns because their bone marrow is immature and rapidly delivering nucleated cells and reticulocytes. For a differential diagnosis of macrocytes, see Figure 6.6.

Differential Diagnosis of Macrocyte

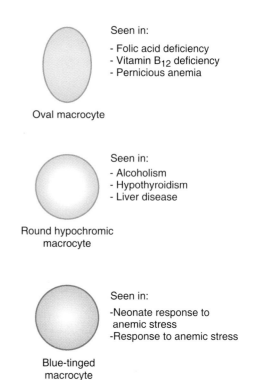

Seen in:
- Folic acid deficiency
- Vitamin B_{12} deficiency
- Pernicious anemia

Oval macrocyte

Seen in:
- Alcoholism
- Hypothyroidism
- Liver disease

Round hypochromic macrocyte

Seen in:
- Neonate response to anemic stress
- Response to anemic stress

Blue-tinged macrocyte

Figure 6.6   Not all macrocytes are the same. This drawing depicts three types of macrocytes, each differentiated by how they are produced with respect to the clinical condition.

CONDENSED CASE

The patient in this study is a 73-year-old woman who has anemia of long standing. She had always been a poor eater. Peripheral smears have consistently shown hypochromia with target and many Howell-Jolly bodies. She has no surgical history and she shows no blood loss through either the gastrointestinal or genitourinary tract. Her lab results are WBC of 2.7×10^9/L, RBC 2.25×10^{12}/L, Hgb 7.8 g/dL, Hct 23%, and MCV 111 fL. **Based on these findings, what is your initial clinical impression?**

Answer

This patient most likely has a megaloblastic anemia. Her age, dietary habits, and complete blood count can lead to that impression. With her dietary history, she may have initially had an iron deficiency condition, and her peripheral smear results seem to verify that. However, it seems as if her condition has shifted toward a vitamin B_{12} or folic acid deficiency. Serum vitamin B_{12} and folic acid assays should be ordered, and a Schilling test may be considered to rule in or rule out an intrinsic factor deficit.

Summary Points

- Macrocytic anemias have an MCV of greater than 100 fL and a normal MCHC.
- Megaloblastic anemias are macrocytic anemias in which vitamin B_{12} and/or folic acid is deficient.
- Not all macrocytic anemias are megaloblastic.
- Vitamin B_{12} and folic acid deficiencies lead to impaired DNA synthesis.
- The bone marrow in megaloblastic anemias is hypercellular with the red cell precursors

showing distinct chromatin and cytoplasmic changes.

- Megaloblastic anemias show ineffective erythropoiesis in the bone marrow: premature destruction of red cell precursors before delivery into the circulation.

- The peripheral smear in megaloblastic anemia shows macrocytes, oval macrocytes, and hypersegmented neutrophils.

- Pancytopenia and reticulocytopenia are prominent features of the megaloblastic processes.

- Patients with megaloblastic anemia may exhibit symptoms of anemia as well as neurological symptoms, such as numbness or difficulty walking.

- Intrinsic factor, secreted by the parietal cells of the stomach, is necessary for vitamin B_{12} to be absorbed.

- Intrinsic factor deficiency can lead to pernicious anemia, a subset of megaloblastic anemia.

- Intrinsic factor deficiency may develop because intrinsic factor is not being secreted or because it is being blocked or neutralized.

- Ninety percent of individuals experiencing pernicious anemia have parietal cell antibodies.

- Folic acid deficiency is the most common vitamin deficiency in the United States.

- Serum B_{12}, folic acid, and red cell folate can be determined by radioimmunoassay.

- Individuals with vitamin B_{12} deficiency will require lifelong therapy.

- Folic acid deficiency requires short-term therapy.

- The Schilling test is used to determine whether there is faulty absorption of vitamin B_{12}. Deficiency is the result of intrinsic factor or malabsorption syndrome.

- There are causes of a macrocytic anemia other than megaloblastic processes.

- Macrocytes may be seen in reticulocytosis, alcoholism, or liver disease.

CASE STUDY

Mrs. C., a 79-year-old woman, presented to the emergency department barely able to walk. She said that she had gotten progressively weaker in the past couple of weeks and that she has noticed that her appetite was failing. She had seen some yellow color to her eyes and skin, and that worried her. She had no desire to eat but she did crave ice. Mrs. C. was thin, emaciated, and pale, and she had difficulty walking and seemed generally confused. A CBC and peripheral smear were ordered, with more tests pending the initial results. The initial results are WBC of 4.5×10^6/L, RBC 2.12×10^9/L, Hgb 7.5 g/dL, Hct 22%, MCV 103 fL, MCH 35.3 pg, MCHC 34.9, and platelet count 105×10^6/L. The peripheral smear showed a mixture of microcytes and macrocytes, with target cells, schistocytes, few oval microcytes, rare hypersegmented neutrophils, and occasional hypochromic macrocytes. Because of mixed blood picture, an iron profile was ordered as well as serum folate and serum B_{12}. **Which conditions show hypersegmented neutrophils?**

Insights to the Case Study

This case study presents a confusing morphological picture because no *one red cell* morphology leads to any single clinical conclusion. The follow-up blood work showed serum iron of 25 μg/dL (reference range, 40 to 150), TIBC 500 μg/dL (200 to 400), red cell folate 100 ng/mL (130 to 268), and serum B_{12} 200 pg/dL (100 to 700). Clearly, there are multiple nutritional deficiencies at work here. Mrs. C. is in a vulnerable age range, prone to poor dietary habits and noncompliance to health or food suggestions. Yet as can be seen from her laboratory values, she is iron and folic acid deficient. Folic acid deficiency is one of the most common vitamin deficiencies in the United States and easy to develop because folic acid stores are moderate and the folic acid daily requirement is high. Add to this her iron deficiency, and you have a set of symptoms and a blood smear picture that represents a mixture of morphologies. She clearly showed a pancytopenia, but she did not show the blatantly elevated MCV. Her elevated MCH could have been a clue to the megaloblastic process because in the megaloblastic anemias, the MCV and MCH are usually high. Her peripheral smear shows microcytes and macrocytes, with a few target cells and an occasional hypersegmented neutrophil. She was immediately started on oral iron and oral B_{12} supplementation, and her physical symptoms began to diminish. Once her mental capacity was cleared, she began nutritional counseling, and she began to receive visits from Meals on Wheels, to ensure that she had a balanced and varied diet.

Review Questions

1. Which bone marrow changes are most prominent in the megaloblastic anemias?
   a. M:E ratio of 10: 1
   b. Hypocellular bone marrow
   c. Asynchrony in the red cell precursors
   d. Shaggy cytoplasm of the red cell precursors

2. Which morphological changes in the peripheral smear are markers for megaloblastic anemias?
   a. Oval macrocytes and hypersegmented neutrophils
   b. Oval and hypochromic macrocytes
   c. Pappenheimer bodies and hypochromic microcytes
   d. Dimorphic red cells and Howell-Jolly bodies

3. Which is the most common vitamin deficiency in the United States?
   a. Vitamin A
   b. Folic acid
   c. Calcium
   d. Vitamin B_{12}

4. Which of the following group of symptoms is particular to patients with megaloblastic anemia?
   a. Pallor and dyspnea
   b. Jaundice and hemoglobinuria
   c. Difficulty in walking and mental confusion
   d. Pica and fatigue

5. Which one of the following substances is necessary for vitamin B_{12} to be absorbed?
   a. Transferrin
   b. Erythropoietin
   c. Intrinsic factor
   d. Cubilin

6. Which of the following clinical findings is indicative of intramedullary hemolysis in megaloblastic processes?
   a. Increased red count
   b. Increased hemoglobin
   c. Decreased bilirubin
   d. Increased LDH

7. Which of the following adequately describes the pathophysiology of the megaloblastic anemias?
   a. Lack of DNA synthesis
   b. Defect in globin synthesis
   c. Defect in iron metabolism
   d. Excessive iron loading

● TROUBLESHOOTING

What Clinical Possibilities Should I Consider in a Patient With an Increased MCV? What Preanalytic Variables May Increase the MCV?

When a patient presents with a macrocytic blood picture, there are several clinical possibilities to consider. The most obvious reason for an increased MCV is a patient with a megaloblastic process. Supporting laboratory data for this possibility would include a pancytopenia, a reticulocytopenia, increased LDH, and a peripheral smear with macro-ovalocytes, hypersegmented neutrophils, and other poikilocytes. Follow-up testing should initially include an assessment of the vitamin B_{12} and folic acid levels, as well as testing for intrinsic factor antibodies.

A second patient population to consider when assessing a macrocytic anemia would be those who have liver disease, alcoholic cirrhosis, hypothyroidism, or chemotherapy. These patients would NOT show a pancytopenia but would show a moderate anemia with slightly increased MCV with round microcytes and perhaps siderocytes. A thorough review of the patient history should give insights into the nature of the macrocytic anemia. An often forgotten but fairly consistent reason for a slightly increased MCV is regenerative bone marrow. Patients who have inherited blood disorders such as sickle cell anemia, thalassemia major, or other hemolytic processes are transfused on a regular basis as part of their disease management. Not only do the transfused cells lend some size variation to their clinical process, but also the chronic anemia in these patients leads to a premature release of reticulocytes, which are immature cells that are larger than normal red cells. When reticulocytes are stained with Wright's stain, polychromatophilic macrocytes appear in the peripheral smear. In a peripheral smear with increased polychromasia, a slightly macrocytic blood picture is often seen. A simple assessment for the reticulocytes will show an increased value, which is contributory to the source of the increased MCV.

The MCV is a highly stable parameter, yet several preanalytic variables can alter the MCV. If a sample fails a delta check as a result of a rise in MCV, several considerations are in order. Sample contamination may increase the red cell size, especially if the sample is drawn through an intravenous line or line that has been flushed with anticoagulant. Another condition capable of raising the MCV is high glucose volume either as a result of a diabetic episode or coma or as a result of blood drawn through the intravenous glucose infusion line. A quick check of the glucose level in the sample should reveal the source of the erratic MCV.

WORD KEY

Achlorhydria • Lack of hydrochloric acid in the gastric contents

Intramedullary hemolysis • Premature hemolysis of red cell precursors in the bone marrow

Myelin • Fatty substance around a nerve

Paranoia • Mental conditions characterized by systematic delusions

Spasticity • Involuntary muscular contractions

Paresthesias • Abnormal tingling or prickling sensation

References

1. Doig K. Anemias caused by defect of DNA metabolism. In: Rodak B, ed. Hematology: Clinical Principles and Applications, 2nd ed. Philadelphia: WB Saunders, 2002; 229.
2. Lotspeich-Steininger CA. Anemias of abnormal nuclear development. In: Steine-Martin EA, Lotspeich-Steininger CA, Koepke CA, eds. Clinical Hematology: Principles, Procedures and Correlations, 2nd ed. Philadelphia: Lippincott, 1998; 156.
3. Morrison HI, Schaubel D, Desmeules M, et al. Serum folate and the risk of fatal coronary heart disease. JAMA 275:1893–1896, 1996.
4. Ishtiaq O, Baqai HZ, Anwer F. Patterns of pancytopenia in a general medical ward and a proposed diagnostic approach. J Ayub Med Coll Abbottabod 16:8–13, 2004.
5. Carmel R. Cobalamin, the stomach and aging. Am J Clin Nutr 66:750–759, 1997.
6. Taghizadeh M. Megaloblastic anemias. In: Harmening D, ed. Clinical Hematology and Fundamentals of Hemostasis, 4th ed. Philadelphia: FA Davis, 2002; 118.
7. Kozyraki R, Kristiansen M, Silahtaroglu A, et al. The human intrinsic factor, vitamin B12 receptor, cubilin: Molecular characterization and chromosomal mapping of the gene to 10 p within the autosomal recessive megaloblastic anemia (MCA 1) region. Blood 91: 3593–3600, 1998.
8. Tejiani S. Pernicious anemia: Vitamin B12 to the rescue. ADVANCE for Medical Laboratory Professionals 10: 16–18, 1998.
9. Ingram CF, Fleming AF, Patel M, et al. The value of intrinsic factor antibody test in diagnosing pernicious anemia. Cent Afr J Med 44:178–181, 1998.
10. Nyhols E, Turpin P, Swain D, et al. Oral vitamin B12 can change our practice. Postgrad Med J 79:218–220, 2003.

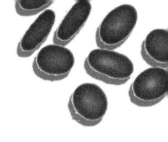

7

Normochromic Anemias: Biochemical and Membrane Disorders and Miscellaneous Red Cell Disorders

Betty Ciesla

The Role of the Spleen in Red Cell Membrane Disorders

Hereditary Spherocytosis

The Genetics and Pathophysiology of Hereditary Spherocytosis

Clinical Presentation in Hereditary Spherocytosis

Laboratory Diagnosis of Hereditary Spherocytosis

Treatment and Management of Hereditary Spherocytosis

Hereditary Elliptocytosis

Common Hereditary Elliptocytosis

Southeast Asian Ovalocytosis

Spherocytic Hereditary Elliptocytosis

Hereditary Pyropoikilocytosis

Hereditary Stomatocytosis and Hereditary Xerocytosis

Glucose-6-Phosphate Dehydrogenase Deficiency

The Genetics of Glucose-6-Phosphate Dehydrogenase Deficiency

Clinical Manifestations of Glucose-6-Phosphate Dehydrogenase Deficiency

Diagnosis of Glucose-6-Phosphate Dehydrogenase Deficiency

Pyruvate Kinase Deficiency

Miscellaneous Red Cell Disorders

Aplastic Anemia

Fanconi's Anemia

Diamond-Blackfan Anemia

Paroxysmal Nocturnal Hemoglobinuria

Cold Agglutinin Syndrome

Paroxysmal Cold Hemoglobinuria

Objectives

After completing this chapter, the student will be able to:

1. Review the functions of the spleen as they relate to red cell membrane integrity.

2. Identify the red cell membrane defect in hereditary spherocytosis.

3. Describe the clinical findings and laboratory data in patients with hereditary spherocytosis.

4. Describe the relevant red cell morphology in patients with hereditary spherocytosis.

5. Describe the osmotic fragility test and its clinical usefulness.

6. Identify the red cell membrane defects in hereditary stomatocytosis, hereditary elliptocytosis, and hereditary pyropoikilocytosis.

7. Compare and contrast the clinical and peripheral smear findings from hereditary stomacytosis, hereditary elliptocytosis, and hereditary pyropoikilocytosis.

8. Define the pathophysiology of the red cell biochemical disorders.

9. Describe the mutations and ethnic distinctions in glucose-6-phosphate dehydrogenase deficiency.

10. Describe Heinz bodies with respect to their appearance in supravital and Wright stain.

11. Define the defect in the rare membrane disorders of hereditary xerocytosis and Southeast Asian ovalocytosis.

12. Discuss the characteristics of aplastic anemia, paroxysmal nocturnal hemoglobinuria, paroxysmal cold hemoglobinuria, Fanconi's anemia, and Diamond-Blackfan syndrome.

THE ROLE OF THE SPLEEN IN RED CELL MEMBRANE DISORDERS

The spleen plays a vital role in red cell health and longevity. Because 5% of cardiac output per minute is filtered through the spleen, this organ has ample opportunity to survey red blood cells for imperfections. Only those red cells that are deemed "flawless" are conducted through the rest of the red cell journey. The four functions of the spleen have been explained in Chapter 2, but when considering red cell membrane defects, it is the splenic filtration function that is the most relevant. As each red cell passes through the spleen, the cell is inspected for imperfections. Now imperfections may take many forms from inclusions to parasites to abnormal hemoglobin products or an abnormal membrane. Inclusions may be removed from the cell, leaving the membrane intact and allowing the red cells to pass through the rest of circulation unharmed. But if the red cell has abnormal hemoglobin (such as seen in thalassemia) or abnormal membrane components, then red cell elasticity and deformability are harmed. Some degree of hemolysis usually results. In the case of spherocytes from hereditary spherocytosis, those red cells are less elastic and therefore the exterior membrane of the cell is shaved off, leaving a smaller, more compact red cell structure, a spherocyte. A spherocyte represents abnormal red cell morphology with a shortened life span and a low surface area to volume ratio (Fig. 7.1).

HEREDITARY SPHEROCYTOSIS

The Genetics and Pathophysiology of Hereditary Spherocytosis

Hereditary spherocytosis (HS) is a well-studied disorder and fairly common among individuals of northern European origin, with an incidence of 1:5000.[1] The mode of inheritance in 75% of individuals is autosomal dominant, while the other 25% have an autosomal recessive presentation. The defect in the disorder is a deficiency of the key membrane protein, spectrin, and, to a lesser degree, a deficiency of membrane protein ankyrin (see Chapter 3) and the minor membrane proteins band 3 and protein 4.2. The red cell membrane disorders have been clearly defined genetically, with five gene mutations implicated in HS: *ANK1* (ankyrin), *SPTB* (spectrin, beta chain), *SLC4A1* (band 3), *EPB42* (protein 4.2), and *SPTA1* (spectrin, alpha chain).[2] Spectrin and ankyrin are part of the cytoskeletal matrix proteins that supports the lipid bilayer of the red cell. These proteins are responsible for the elasticity and deformability of the red cell, crucial properties, because the average red cell with a diameter of 6 to 8 μm must maneuver through circulatory spaces of much smaller diameter. The normal red cell is capable of stretching 117% of its surface volume (see Chapter 3) *only* if spectrin and ankyrin are in the proper amount and fully functioning. The red cell membrane in patients with HS is stretchable, but it is less elastic and can only expand 3% before it ruptures.[3] The spleen is a particularly caustic environment for spherocytes, with its low pH, low ATP, and low glucose. Spherocytic red cells also exhibit problems with membrane diffusion. The active passive transport system of *normal* red cells allows ions and gasses to pass across the red cell membrane in a balanced and harmonious fashion. As a result of the defective membrane proteins, the active passive transport system is disrupted and spherocytes accumulate sodium at a higher rate than for normal red cells in the splenic microenvironment. They are less able to tolerate changes in their osmotic environment before they swell and lyse.[4] Once an individual with HS has been splenectomized, red cell survival is more normal, giving fewer complications from chronic hemolysis. There is no evidence of spherocytes in the bone marrow environment indicating that this phenomenon occurs strictly at the level of the peripheral circulation.

Clinical Presentation in Hereditary Spherocytosis

Clinical presentations in HS are heterogeneous and range from disorders of lifelong anemia to those with subtle clinical and laboratory manifestations. Typically the patient with HS will manifest with anemia, **jaundice,** and splenomegaly. Splenomegaly of varying degrees will be the most common presenting symptom, followed by a moderate anemia and recurrent jaundice,

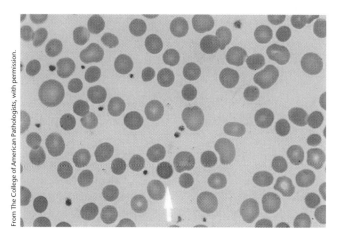

Figure 7.1 Spherocyte. Note the density of the cell with respect to the other red cells in the background.

From The College of American Pathologists, with permission.

usually in younger children.[5] Older individuals will have a well-compensated hemolytic process with little or no anemia. Compensated hemolytic processes indicate that the bone marrow production and destruction have reached equilibrium and that the peripheral indicators of hemolysis may not be present. Reticulocytosis will be a standard feature of individuals with HS as evidenced by polychromatophilic macrocytes on the peripheral smear and reticulocyte counts ranging from 3% to 10%.[6] The peripheral smear will also show spherocytes in most patients with HS; however, the number of spherocytes varies considerably from field to field. Spherocytes are a *distinctive* morphology and are recognized as dense, small, round red cells lacking central pallor. With careful observation, the trained eye should be able to isolate and recognize spherocytes from the normal red cell population on the peripheral smear.

Patients with HS will show a moderate anemia, and 50% will show an elevated MCHC of 36% or greater, a significant finding in the CBC. The MCV will be low normal and RDW will be slightly elevated. Taken together, an increased MCHC combined with an elevated RDW adds strong predictive value in screening for HS.[7] Increased bilirubin is a frequent finding, owing to continued hemolysis, and younger patients tend to form gallstones. **Cholelithiasis,** or the presences of gallstones, is a common complication of patients with HS[8] and occurs with greatest frequency in adolescents and young adults.

Documentation of spherocytes on a peripheral smear considerably raises the index of suspicion of a hemolytic process. Spherocytes, however, result from four mechanisms: HS (already discussed), autoimmune hemolytic anemia, thermal damage, or natural red cell death (Fig. 7.2). Spherocytes produced from an autoim-

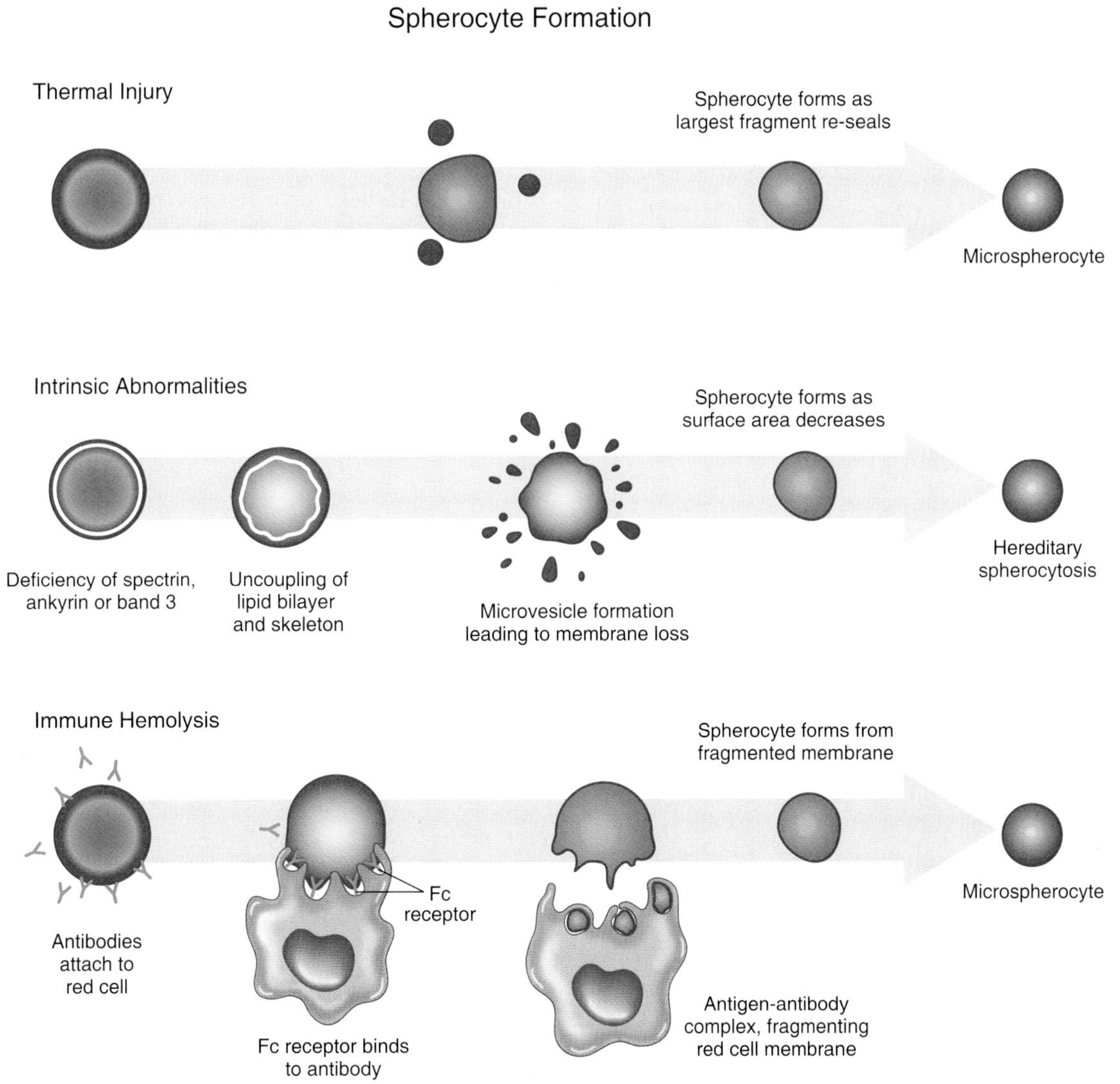

Spherocyte Formation

Figure 7.2 Three mechanisms of spherocyte formation.

Adapted From Glassy E. Color Atlas of Hematology: An Illustrated Guide Based on Proficiency Testing. Northfield, IL: College of American Pathologists, 1998, with permission.

mune process are the result of an antibody being attached to the red cell and then removed or sheared as the coated red cell passes through the spleen. As this occurs, the exterior membrane of the red cell is sheared and a spherocyte produced. A more moderated spherocyte-producing process is senescence, or natural red cell death. As the cell ages, it progressively loses membrane, leading to the production of spherocytes. However, in the normal peripheral smear, spherocytes are not seen because they are removed by the spleen under normal circumstances of cell death.

Laboratory Diagnosis of Hereditary Spherocytosis

The laboratory diagnosis of HS is relatively easy in an individual with elevated MCHC, RDW, and the presence of spherocytes. Because most individuals have mild or moderate disease and share a common clinical laboratory picture, additional laboratory testing is usually not necessary. The confirmatory tests, though, are labor intensive and usually not offered as part of a regular laboratory menu of test items. The osmotic fragility test, incubated and unincubated, is the test of choice to confirm a diagnosis of HS. Red blood cells from patients suspected of having HS are subjected to varying salt solutions ranging from isotonic saline (0.85% NaCl) to distilled water (0.0% NaCl). Under isotonic conditions, normal red cells reach equilibrium and have little hemolysis. As the solutions become more hypotonic (less salt and more water), hemolysis occurs and is observed at the initial appearance of hemolysis and after complete hemolysis. The level of complete hemolysis is usually the only data reported on the patient sample. Normal red cells initially hemolyze at 0.45% NaCl. Red cells from patients with HS have a decreased surface to volume ratio and an increased osmotic fragility. They are less able to tolerate an influx of water and therefore lyse at 0.65% (Fig. 7.3). An increased osmotic fragility curve will be seen in conditions other than HS such as autoimmune hemolytic anemia or any of the acquired hemolytic processes. Conditions such as thalassemia and iron deficiency anemia will show a reduced osmotic fragility (hemolysis at 0.20%) owing to the high number of target cells, a red cell morphology with a capacity to intake a high influx of water before hemolysis.

Treatment and Management of Hereditary Spherocytosis

It should come as no surprise that because the spleen is the offending organ in HS, splenectomy is often suggested as a remedy for moderate to severe hemolysis in

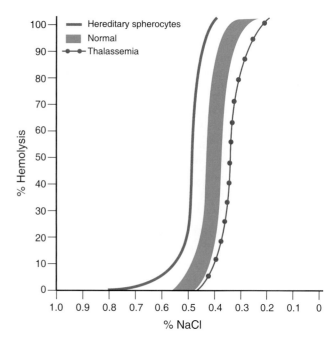

Figure 7.3 Osmotic fragility curves. Normal patient's plot is shown in the shaded area. The curve to the *right* shows a decreased fragility as seen in patients with sickle cell anemia. The curve to the *left* shows an increased fragility as seen in patients with hereditary spherocytosis.

this disease. Removal of the spleen will diminish the anemia by allowing the spherocytes to remain in the circulation longer, thus reducing the need for blood transfusion, and in some cases minimizing gallbladder disease. Splenectomy is a procedure that demands serious consideration before approval. Splenectomy in younger children poses serious risks to those children by making them more vulnerable to infections with encapsulated organisms. **Prophylactic** penicillin should be offered postsurgery to this age group, or a partial splenectomy surgical procedure should be considered. Partial splenectomy is known to reduce hemolysis while preserving important immune splenic function.[9] If symptoms return as a result of remaining splenic tissue, a total splenectomy may be considered once the patient has the appropriate management and support.

HEREDITARY ELLIPTOCYTOSIS

Hereditary elliptocytosis (HE) is a highly variable red cell membrane disorder with many clinical subtypes. Its occurrence is 1:4000 in the population, affecting all racial and ethnic groups.[10] The inheritance is usually autosomal dominant. At the heart of this membrane defect is a disordered or deficient spectrin and proteins commonly associated with the alpha and beta spectrin regions. A decreased thermal stability occurs in each of the clinical subtypes.

Elliptocytes are present to varying degrees in each of the following subtypes, and their red cell deformability is affected with degrees of hemolysis. Four clinical subtypes are discussed: common HE, Southeast Asian ovalocytosis, spherocytic HE, and hereditary pyropoikilocytosis.

Common Hereditary Elliptocytosis

The clinical variants under this subheading range from those individuals who are silent carriers to those who are transfusion dependent. Individuals with the silent carrier state of HE are hematologically normal but are known to be related to individuals with HE and hereditary pyropoikilocytosis through family studies. Common HE has two clinical presentations. In mild common HE, 30% to 100%[1] of the cells are elliptical and most patients show no clinical symptoms (Fig. 7.4). Some patients may show slight hemolysis with elliptocytes and fragmented cells. The more severe variant of common HE, common HE with infantile pyropoikilocytosis, shows fragmented and bizarre red cell shapes from birth with a moderate hemolytic component and jaundice. As the patient ages, the disease converts to a mild HE in presentation (Table 7.1).

Southeast Asian Ovalocytosis

A common red cell condition in many of the Melanesian and Malaysian populations, the red cells of this particular subgroup are spoon-shaped and appear to have two bars across their center. Hemolysis may or may not be present, and this shape may give mild protection against all species of malaria.[11] The red cells with this disorder are strongly heat resistant and rigid and are able to maintain their shape under temperatures that cause normal red cells to crenate or burst. This auto-

Table 7.1 ◉ Variants of Common Hereditary Elliptocytosis
• Silent carrier
• Mild common HE, either chronic hemolysis or moderate hemolysis
• Common HE with severe infant pyropoikilocytosis shows moderate hemolysis

somal dominant disorder has a well-defined band 3 molecular defect (Fig. 7.5).

Spherocytic Hereditary Elliptocytosis

This defect is a cross between HE and HS. The red cells of affected individuals will show more spherocytes and oval elliptocytes. This defect is common in individuals with northern European ancestry and shows a mild hemolysis and red cells of increased osmotic fragility. Gallbladder disease is a common feature, and splenectomy may be indicated if the hemoglobin drops quickly.

Hereditary Pyropoikilocytosis

This rare recessive disorder of the red cell membrane affects African American individuals primarily. Two mechanisms are at work in the red cells of HPP: a reduced assembly of alpha and beta spectrin on the membrane and increased susceptibility of mutant spectrin to degrade.[12] Hemoglobin values are extremely low, less than 6.5 g/dL, and the red cell morphology is incredibly bizarre with red cell budding, rare elliptocytes, and spherocytes. What makes these defective red cells unique is their heat sensitivity. Normal red cells will

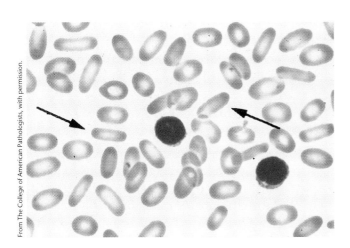

From The College of American Pathologists, with permission.

Figure 7.4 Elliptocytes. Note these cells are pencil shaped.

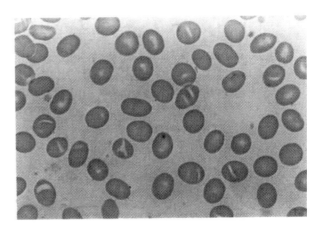

Figure 7.5 Photomicrograph of Southeastern Asian ovalocytosis.

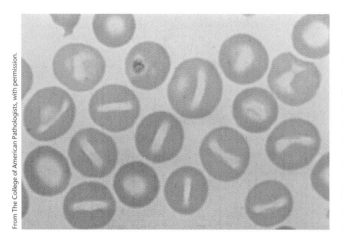

From The College of American Pathologists, with permission.

Figure 7.6   Stomatocytes.

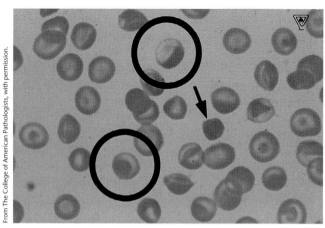

From The College of American Pathologists, with permission.

Figure 7.7   Hereditary xerocytosis.

show **crenation** and hemolysis at 49°C, but red cells from patients with HPP will fragment at 46°C. Some may even fragment at 37°C, body temperature, with prolonged heating. Individuals with this disorder will have severe hemolysis, poor growth, and facial abnormalities due to the expanded bone marrow mass. The MCV is extremely low with a range of 50 to 75 fL.[13]

HEREDITARY STOMATOCYTOSIS AND HEREDITARY XEROCYTOSIS

Hereditary stomatocytosis is a rare hemolytic disorder in which the red cells have an intrinsic defect related to sodium and potassium permeability. The defect, which is autosomal dominant, is identified as a deficiency in the membrane protein, stomatin, thought to regulate ions across the red cell channel.[14] Because of this transport lesion, the intracellular sodium content increases, leading to increased water content and a mild decrease in intracellular potassium. The red cell swells and take on a morphology that appears as if the red cells have slits or bars in the center, as if the cell is "smiling." Peripheral smears show 10% to 30% stomatocytes (Fig. 7.6) with an elevated MCV and decreased MCHC. Patients will show a mild, moderate, or marked anemia that can be corrected by splenectomy, a dangerous procedure in this disorder because many patients have thrombotic complications.[15] Stomatocytes may also be seen in individuals with Rh null disease—those individuals who lack Rh antigens. These patients show a moderate anemia with a combination of spherocytes and stomatocytes.

Hereditary xerocytosis (Fig. 7.7) is a rare autosomal dominant condition in which red cells have an increased surface-to-volume ratio, leading to moderate to severe anemia, a decreased osmotic fragility, and high MCHC.[16]

Red cells are markedly dehydrated and show an irreversible potassium loss and formation of xerocytes, a peculiar red cell morphology where the hemoglobin of red cells seems puddled at one end of the red cell. The etiology of this disorder is unknown.

GLUCOSE-6-PHOSPHATE DEHYDROGENASE DEFICIENCY

There are a limited number of inherited disorders of red cells related to biochemical deficiencies. Glucose-6-phosphate dehydrogenase (G6PD) deficiency represents a fascinating and far-reaching disorder that has at its core a metabolic misstep. G6PD is the catalyst in the first stages of the oxidative portion of the red cell's metabolism and a key player is the phosphogluconate pathway, whose role it is to keep glutathione in the reduced state. Glutathione is the chief red cell antioxidant and serves to protect the red cell from oxidant stress due to peroxide buildup and other compounds or drugs. The pathway to reduced glutathione is initiated when NADP (nicotinamide adenine dinucleotide phosphate) is converted to NADPH by the action of G6PD, an essential enzyme in the hexose monophosphate shunt. Once this occurs, NADPH converts oxidized glutathione to reduced glutathione and the red cell is protected.

The Genetics of Glucose-6-Phosphate Dehydrogenase Deficiency

G6PD deficiency is the most common human enzyme deficiency in the world, present in over 400 million people.[17] This is a staggering number of affected individuals, yet this disease has an extraordinarily low profile for reasons we will soon understand. G6PD was discovered in America in 1950, when healthy black soldiers developed hemolysis as a result of primaquine antimalarial drugs. The populations most affected are in West Africa, the Middle East, Southeast Asia, and other Mediterranean ethnicities. G6PD is inherited as an X-linked recessive disorder with mother-to-son transmission. Women are conductors of the aberrant genes, and if they pass this gene to their male children, the child will inherit the disease. In heterozygous females, two populations of cells have been observed: a normal cell population and a G6PD cell population. The expression of G6PD deficiency is highly variable among heterozygotes and may at times cause disease. Homozygous females will manifest the disease. The human purified G6PD gene has 531 amino acids and is located near the genes for factor 8 and color blindness. Over 400 variants have been named, and many of the variants are caused by amino acid substitutions.[18] There are five known genotypes: two are normal and three are abnormal with varying amounts of hemolysis (Table 7.2). G6PD-deficient individuals are also afforded protection during malarial infections.[19] For a Web-accessible database that details locus-specific mutations, see http://www.bioinf.org.uk/g6pd/.

Clinical Manifestations of Glucose-6-Phosphate Dehydrogenase Deficiency

Acute Hemolytic Anemia

Four clinical conditions are associated with G6PD deficiency: drug-induced acute hemolytic anemia, favism, neonatal jaundice, and congenital nonspherocytic anemia. Classically, individuals with G6PD are hematologically normal and totally unaware that they possess a variant G6PD genotype. For whatever reason, they become exposed to a drug or have an infection and develop a self-limited but frightening hemolytic episode. Eventually, their G6PD status is investigated,

and if a diagnosis is made, it becomes part of their medical record. Affected individuals are then made aware of a growing list of drugs that may cause hemolysis if injected or ingested. In a drug-induced process or an infection-induced hemolytic process, the patient experiences nausea, abdominal pain, and rapidly decreasing hematocrit within a 24- to 48-hour period. The level of hemolysis is alarming as the hemoglobin and hematocrit drop quickly and the intravascular lysis manifests as hemoglobinuria in which the urine has the color of Coca Cola, port wine, or strong tea.[20] The LDH and reticulocytes are increased, while the anemia is normochromic and normocytic with the bone marrow showing erythroid hyperplasia. The peripheral smear shows marked polychromasia and a few bite cells. Bite cells (Fig. 7.8) are formed as Heinz bodies and are pitted from the red cells by the spleen. Heinz body inclusions (Fig. 7.9) are large inclusions (0.2 to 3 μm) that are rigid, distort the cell, and hang on the cell periphery (see Chapter 3). These inclusions are formed from denatured or precipitated hemoglobin that occurs in the G6PD-deficient individual on exposure to the oxidizing agent, because the lack of the G6PD enzyme causes oxidative destruction of the red cell. Heinz bodies are not visible on Wright's stain but may be seen when blood cells are stained with supravital stains such as crystal violet. The formation of Heinz bodies may be induced experimentally with phenylhydrazine. As the inclusion-laden red cells pass through the spleen, the Heinz bodies are pitted from the cell surface and what remains are bite or helmet cells (Fig. 7.10). Heinz bodies and subsequently bite cells are a transitory finding in G6PD-deficient individuals. The absence of this particular morphology cannot be used as a definitive argument against this diagnosis. Fortunately, for individuals who have a drug-induced hemolytic event, the hemato-

Table 7.2 ●	Genotypes of G6PD
GdB+	Normal genotypes
GdA+	Normal genotype but mutated gene
GdA−	Abnormal genotype in 11% of American black males
Gd Med	Abnormal genotype seen in whites, those of Mediterranean origin, Kurdish Jews
Gd Canton	Abnormal genotype seen in Thailand, Vietnam, other Asian populations

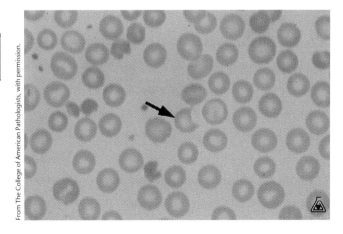

From The College of American Pathologists, with permission.

Figure 7.8   Bite cells.

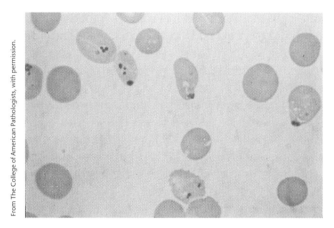

From The College of American Pathologists, with permission.

Figure 7.9   Heinz bodies.

Table 7.3 ● Modified List of Compounds That May Cause Hemolysis in G6PD-Deficient Individuals

- Aspirin
- Phenacetin
- Chloroquine
- Chloramphenicol
- Sulfacetamide
- Naphthalene
- Vitamin K

logical consequences are self-limiting; however, individuals with G6PD variants must be cautioned about their drugs or chemicals known to provoke a hemolytic episode in susceptible individuals (Table 7.3).

Favism

The second most severe clinical condition is favism. Favism is usually found in individuals of the G6PD Mediterranean or Canton type. Hours after ingesting young fava beans or broad beans, the individual usually becomes irritable and lethargic. Fever, nausea, and abdominal pain follow, and within 48 hours gross hemoglobinuria may be noted. Heinz bodies may or may not be observed. Patients present with a normochromic, normocytic process with polychromasia, decreased haptoglobin, and increased bilirubin. There have been incidents of favism from individuals inhaling fava beans pollen or from babies nursed by a mother

who unknowingly transmitted fava bean metabolites in their milk. Fava beans, however, trigger hemolytic episodes in only 25% of those deficient individuals.

Neonatal Jaundice

Neonatal jaundice (NNJ) related to G6PD deficiency occurs within 2 to 3 days after birth. In contrast to hemolytic disease of the newborn, patients with neonatal jaundice show more jaundice than anemia. Early recognition and management of the rising bilirubin are essential to prevent neurological complications (such as kernicterus) in these infants. Data on infants from Malaysia, the Mediterranean, Hong Kong, and Thailand have shown the incidence of NNJ to be quite frequent. Of note also is the increased sensitivity of these individuals to vitamin K substitutes, triple dye used to treat umbilical cords, and camphorated powder. These substances may cause a deterioration of the hematological

Adapted From Glassy E. Color Atlas of Hematology: An Illustrated Guide Based on Proficiency Testing. Northfield. IL: College of American Pathologists, 1998, with permission.

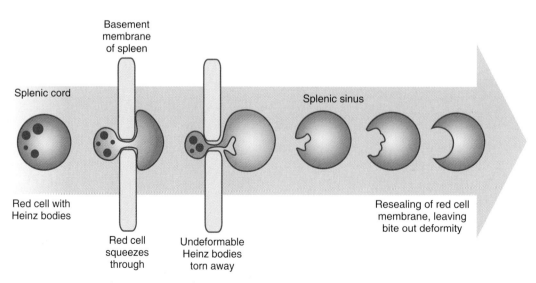

Figure 7.10   Schematic representation of bite cell formation.

state. Phototherapy (intense light therapy) and transfusion support are used to treat affected infants.

Congenital Nonspherocytic Hemolytic Anemia

The final clinical condition is congenital nonspherocytic hemolytic anemia (CNSHA). Patients who have this condition have a history of neonatal jaundice complicated by gallstones, enlarged spleen, or both and may be investigated for jaundice or gallstones in their adult life. The anemia varies in severity from minimum to transfusion dependent. Splenectomy may be considered provided the appropriate management is in place, that is, prophylactic therapy and management. The clinical picture suggests a chronic hemolysis that is mainly extravascular with hyperbilirubinemia, decreased haptoglobin, and increased reticulocytes.

Diagnosis of Glucose-6-Phosphate Dehydrogenase Deficiency

The detection of G6PD deficiency in an individual is complicated by the many genetic variants, the heterozygosity of the disorder, and the fact that young red cells show an increased enzyme level just by virtue of age. Several technical considerations must be kept in mind when determining a person's enzyme status. Appropriate timing of the test is critical for accurate results. If G6PD deficiency is considered during an acute hemolytic episode, reticulocytes will be pouring from the bone marrow into the peripheral circulation. Therefore, testing should be performed once the hemolytic episode has resolved and the counts have returned to normal. Enzyme assay of older red cells are recommended. The entire picture, including clinical presentation, CBC, peripheral smear, and the enzyme status, must be analyzed before a diagnosis is made.

PYRUVATE KINASE DEFICIENCY

Pyruvate kinase deficiency (PK) is a rare enzyme disorder of the Embden-Meyerhof pathways. Red cells lacking this enzyme are unable to generate adenosine triphosphate (ATP) from adenosine diphosphate (ADP) for red cell membrane function. The result is rigid, inflexible cells that are sequestered by the spleen and hemolyzed. Both sexes are affected in this autosomal recessive disorder. There is a high incidence in individuals of northern European origin and in the close-knit Amish population of Mifflin County, Pennsylvania.[21] Patients show a moderate hemolysis with hematocrits of between 18% and 36%,[22] with little abnormal morphology on the peripheral smear, save for

marked polychromasia and a few nRBCs. A fluorescent screening test is used followed by a specific assay for PK activity.

MISCELLANEOUS RED CELL DISORDERS

Aplastic Anemia

Aplastic anemia is one of a group of hypoproliferative disorders in which there is cellular depletion and a reduced production of all blood cells, pancytopenia. Discovered in 1888 by Dr. Paul Ehrlich, this syndrome is usually idiopathic but thought to be a result of two possible mechanisms: an antibody directed against an antigen on stem cells or an immune mechanism that is at play, in which T lymphocytes suppress stem cell proliferation.[23] Several situations seem to predispose an individual to an aplastic episode:

a. Radiation
b. Chemotherapy or chemicals
c. Benzene either directly or indirectly and
d. Viruses, especially Epstein-Barr and hepatitis B and C

Clinical characteristics of this syndrome include a decreased marrow cellularity, pancytopenia, and reticulocytopenia. Aplastic anemia is an insidious process, and the syndrome progresses in a slow but orderly fashion with symptoms reflective of the depressed cellular elements. When red cells significantly deplete, patients will show fatigue, heart palpitations, and dyspnea. As platelets deplete, **ecchymosis** and mucosal bleeds develop and white count depletion leads to infections. In many cases, the peripheral smear shows lymphocytosis. Treatment for this normochromic normocytic anemia includes transfusion support and steroids, with a few patients recovering spontaneously.

Occasionally, stem cell transplantation is used to treat severe aplastic anemia presentation.[24]

Fanconi's Anemia

Characterized by Dr. Fanconi in 1927, Fanconi's anemia is a rare autosomal recessive disorder affecting physical characteristics as well as bone marrow development. Over 400 cases have been reported worldwide, and there is a database, the International Fanconi Anemia Registry, that provides current information concerning this disorder. There are numerous chromosomal abnormalities in this disorder, as well as defective DNA repair and many chromosomal breaks.[25] The bone marrow often shows a macrocytic process with thrombocytopenia and leukopenia, developing before red cell depletion. Hemoglobin F values are increased. The physical characteristics of a Fanconi's anemia patient reveal short stature, hyperpigmentation on the trunk and neck, microcephaly, broad nose, and structural abnormalities of the kidney.[26] Life span is shortened with a mean survival of 16 years, and these individuals have a tendency toward the development of leukemia and other cancers. Treatment is supportive as complications from aplasia develop. The only curative therapy is a bone marrow transplant.

Diamond-Blackfan Anemia

Diamond-Blackfan anemia, discovered in 1938 by Dr. Diamond and Dr. Blackfan, shows dominant and recessive inheritance patterns. This congenital hypoplastic disorder is usually diagnosed in early infancy; 80% of individuals are severely anemic by age 6 months.[27] Several physical abnormalities have been observed, including short stature, low birth weight, head and facial abnormalities, and a tendency for children with Diamond-Blackfan anemia to look more like each other than family members. The bone marrow is usually lacking in red cell precursors with a slightly decreased number of leukocytes. The average hemoglobin is 7 g/dL and hemoglobin F is increased. Treatment includes steroids and transfusional support with careful attention to the possibility of hemosiderosis. Twenty-five percent of patients spontaneously recover.[28]

Paroxysmal Nocturnal Hemoglobinuria

The rare hemolytic anemia paroxysmal nocturnal hemoglobinuria (PNH) is notable because the increased susceptibility of the red cells to complement lysis is directly related to a clonal membrane defect. Classically, red cells are destroyed while patients sleep because of their increased sensitivity to complement lysis, and upon arising the patient notices bloody urine or hemoglobinuria. PNH occurs because of a somatic mutation in the hematopoietic stem cells designated as phosphatidylinositol glycan class A (PIGA). The X-linked mutation PIGA is essential for the synthesis of the glycosylphosphatidylinositol (GPI)-anchored proteins present in all cell lines. As a result of this mutation, nine cell surface proteins are missing from cells.[29] Two proteins in particular, CD55 decay accelerating factor and CD59 membrane inhibitor, offer protection to red cells against lysis by complement. Therefore, intravascular lysis is a primary manifestation of red cells missing these proteins. The intensity of lysis in the form of hemoglobinuria has been described by patients as having urine samples that range in color from strong tea to tar.

PNH patients have a variable presentation with an unexpected onset in 30% of cases. Marrow failure is part of the clinical picture, yet its onset and its prevalence are not yet fully appreciated.[30] Patients may have a mild to severe anemia. Most are pancytopenic with reticulocyte levels that are elevated but not appropriate with respect to the level of anemia. Neutropenia is always present, but there is usually the absence of stainable iron due to continued lysis. Many patients have a tendency toward thrombosis, especially in unusual sites like the dermal vessels, brain, liver, and abdomen.[31] In these patients, anticoagulant therapy may need to be considered, because thrombosis can account for considerable mortality. Treatment for patients with PNH includes transfusion support and, in selected younger patients, bone marrow transplant.[32] Iron therapy may also be included once the patient's iron status has been assessed. A new drug, eculixumab, blocks complement activity by binding to C5 and thus preventing hemolysis. This new monoclonal antibody treatment is well tolerated and has been effective in clinical trials in improving hemolysis and relieving symptoms.[33] Screening procedures usually employed in the diagnosis of PNH are the sugar water test, the Ham's test, and flow cytometry.

The Sugar Water Test

In the sugar water test, a 50% solution of the patient's washed EDTA red cells are mixed with ABO/Rh-compatible serum and sugar solution is added. The solutions are incubated for 30 minutes and then centrifuged. The percent hemolysis is determined by spectrophotometer. Normal cells show less than 5% hemolysis and suspect cells will show between 10% and 80% hemolysis.

The Ham's Test

The Ham's test is used to confirm a diagnosis of PNH. The patient's serum is acidified using 0.2N HCl. A 50% solution of the patient's cells is added to tubes containing the patient's acidified serum, unacidified serum, and normal ABO-compatible serum. A normal red cell control is run. Normal red cells will not hemolyze, but cells from patients with PNH will hemolyze with acidified serum from the patient and from normal ABO-compatible serum (Fig. 7.11).

(**Note**: These tests are rarely performed in the laboratory, because so few individuals have PNH, but they are simple and direct and yield some value.)

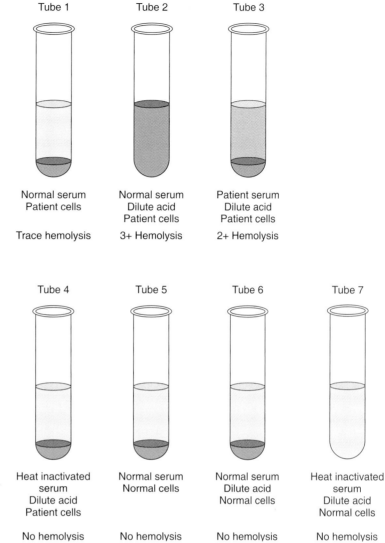

Figure 7.11 Ham's test. Note varying degrees of hemolysis in tubes 1, 2, and 3. Hemolysis occurs in tubes containing patient cells, patient serum, and acidified serum. Hemolysis does not occur in tubes with heat-inactivated serum and control cells, because heat inactivates complement.

Tube 1
Normal serum
Patient cells

Trace hemolysis

Tube 2
Normal serum
Dilute acid
Patient cells

3+ Hemolysis

Tube 3
Patient serum
Dilute acid
Patient cells

2+ Hemolysis

Tube 4
Heat inactivated
serum
Dilute acid
Patient cells

No hemolysis

Tube 5
Normal serum
Normal cells

No hemolysis

Tube 6
Normal serum
Dilute acid
Normal cells

No hemolysis

Tube 7
Heat inactivated
serum
Dilute acid
Normal cells

No hemolysis

Flow Cytometry in the Diagnosis of PNH

Currently, flow cytometry procedures are available that can test white cells for the presence or absence of GPI-linked proteins. White cells can be examined for reactivity to anti-CD48, CD55, and CD59, all of which are anchored proteins.[34] A new diagnostic procedure, FLAER (fluorescent-labeled aerolysin) has proved effective in detecting smaller populations of abnormal leukocytes in PNH.[35] This technique may prove useful in determining PNH cell clones in individuals presenting with varying levels of bone marrow failure.

Cold Agglutinin Syndrome

Cold agglutinin syndrome (CAS) is another of the rare hemolytic disorders that affect primarily individuals over 50 years of age. Also known as cold hemagglutinin disease (CHAD), the hemolysis in this disorder is

caused by an IgM autoantibody of wide thermal range. Complement is fixed on the red cells during cold temperatures, 0° to 5°C and then red cells agglutinate and hemolyze as body temperature rises, 20° to 25°. Patients experience acrocyanosis or numbness and a bluish tone to the fingertips and toes and will experience weakness, pallor, and weight loss. The lysis is intravascular with a positive direct **antiglobulin test** (with polyclonal antihuman globulin reagent or anti-C3d). Some hemoglobinuria may be present. If the antibody is strong, the CBC will need correcting because the antibody coats the red cells, causing agglutination and falsely elevated red cell indices and hematocrit. The sample should be warmed at 37°C for 15 to 30 minutes and then recycled through the instrument for accurate results. After warming, all parameters should be accurate. Treatment is circumstantial, depending on the level of hemolysis; many individuals change location and opt for warmer climates to avoid hemolytic episodes altogether.

Paroxysmal Cold Hemoglobinuria

Paroxysmal cold hemoglobinuria (PCH) is a rare hemolytic anemia caused by anti-P, which attaches to the red blood cells at lower temperature and then activates complement at warmer temperatures. Lysis occurs at body temperature. The lysis is intravascular and severe, with hemoglobinemia, hemoglobinuria, and increased bilirubin. The symptoms are similar to a hemolytic transfusion reaction with back pain, fever, chills, and abdominal pain. Some patients may require transfusion.[33] The screening test for PCH is the Donath-Landsteiner test, which is rarely performed in the clinical laboratory.

The Donath-Landsteiner Test

The patient's anticoagulated blood sample is split into two parts. The first aliquot is the control and should be incubated at 37°C for 1 hour. The second aliquot is placed at 4°C for 30 minutes and then incubated at 37°C for 30 minutes. Both aliquots should be centrifuged and then observed for hemolysis. The control should show no hemolysis. If the second aliquot shows hemolysis, that is evidence for PCH.

CONDENSED CASE

A 2-year-old African American boy was seen in the sick baby clinic with vomiting, fever, and red-colored urine staining his diapers. His initial lab results showed hemoglobin of 5 g/dL and hematocrit of 15%. The most remarkable chemistry value was an LDH of 500 IU/L (reference range, 0 to 100 IU/L), which is extremely elevated. His peripheral smear revealed polychromasia and occasional bite cells.

When the mother was questioned as to whether the baby had ingested anything out of the ordinary, she stated that the baby has been chewing on mothballs in her closet. The baby was transported to the intensive care unit.

What is happening to the baby?

Answer

The baby is suffering from severe intravascular lysis as evidenced by the LDH value and the extremely low hemoglobin and hematocrit. Most likely, the baby has G6PD deficiency brought on by chewing on naphthalene, the active ingredient of mothballs. Naphthalene is an oxidizing drug and in this case has put the baby's red cells under oxidant stress. Occasional bite cells in the smear suggest the formation of Heinz bodies and their subsequent removal by the spleen.

Summary Points

- The spleen plays a vital role in red cell health and longevity.
- HS is an autosomal dominant disorder of several membrane proteins, the key protein being spectrin.
- Spherocytes are less deformable and are more osmotically fragile.
- Patients with hereditary spherocytes show splenomegaly, jaundice, and increased tendency for gallstone disease.
- The osmotic fragility test is a labor intensive but valuable test to assess red cell viability in different hypotonic salt solutions.

- HE is a membrane disorder of spectrin showing decreased thermal stability.
- There are several clinical variants of HE, including common HE, Southeast Asian ovalocytosis, and spherocytic HE.
- Hereditary pyropoikilocytosis is a recessive membrane disorder with a bizarre red cell morphology that shows hemoglobin budding.
- Hereditary stomatocytosis is a membrane disorder in which red cells have an intrinsic defect to sodium and potassium permeability.
- G6PD deficiency is the most common enzyme deficiency in the world.

- G6PD is an X-linked recessive disorder with over 400 variants.

- The drug- or infection-induced hemolysis in G6PD is intravascular, brisk, and self-limiting.

- Most individuals with G6PD deficiency are totally unaware of their hematological condition until they are challenged by a drug that produces oxidant stress.

- Pyruvate kinase deficiency is a enzyme deficiency of the Embden-Meyerhof pathway.

- Aplastic anemia is a hypoproliferative disorder in which there is cellular depletion and a reduced production of blood cells.

- Fanconi's anemia and Diamond-Blackfan syndromes are rare hypoproliferative disorders with congenital malformations.

- PNH is a hemolytic anemia that is caused when nine red cell surface proteins are absent and red cells become increasingly sensitive to complement lysis.

- CAS is a disease of the elderly and caused by an IgM autoantibody of wide thermal range.

- Paroxysmal cold hemoglobinuria is an extremely rare hemolytic disorder caused by anti-P of a wide thermal range.

CASE STUDY

A 28-year-old man presents to the emergency department with a complaint of abdominal pain. He appeared quite ill with nausea, cold sweats, and tachycardia. He had taken aspirin when he started feeling sick. The patient appeared slightly jaundiced and upon further questioning admitted that his urine has been dark and discolored that day. The preliminary impression was of acute appendicitis.

Pertinent Hematology Results (refer to cover for normal values)

WBC	6.3×10^9/L
RBC	1.00×10^{12}/L
Hgb	4.4 g/dL
Hct	12.6%
MCV	126 fL
MCH	43.9 pg
MCHC	34.8%

The white cell differential was essentially normal; however, the red cell morphology was abnormal, showing basophilic stippling, slight polychromasia, moderate teardrop cells, and occasional schistocytes and ovalocytes.

Pertinent Chemistry Results

Direct bilirubin	0.7 mg/dL	(0.0 to 0.4 mg/dL)
Total bilirubin	7.9 mg/dL	(0.1 to 1.4 mg/dL)
Indirect bilirubin	7.2 mg/dL	(0.1 to 0.8 mg/dL)
SGOT	567 IU/L	(0 to 100 IU/L)
LDH	2844 IU/L	(0 to 100 IU/L)

Insights to the Case Study

This case is an example of a patient with G6PD deficiency. He has suffered a violent hemolytic episode as a result of exposure to drugs—aspirin in this case. This previously healthy individual has no idea that he has an abnormal G6PD variant. He is very ill, and his red count, hemoglobin, and hematocrit are extremely depressed. Notice that his MCV is macrocytic and his MCH and RDW are also elevated. The indirect bilirubin, SGOT, and LDH are each increased, and these serum chemistry elevations are indicative of a hemolytic episode of monumental proportions.

The MCV is increased due to increased reticulocytosis that manifests in the peripheral circulation as polychromasia and nRBCs, as seen in this patient's peripheral smear. A Heinz body preparation was performed by allowing equal volumes of EDTA blood to mix with crystal violet stain for 20 minutes. Several Heinz bodies were observed in this preparation. The hemolysis in G6PD deficiency is primarily intravascular as noted by the hemoglobinuria and hemoglobinemia. However, because most individuals have enlarged spleens, not all of the cell lysis is of the intravascular type; some will be extravascular. Most individuals who have G6PD deficiency remain in a steady state and are hematologically normal; they hemolyze only when exposed to an oxidative drug. Fortunately, for these individuals, these events are self-limiting and, while troubling, their hematological status will return to normal.

Review Questions

1. Which of the following inclusions cannot be visualized by the Wright-stained peripheral smear?
   a. Basophilic stippling
   b. Hemoglobin H inclusion bodies
   c. Howell-Jolly bodies
   d. Heinz bodies

2. Which of the following functions most affect spherocytes as they travel through the circulation?
   a. They tend to form inclusion bodies.
   b. They are less deformable and more sensitive to the low glucose in the spleen.
   c. They tend to be sequestered in the spleen because of abnormal hemoglobin.
   d. They form siderotic granules and cannot navigate the circulation.

3. Many individuals with hereditary spherocytosis are prone to jaundice because of:
   a. EBV
   b. pathologic logical fractures
   c. gallstone disease
   d. skin pigmentation

4. Which of the following are characteristics of hereditary pyropoikilocytosis?

   a. Elliptocytes with spherocytes intermixed in the peripheral smear
   b. Spherocytes with polychromasia and low MCV
   c. Elliptocytes, spherocytes, and budding red cells
   d. Mostly elliptocytes with few other morphologies

5. Which red cell morphology is formed as a result of Heinz bodies being pitted from the red cell?
   a. Acanthocytes
   b. Bite cells
   c. Burr cells
   d. Stomatocytes

6. Which of the following hemolytic disorders has red cells that are especially sensitive to lysis by complement?
   a. Paroxysmal nocturnal hemoglobinuria
   b. Fanconi's anemia
   c. Aplastic anemia
   d. Hereditary spherocytosis

7. In the osmotic fragility test, normal red cells hemolyze at which level?
   a. 0.65%
   b. 0.45%
   c. 0.20%
   d. 0.30%

● TROUBLESHOOTING

What Kinds of Clinical Situations Come to Mind When the MCHC Is Above 36.0%?

A 72-year-old man was seen in the emergency department for gastrointestinal bleeding and sepsis, and was subsequently admitted. He had the usual emergency department tests ordered: chemistry panel, PT/aPTT, urinalysis, and CBC. His CBC showed:

WBC	10.8×10^9/L
RBC	3.58×10^{12}/L
Hgb	10.7 g/dL
Hct	30.5%
MCV	85.3 fL
MCH	29.8 pg
MCHC	34.9%
PLT	16×10^9/L
RDW	13.7%

During his 3-day stay, the patient's red cell indices began to fluctuate (MCH and MCHC) and his hemoglobin results showed variability. The CBC results on day 3 were:

WBC	15.9×10^9/L
RBC	2.80×10^{12}/L
Hgb	9.3 g/dL
Hct	23.9%
MCV	85.5 fL
MCH	33.4 pg
MCHC	39.0%**
PLT	79×10^9/L
RDW	15.1%

Several indices in the CBC were flagged (asterisks) and warranted further investigation. At first, when the technologists noticed these increases, several scenarios came to mind: 1) cold agglutinins, 2) lipemia, or 3) spherocytes. The technologist followed standard operating procedures (SOP) for an elevated MCHC. First, the sample was warmed in a 37°C water bath for 30 minutes and then reanalyzed on the Coulter LH750. The results remained unchanged. At times, cold agglutinins require longer incubation in a water bath to correct. This was not the case with this particular specimen, since it was incubated for 30 minutes longer. The MCHC refused to budge even after longer incubation. When a sample is incubated for 30 minutes or

longer, cells settle away from the plasma and the technologist can observe the plasma for the presence of lipemia. The observations revealed a slight increase (or cloudiness), but not true lipemia, which interferes with the MCHC. The final step was to look for spherocytes on the peripheral smear. The smear was negative for spherocytes. At this point the technologist could not account or explain the MCHC, and reported the results commenting under the MCHC: no hemolysis, no presence of cold agglutinins, and no spherocytes.

WORD KEY

Antiglobulin test • Test used in immunohematology to determine if a patient has made an alloantibody present in the serum or an antibody that is coating the red cells

Cholelithiasis • Gallbladder disease

Crenation • Term used to describe the edges of red cells that seem to have ridges

Ecchymosis • bruising

Jaundice • Yellowish color usually seen in the mucous membranes of the eyes and noticed as an overall skin color

Prophylactic • Preventive

References

1. Lux SE, Becker PS. Disorders of the red cell membrane skeleton: Hereditary spherocytosis and hereditary elliptocytosis. In: Scriver CR, Baudet AB, Sly US, et al, eds. The Metabolic Basis of Inherited Disease, 6th ed. New York: McGraw-Hill, 1989; 2367.
2. Iolascon A, Perrotta S, Stewart GW. Red blood cell membrane defects. Rev Clin Exp Haematol 7:22–56, 2003.
3. Evans EA, Waugh R, et al. Elastic area compressibility modules of red cell membrane. Biophys J 16:585, 1976.
4. Vives Corrons JL, Besson I. Red cell membrane Na+ transport system in hereditary spherocytosis relevance to understanding the increased Na+ permeability. Ann Hematol 80:535–539, 2001.
5. Panigrahi I, Rhadke SR, Agarwal A, et al. Clinical profile of hereditary spherocytosis in North India. J Assoc Phys India 50:1360–1367, 2002.
6. Payne MS. Intracorpuscular on defects leading to increased erythrocyte destruction. In: Rodak B, ed. Hematology: Clinical Principles and Applications, 2nd ed. Philadelphia: WB Saunders, 2002; 267.
7. Michaels LA, Cohen AR, Zhao H, et al. Screening for hereditary spherocytosis by use of automated erythrocytes indices. J Pediatr 13:957–960, 1997.
8. Tamary H, Aviner S, Freud E, et al. High incidences of early cholelithiasis detected by ultrasonography in children and young adults with hereditary spherocytosis. J Pediatr Hematol Oncol 25:952–954, 2003.
9. deBuys Roessingh AS, de Laguasie P, Rohrlich P, et al. Follow up of partial splenectomy in children with hereditary spherocytosis. J Pediatr Surg 37:1459–1463, 2002.
10. Gallagher PG, Forget BD, Lux SE. Disorders of the erythrocyte membrane. In: Nathan DG, Oski SH, eds. Nathan and Oski's Hematology of Infancy and Childhood, 5th ed. Philadelphia: WB Saunders, 1998; 544–664.
11. Cattani JA, Gibson FD, Alperes MP, et al. Hereditary ovalocytosis and reduced susceptibility to malaria in Papua New Guinea. Trans R Soc Trop Med Hyg 705–709, 1987.
12. Hanspal M, Hanspal JS, Sahr KE, et al. Molecular basis of spectrin deficiency in hereditary pyropoikilocytosis. Blood 82:1652–1660, 1993.
13. Palek J. Hereditary elliptocytosis and related disorders. Clin Hematol 14:45, 1985.
14. Fricke B, Argent AC, Chetley MC, et al. The "stomatin" gene and protein in overhydrated hereditary stomatocytosis. Blood 102:2268–2277, 2003.
15. Stewart GW, Amess JA, Eber SW, et al. Thromboembolic disease after splenectomy for hereditary stomatocytosis. Br J Hematol 93:303–310, 1996.
16. Glader BE, Fortier N, et al. Congenital hemolytic anemia associated with dehydrated erythrocytes and increased potassium ions. N Engl J Med 291:491, 1974.
17. Fiorelli G, Martinez di Montemuros F, Capellini MD. Chronic non-spherocytic hemolytic disorders associated with glucose 6 phosphate dehydrogenase variants. Baillieres Best Pract Res Clin Haematol 13:39–55, 2000.
18. Beutler E. Red cell enzyme defects. Hematol Pathol 4:103–114, 1990.
19. Mehta A, Mason PJ, Vulliam TJ. Glucose 6 phosphate dehydrogenase. Baillieres Best Pract Res Clin Haematol 13:21–38, 2000.
20. Lazzato L. G6PD deficiency and hemolytic anemias. In: Nathan DG, Oski FA, eds. Nathan and Oski's Hematology of Infancy and Childhood, 4th ed. Philadelphia: WB Saunders, 1993; 679.

21. Valentine WN, Koyichi RT, Paglia DE. Pyruvate kinase and other enzyme deficiency disorders of the erythrocyte. In: Scriver CR, Beaudet AL, Sly WS, Valle D, eds, The Metabolic Basis of Inherited Diseases, 6th ed. New York: McGraw-Hill, 1989; 1606–1628.

22. Brown BA. Hematology: Principles and Procedures, 6th ed. Philadelphia: Lea and Febiger; 1993; 298.

23. Gordon-Smith EC, Marsh JC, Gibson FM. Views on the pathophysiology of aplastic anemia. Int J Hematol 76 (Suppl 12):163–166, 2002.

24. Trigg ME. Hematopoietic stem cells. Pediatrics 113 (Suppl 4):1051–1057, 2004.

25. Bagby GC Jr. Genetic basis of Fanconi's anemia. Curr Opin Hematol 10:68–73, 2003.

26. Schroeder-Kurth TM, Auerbach AD, Obe G. Fanconi Anemia: Clinical, Cytogenetics and Experimental Aspects. Berlin: Springer-Verlag, 1989; 264.

27. Alter BP, Young NS. The bone marrow failure syndromes. In: Nathan DG, Oski FA, eds. Nathan and Oski's Hematology of Infancy and Childhood, 4th ed. Philadelphia: WB Saunders, 1992; 263.

28. Krijanovski OI, Seiff CA. Diamond-Blackfan anemia. Hematol Oncol Clin N Am 11:1061, 1997.

29. Lawrence LW, Harmening DM, Green R. Hemolytic anemia: Extracorpuscular defects and acquired intracorpuscular defects. In: Harmening D, ed. Clinical Hematology and Fundamentals of Thrombosis, 4th ed. Philadelphia: FA Davis, 2002; 202.

30. Young NS. Paroxysmal nocturnal hemoglobinuria: Current issues in pathophysiology and treatment. Curr Hematol Rep 4:103–109, 2005.

31. Hillmen P, Lewis SM, Bressler M, et al. Natural history of PNH. N Engl J Med 333:1253–1258, 1995.

32. Meyers G, Parker CJ. Management issues in paroxysmal nocturnal hemoglobinuria. Int J Haematol 77:125–132, 2003.

33. Hill A, Hillmen P, Richards SJ, et al. Sustained response and long-term safety of eculizumab in paroxysmal nocturnal hemoglobinuria. Blood 106:2559–2565, 2005.

34. Schubert J, Alvarado M, Uciechowski P, et al Diagnosis of paroxysmal nocturnal haemoglobinuria using immunophenotyping of peripheral blood cells. Br J Haematol 79:487–492, 1991.

35. Brodsky RA, Mukhina GL, Li S, et al. Improved detection and characterization of paroxysmal nocturnal hemoglobinuria using fluorescent aerolysin. Am J Clin Pathol 114:459–466, 2000.

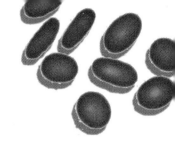

8 The Normochromic Anemias Caused by Hemoglobinopathies

Betty Ciesla

General Description of the Hemoglobinopathies

Sickle Cell Anemia

Genetics and Incidence of Sickle Cell Anemia

Pathophysiology of the Sickling Process

Clinical Considerations for Sickle Cell Anemia

Disease Management and Prognosis

Laboratory Diagnosis

Sickle Cell Trait

Hemoglobin C Disease and Trait and Hemoglobin SC

Variant Hemoglobins of Note

Hemoglobin S-beta thalassemia

Hemoglobin E

Hemoglobin D$_{Punjab}$/Hemoglobin G phila

Hemoglobin O$_{Arab}$

Objectives

After completing this chapter, the student will be able to:

1. Recall the general characteristics of the hemoglobinopathies.
2. Describe the pathophysiology of the sickle disorders.
3. Identify the amino acid substitution in sickle cell disorders.
4. Identify the amino acid substitution in hemoglobin C disease.
5. Describe the inheritance patterns of the sickle disorders.
6. List the clinical and laboratory features of sickle cell anemia, sickle cell trait, hemoglobin C disease, hemoglobin C trait, and hemoglobin SC disease.
7. Review the physiological conditions that most typically affect individuals with sickle cell anemia.
8. List conditions that may precipitate a sickle cell crisis.
9. Recognize normal hemoglobin patterns on hemoglobin electrophoresis at pH 8.6 and 6.2.
10. Recognize abnormal hemoglobin patterns on electrophoresis at pH 8.6 and 6.2.
11. Describe the treatment protocol for patients with sickle cell anemia.
12. Differentiate the clinical and laboratory features of other abnormal hemoglobins such as hemoglobin E, O$_{Arab}$, D, and G$_{phila}$.
13. List the key features of sickle hemoglobin in combination with thalassemias.
14. Calculate the white blood cell correction formula when nucleated red blood cells (nRBCs) are noted in the peripheral smear.
15. Summarize the general principles of acid and alkaline electrophoresis and isoelectric focusing.

GENERAL DESCRIPTION OF THE HEMOGLOBINOPATHIES

Disorders of the globin chain of the hemoglobin molecule have stirred the curiosity of scientists and hematologists for generations. When Linus Pauling discovered in 1949 that the altered hemoglobin migration pattern of sickle cell patients was due to a change in globin, the excitement among the scientific community was palpable. Dr. Pauling won The Nobel Prize for his discovery. Here was a description of the first molecular disease. Because proteins form the basis of the globin chain, there must be some abnormality *in* the chain to account for what was seen in the hemoglobin electrophoresis of sickle cell anemia individuals. Ingram et al.[1] discovered the specific amino acid substitution located on the globin chain (valine substituted for glutamic acid or glutamine) and the specific abnormal codon responsible for this substitution has been characterized. In molecular terms, the nucleotide triplet guanine-adenine-guanine codes for the amino acid glutamine in the sixth position of the normal beta chain. In sickle cell patients, adenine is replaced by thymine coding for the amino acid valine. When valine is substituted for glutamine, an abnormal hemoglobin, hemoglobin S, is produced. Presently over 600 hemoglobin variants exist worldwide and most are beta chain disorders.[2] To appreciate the magnitude of this statement, a brief review of the hemoglobin molecule is in order. All normal adult hemoglobins consist of two alpha chains, which have 141 amino acids in sequence, complemented by two non-alpha chains: beta, gamma, or delta. The non-alpha globin chains have 146 amino acids with amino acids linked together in sequence. Hemoglobinopathies occur as a result of one of four abnormal functions[3]:

1. A single amino acid substitution in one of the chains, usually the beta chain (i.e., sickle cell trait or disease)
2. Abnormal synthesis of one of the amino acid chains (i.e., thalassemia)
3. Fusion of hemoglobin chains (i.e., hemoglobin Lepore).

4. Extension of an amino acid chain (i.e., hemoglobin Constant Spring)

Single amino acid substitutions in the beta chain account for most of the hemoglobinopathies that present with a hemolysis and clinical symptoms.

SICKLE CELL ANEMIA

Genetics and Incidence of Sickle Cell Anemia

The genetics of sickle cell anemia are not complicated. Sickle cell anemia is a beta chain variant and inheritance of the beta chains is located on chromosome 11. Chromosome 11 has one location on each chromosome for the inheritance of a normal beta chain or an abnormal beta chain; therefore, the sickle cell anemia is **autosomal** codominant, inherited in simple Mendelian fashion (Fig. 8.1). At present, there are 80,000 Americans who have sickle cell disorders spread among 65% with sickle cell disease, 24% with hemoglobin SC disease, and 10% with sickle cell beta thalassemia.[4] Individuals born with sickle cell trait were not included in the percentages. African American babies born with sickle cell disease occur with a frequency of 1:375. The sickle gene is especially prominent in African populations near areas endemic for malaria including Central and West Africa, some parts of the Mediterranean, Asia, and India. The sickle gene is seen frequently in African American populations and with increasing frequency in nonblack populations.[5] The presentation of symptoms in individuals with sickle cell anemia is highly variable, a direct result of the different haplotypes of hemoglobin S that are inherited. Each haplotype differs from the other by possessing different sequences of some nucleotides in the DNA strands, but they are all located in the same gene cluster. There are four primary haplotypes of the sickle beta gene: Asian, Senegal, Benin, and Bantu.[6] Haplotypes may be inherited homzygouosly or heterozygously. Each of these haplotypes differs in the amount of hemoglobin F the red cell possesses. Higher hemoglobin F concentrations mean a less severe clinical presentation. The Asian haplotype is seen in

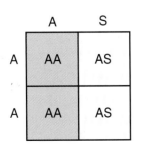
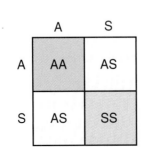
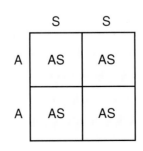

Figure 8.1 Mendelian genetics by Punnett square. Three scenarios are presented; AA × AS, AS × AS, and AA × SS. Note the percentage of trait individuals (AS) as opposed to those affected individuals (SS).

Table 8.1 ⊙ Haplotypes of the Sickle Cell Gene	
Haplotype	**Location**
Asian	Saudi Arabia, Asia
Senegal	West Africa Coast
Benin	West Africa, Mediterranean
Bantu	Central South Africa
Senegal/Bantu have Hgb F levels between 5% and 20%/Benin <10%/Asian >20%	Benin is the haplotype from the most seriously affected patients

Saudi Arabia and Asia; the Senegal haplotype, the west African coast; the Benin haplotype, West Africa; and the Mediterranean and Bantu haplotype, Central and South Africa (Table 8.1). Levels of hemoglobin F greater than 10% serve to lessen the clinical severity for sickle cell anemia patients.[7]

Pathophysiology of the Sickling Process

The beta chain has a carefully sequenced group of amino acids with glutamine or glutamic acid in the sixth position from the terminal end. If a person inherits the sickle gene, then valine is substituted for glutamic acid in the sixth position of the beta chain and the abnormal hemoglobin S is present in the person's red cells. Homozygous inheritance results in sickle cell disease, with most of the hemoglobin being hemoglobin S. Heterozygous inheritance results in sickle cell trait, in which hemoglobin S and hemoglobin A are present. The inheritance of one single abnormal amino acid means that the individual inherits hemoglobin S ($\alpha_2\beta_2^{6glu\rightarrow val}$) and sets in motion a myriad of events that alter the patient's quality of life and life span. Lives change when sickle cell disease is present, and the changes are dramatic and at times overwhelming. As we have already determined, it is essential for the hemoglobin in the red cells to remain soluble and pliable as the red cell passes through the oxygenated and deoxygenated rigors of circulation. Red cells possessing hemoglobin S as the majority hemoglobin are insoluble or rigid in areas of low oxygen concentration like the spleen, liver, kidneys, joints, and extremities. Instead of having a fluid hemoglobin content, hemoglobin S forms liquid tactoids or polymers of hemoglobin that appear as long, thin bundles of fibers under electron microscopy.[8] Because of this, affected red cells become rigid and inflexible and form an irreversibly sickled cell (ISC) with

a pointed projection. These misshapen and inflexible red cells obstruct small vessels and adhere to vascular endothelium, increasing the viscosity of the blood as circulation is slowed. Less oxygen is available to the tissues, the pH of the blood drops, and this combination of events quickly escalates the sickling process. Sickling is also induced by hypoxia, acidosis, dehydration, fever, and exposure to cold. Once red cells exit the spleen, they may return to the oxygenated environment of the lung and may be able to revert to the discoid shape or wheat shape (RSC). But for many hemoglobin S red cells, repeated sickling terminates their life span and they are trapped in the splenic graveyard. The extent to which a red cell will sickle depends on the amount of hemoglobin S, the amount of hemoglobin F, and the physiological conditions present that may advance sickling.

Clinical Considerations for Sickle Cell Anemia

Patients with sickle cell anemia are usually diagnosed through neonatal screening programs or between 6 months and 2 years of age. Prior to this time, red cells are protected from sickling with high levels of hemoglobin F, because the switch from the production of hemoglobin F to hemoglobin A occurs between 3 and 6 months of age. Young children will manifest with symptoms of chronic hemolytic anemia, failure to thrive, infection, or dactylitis, painful swelling of hands and feet by sickled cells in the microcirculation. Basic clinical considerations for sickle cell patients fall under five categories:

- Chronic hemolytic anemia
- Recurrent painful attacks
- Bacterial infections
- Deterioration of tissue and organ function
- Shortened life expectancy

Taken together, these conditions represent a complicated set of guideposts for medical management of a patient with sickle cell disease. Primary care physicians who treat sickle cell patients must be familiar with these particular complications. Each patient will have a unique presentation of their sickle state. Some will have a lifetime of complications and hospitalizations, and others will not be affected until later in life. Nevertheless, possessing hemoglobin S homozygously is not to be ignored or trivialized.

The Anemia

Most patients with sickle cell anemia have a chronic hemolytic process, characterized by a hypercellular bone marrow, red cells that live only 10 to 20 days,[9] a marked reticulocytosis (8% to 12%), increased bilirubin, and cholelithiasis. The anemia is usually compensated with hematocrits in the range of 20% to 25%, and patients do well even with these low numbers. Complications occur in the form of aplastic anemia or splenic sequestration crisis. Acute aplastic anemia may develop as a result of infection, usually parvovirus, when the already overworked bone marrow simply fails to produce cells. The hematocrit may fall by 10% to 15% per day.[10] Transfusion is essential because there is no backup therapy for bone marrow aplasia and death may occur without transfusion intervention.

The Spleen

This organ bears the burden of the sickle process. Many patients will have an initial splenomegaly, but by 5 to 6 years of age,[11] this organ drastically changes. Functional asplenia occurs within the first 2 years as the spleen loses its ability to clear abnormalities from red cells. Howell-Jolly bodies and other inclusions are evident in the peripheral smear, and there is increased incidence of severe infections, due to the weakened immune function of the spleen. Repeated **infarctions** and congestion of the spleen will lead to autosplenectomy, producing a fibrosed and shriveled organ. This scarred organ is dysfunctional, lacking the basic and most important splenic functions. Two consequences may develop: overwhelming sepsis and splenic sequestration. In an historical study performed in 1986, the incidence of infection dropped 85% with the use of oral penicillin compared with a **placebo** study in patients of the same age range.[12] *Streptococcus pneumoniae* infections are especially grave in this age group, yet other encapsulated organisms, such as *Haemophilus influenzae* and *Neisseria meningitidis,* pose serious hazards. Acute splenic sequestration is most often a complication of young children. The onset is sudden, as large volumes of blood pool in the spleen. Distention of the abdomen and **hypovolemic** shock occur because of the rapid pooling. Recovery is not guaranteed as often the condition goes unrecognized and treatment is delayed.

The Lungs

Sickling can occur in any organ of the body, yet the lungs are particularly susceptible to occlusions in the microenvironment of the pulmonary space. During the course of disease, patients may experience clinical lung conditions that are chronic or acute. Often, minute pulmonary infarctions may go undetected, but over time these may lead to impaired pulmonary function and pulmonary hypertension in 20% to 40% of patients, which carries a high risk of death.[13] Children with sickle cell anemia are 100 times more susceptible to pneumonia than are other members of the pediatric population.[14] Acute chest syndrome is characterized by fever, chest pain, hypoxia, and pulmonary infiltrates. These patients are critically ill with an average hospitalization of 10 days. Older patients tend to have a more severe course of disease. Multiple causes are suggested, including pneumonia and other infectious agents and possible fat **embolism**, although pulmonary infarction underlies each of these possibilities. Acute chest syndrome represents the leading cause of death and hospitalization in patients with sickle cell disease and should be considered in any sickle individual who is admitted for pain.[15]

Vaso-occlusive Episodes and Complications

Painful crisis is the trademark of patients with sickle cell disease. In African cultures, the descriptive words associated with this condition translate as "body biting" or "body chewing."[16] Tissue infarctions and sickling in small vessels produce several painful target points. Patients do not experience crisis episodes on a daily basis; for the most part they are able to live reasonably normal lives. Yet, several features may predispose to a crisis event including fever, dehydration, cold, and stress. When a crisis occurs, the pain is described as gnawing, throbbing, and overwhelming with few moments of relief. If the crisis is centered in the bones, patients experience tenderness, warmth, and swelling and some bone necrosis. Infarctions at the joint level lead to swelling, pain, and loss of mobility. What may also result from joint infarction and poor circulation in the limbs are large, pitting ulcers that are slow to heal and difficult to treat. The pain of sickle cell crisis is intense and unrelenting and only temporarily relieved by analgesics. Clinicians may need to reevaluate the protocols and analgesics necessary for pain management in the child and adult sickle population, with a goal of providing some relief and comfort.[17]

Priapism, Retinopathy, and Stroke

Priapism, an unfortunate complication of vaso-occlusion, is the persistent painful erection of the penis that usually occurs around 15 years of age, the age of puberty. The condition may persist for hours, days, or even weeks with analgesics and sedation as the main course of treatment. Repeated episodes may resolutely alter sexual activity or the desire for sexual activity and lead to erectile dysfunction. There is a high incidence of priapism in males with sickle cell anemia, 35%, yet this complication needs additional attention in the overall management of this disease.[18]

Retinopathy refers to the ophthalmological complications that sickle patients experience resulting from sickling lesions and stasis of small blood vessels during the course of their disease. These may begin at 10 years of age and can include retinal detachment, retinal lesions, and possibly blindness.[19] Eye assessments need to be conducted regularly for sickle cell patients, so that appropriate treatment can be initiated and implemented.

Strokes are an infrequent complication of sickle cell anemia, affecting only 7% of children, yet they may yield serious and unpredictable setbacks to this patient group. Young patients who experience a stroke may have some degree of paralysis, coma, or seizure.[20] Preventive measures include identifying children at risk through transcranial Doppler imaging, which may disclose the narrowing of arteries causing a blockage and hypoxia to the brain.[21] An additional strategy is to maintain hemoglobin S levels close to 30% through transfusion therapy. This method has been shown to reduce the recurrence of strokes or prevention of first-time events from 80% to 10%.[22]

Disease Management and Prognosis

Although sickle cell anemia was first described by Dr. Herrick in 1910, interest in sickle cell disease was sluggish and progress for patients with sickle cell anemia was tentative at best. Two events have signaled a significant advance in the disease profile: the passage of the national Sickle Cell Anemia Control Act of 1972 and the establishment of the Cooperative Study of Sickle Cell Disease (CSSCD) in 1979 under the auspices of the National Heart, Lung, and Blood Institute. The study aims to provide a central database to analyze treatment trends, social issues faced by patients, and disease data. Several key issues have been gleaned from 16 years of data[23]:

1. Hospital visits are not the norm and are used only for crisis emergencies.
2. From 5% to 10% of patients account for 40% to 50% of hospital visits.
3. The average age of death for men was 42 years, and women, 48 years.
4. Longer-lived patients had a higher level of hemoglobin F.

Management of patients with sickle cell anemia revolves around prevention of complications and aggressive treatment if they occur. For children, prophylactic antibiotics and pneumococcal vaccines are encouraged, as well as stroke prevention techniques already outlined. Patients may need transfusions every 3 to 5 weeks to maintain a hemoglobin of 9 to 11 g/dL and a hemoglobin S concentration of less than 50%,[4] optimum standards to avoid complications. While a worthy goal, this treatment may lead to iron overload and the development of alloantibodies that could make future transfusions difficult. Both of these occurrences need to be carefully monitored by laboratory screening. Serum ferritin levels and antibody screening should be done routinely on this patient group. Perhaps one of the most auspicious developments for sickle cell patients was use of the drug hydroxyurea. Hydroxyurea increases the level of hemoglobin F in sickle cells, thereby reducing vaso-occlusive episodes and dramatically improving clinical outlooks in this patient group. First proposed by Samuel Charache in 1995, hydroxyurea was found to be successful in reducing crisis intervals and acute chest syndrome at a reasonable drug dose and with few reversible side effects.[24] This was a major breakthrough for this needy patient group and the multicenter clinical study was halted earlier than usual to offer this promising drug to more patients. At long last, sickle cell patients had a reason to be optimistic about their future. An additional, albeit more complex treatment is bone marrow transplantation from a well sibling or allogeneic match. Limited studies have suggested this as a viable alternative, but the procedure itself has considerable risks.

Patients with sickle cell anemia have considerable needs on multiple levels. For this reason, a thoughtful management plan should be developed and attended to so that this patient group may maximize their quality of life. Table 8.2 is presented as a table of interest for the reader. Additional help and advocacy can be obtained from the Sickle Cell Disease Association of America (www.sicklecelldisease.org) located in Baltimore, Maryland.

Laboratory Diagnosis

Patients with sickle cell anemia will have a lifelong normochromic, normocytic anemia with decreased hemoglobin (between 6 and 8 g/dL), hematocrit, and red cell count. The reticulocyte count is always elevated leading to a slightly increased MCV in many cases. Bilirubin and LDH are increased, while haptoglobin is decreased, indicating extravascular hemolysis. During crisis

Table 8.2 ◉ Clinical Management Scheme for the Sickle Cell Patient

Set 1: 0 to 5 years monitor for
- Penicillin prophylaxis
- Splenic sequestration
- Fever or infection
- Stroke
- Pain
- Dental care
- Complete blood count
- Red cell antigen typing
- Pneumococcal vaccine

Set 2: 5 to 10 years monitor for
- Pain
- Dental care
- Add urinalysis and liver function test to lab
- Pulmonary function
- Chest radiograph
- Ultrasound
- Ophthalmologic examination

Set 3: 10 years and beyond
- Include all from Set 2
- Family planning/self-help groups
- Leg ulcers

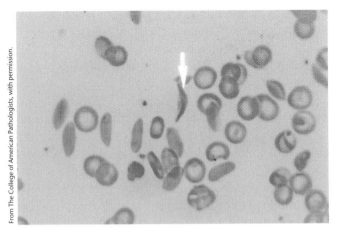

From The College of American Pathologists, with permission.

Figure 8.2 Irreversibly sickled cells. Note one pointed projection.

episodes, the peripheral smear will show marked polychromasia, many nRBCs, target cells, and the presence of irreversible and reversible sickle cells (Fig. 8.2). Peripheral smears from sickle cell patients not in crisis show minimal changes, a few oat-shaped reversible sickle cells, and some polychromasia (Fig. 8.3). White cell counts may need to be corrected for nRBCs by applying the correction formula if automated instrumentation lacks this correction function (Fig. 8.4).

First-level screening procedures for adults include the dithionite solubility, a solubility test based on the principle that hemoglobin S precipitates in high-molarity buffered phosphate solutions. The amount of hemoglobin S is insignificant in this screening procedure because the purpose of this procedure is to detect the presence of hemoglobin S in the test sample. The end point is easy to read as a turbid solution in the presence of hemoglobin S and a clear solution if hemoglobin S is not present (Fig. 8.5). Newborn screening for hemoglobinopathies occurs in most states and for all ethnic groups in the United States, and provides the opportunity for early diagnosis and intervention for sickle cell anemia patients, key ingredients for successful disease

management. Most newborn blood samples are obtained by heel stick and the blood is applied onto dried filter paper ready to be processed for analysis, but cord blood samples are also acceptable. The samples are then analyzed by hemoglobin electrophoresis at either alkaline or acid pH or both, isoelectric focusing, or high-performance liquid chromatography. If electrophoretic techniques are used, two bands, hemoglobin F and hemoglobin S, will be seen in patients with sickle cell anemia because hemoglobin F is predominant in neonates. The healthy neonate will show two bands at hemoglobin A and hemoglobin F, while the individual with sickle cell trait will show three bands: one at F, one at A, and one at S. Table 8.3 shows the relative concentration of hemoglobins A and F at different ages. Challenges in neonatal screening involve identifying unexpected bands as well as small amounts of hemoglobin A or S.[25]

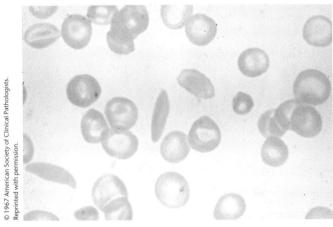

© 1967 American Society of Clinical Pathologists. Reprinted with permission.

Figure 8.3 Reversible sickle cell. Note the blunted ends of the sickle cell.

$$\frac{\text{Correct white count} = \text{original white count}}{100 + n\text{RBCs}} \times 100$$

Figure 8.4 White cell corrections based on number of nRBCs.

Hemoglobin Electrophoresis

Hemoglobin electrophoresis is a time-honored quantitative procedure for isolating hemoglobin bands. This technique is based on the principle that hemoglobins migrate at different positions depending on pH, time of migration, and media used. Cellulose acetate and citrate agar are the media most often selected. Hemoglobin is isolated from a patient sample using a variety of lysing agents such as saponin or water. A small amount of sample is applied to the media and electrophoresed for the prescribed amount of time, and then each band is quantified using densitometry. Figure 8.6 is a comparison of cellulose acetate and citrate agar electrophoresis. What will become immediately noticeable for both media is that several bands have the same migration point. In analyzing each group of patterns, several features must be kept in mind to properly identify the abnormal hemoglobin (Table 8.4). On cellulose acetate at alkaline electrophoresis, hemoglobins E, C, O_{Arab}, and A_2 migrate in the same position and hemoglobins S, D, and G travel together. On citrate agar at acid pH, hemoglobins A, O, A_2, D, G, and E migrate to the same point. Yet, this medium provides excellent separation for hemoglobins S and D and hemoglobins C from E. In practice, most laboratories use a screening technique followed by a known quantitative method that has been

Table 8.3 ● Normal Hemoglobin A and Hemoglobin F Concentrations by Age		
Age	**Hgb F (%)**	**Hgb A (%)**
1 day	77.0 ± 7.3	23 ± 7.3
Up to 12 months	1.6 ± 1.0	98.4 ± 1.0
Adult	<2.0	98

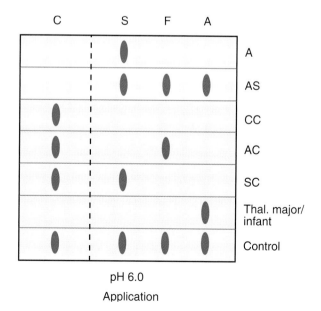

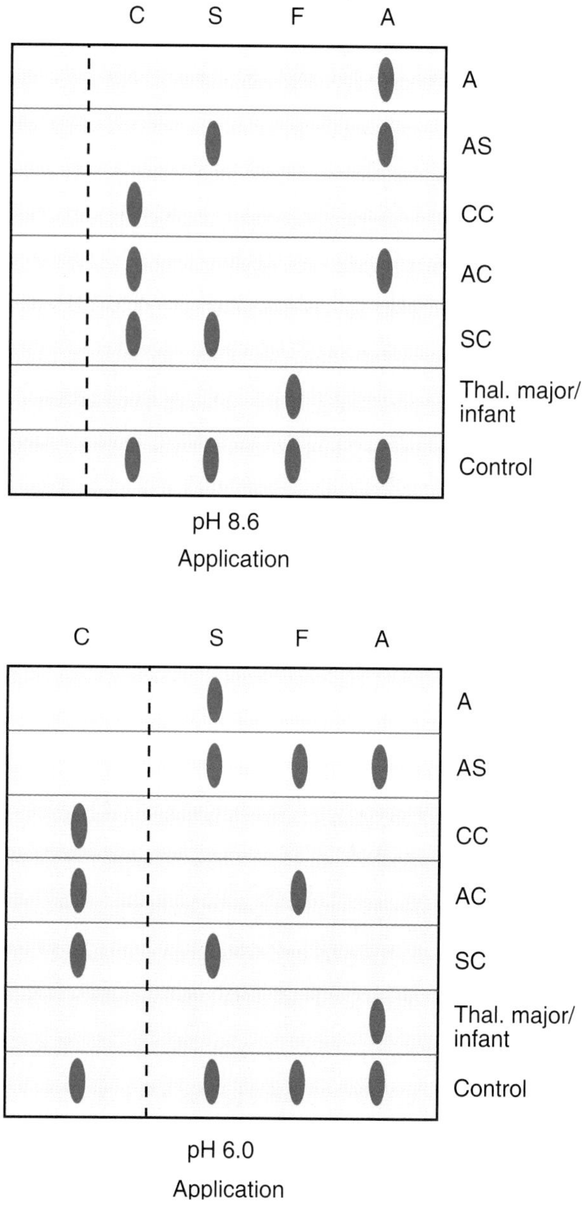

Figure 8.6 Hemoglobin electrophoresis at pH 8.6 and pH 6.2.

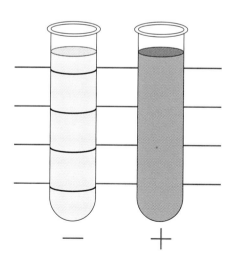

Figure 8.5 Sickle solubility test. An insoluble solution indicates the presence of Hemoglobin S. Clear solution is from a normal patient.

Table 8.4 ◉ **Points to Consider When Analyzing Alkaline Electrophoresis**

- What is the MCV of your patient?
- What is the strength of the band?
- What is the age of your patient?
- Does your patient have a transfusion history?

carefully developed for their hospital setting. Equipment costs, technologist time, and the number of samples to be evaluated factor into the decision as to whether the quantitative technique will be performed on site or sent out to a reference laboratory.

Isoelectric Focusing

Isoelectric focusing (IEF) is the method of choice for most newborn screening in the United States. This refined electrophoretic procedure uses a pH range of between 3 and 10 in polyacrylamide gel. Within this pH range, hemoglobins will achieve their isoelectric point, their point of no net negative charge, and they will focus into sharp distinct bands. Because each hemoglobin is a protein with a distinct amino acid composition, clearly defined points are achieved. This procedure is especially useful when small amounts of abnormal hemoglobin need to be detected.[26] The cost of equipment for IEF is prohibitive in most community hospital settings, but this technique has great value for large-batch analysis such as newborn screening performed in state health laboratories.

Sickle Cell Trait

Sickle cell trait is achieved through heterozygous inheritance of hemoglobin S, in which an individual possesses hemoglobin A at approximately 60% and hemoglobin S at approximately 40%. These individuals are hematologically normal. The prevalence of sickle cell trait is 8% to 10% in the African American population. Approximately 2.5 million people in the United States carry the sickle gene.[27] Population penetrance in parts of western Africa are as high as 25% to 30%, and the protection against malaria is considered to be a large factor for the frequency of this gene in parts of Africa. Several circumstances may put a sickle cell trait individual in jeopardy of having a crisis episode, such as air travel in an unpressurized cabin and high altitudes. Other than this, sickle trait individuals lead normal lives. In a perfect world, every African American individual would know their hemoglobin S status, because a union with another individual carrying sickle cell trait could produce a child affected with sickle cell anemia (1 in 4 chance). Generally, all health educators should encourage their African American students to be tested for the presence of sickle cell gene as part of their normal health screening.

HEMOGLOBIN C DISEASE, TRAIT, AND HEMOGLOBIN SC

Hemoglobin C has a substitution of lysine for glutamic acid ($\alpha_2\beta_2^{glu \rightarrow lys}$) in the sixth position of the N-terminal end of the beta chain. If hemoglobin C is inherited homozygously, the individual has hemoglobin C disease; if heterozygously, then hemoglobin C trait. Hemoglobin C disease has *milder* clinical symptoms than sickle cell anemia and has a much lower prevalence in the African American population (only 2% to 3%). In northern Ghana, however, the incidence of this particular hemoglobin is 17% to 28%.[2] The anemia is normochromic and normocytic, yet there is some increase in the MCHC because red cells from homozygous individuals are denser. Most homozygous individuals show a moderate anemia with a hemoglobin value of between 9 and 12 g/dL. There is a moderate reticulocytosis and splenomegaly. The red cell life span is 38 days, yet few patients exhibit any symptoms. Of particular interest is the possible presence of crystalline structures in the red cells that appear as blocks or "bars of gold" (Fig. 8.7). These peculiar crystals obstruct the microvasculature but melt in the splenic microenvironment. Consequently, splenic function is preserved and little pitting occurs. Target cells (50% to 90%) are the predominant

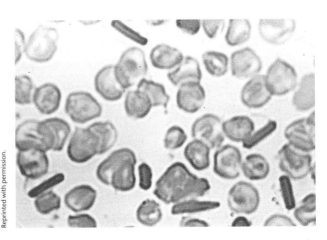

• **Figure 8.7** Hemoglobin CC. Note the presence of crystals shaped like "bars of gold" and many target cells.

red cell morphology, and variations of targeting may include folded or "pocketbook"-shaped cells. Spherocytes may be present. Alkaline electrophoresis will show a single slow moving band in the same position as hemoglobin A$_2$.

The heterozygous condition is termed hemoglobin A-C trait, with a ratio of 60% hemoglobin A and 40% hemoglobin C on alkaline electrophoresis. There are no clinical complications for individuals with this condition, and they may never be noticed except for the presence of 40% target cells on their peripheral smear, an extremely abnormal finding (see Fig. 3.16). Individuals who inherit hemoglobin C should be aware of their hemoglobin status and that of prospective mates.

Hemoglobin SC disease is a combination of two abnormal hemoglobins, hemoglobin S and hemoglobin C. Affected individuals have a moderate anemia, with an average hemoglobin of 8 to 10 g/dL, with a slight reticulocytosis. Red cell life span is reduced to approximately 29 days. Although the disease is less severe than sickle cell anemia, an individual may experience a painful crisis. Pregnant individuals may be severely affected. The peripheral smear shows high numbers of target cells; few reversible sickled cells, and folded cells, with a peculiar crystal shaped like the Washington Monument or a gloved hand showing in some cells (Fig. 8.8). The hemoglobin distribution on alkaline electrophoresis is 50% hemoglobin S and 50% hemoglobin C.

VARIANT HEMOGLOBINS OF NOTE
Hemoglobin S-Beta Thalassemia

This combination hemoglobin may produce a clinical picture as severe as sickle cell anemia, with virtually no hemoglobin A present. The anemia will be microcytic hypochromic, showing the influence of the thalassemia gene, with nRBCs, target cells, polychromasia, and sickle cells. The RDW will be increased as well as the reticulocyte count. As opposed to the usual presentation of sickle cell anemia, splenomegaly is usually present. The severity of the condition overall depends on the beta thalassemia genotype inherited; patients inheriting B^0 have a more severe presentation. On alkaline electrophoresis, two bands are present, one at the location of hemoglobin S and one at the location of hemoglobin A$_2$.

Hemoglobin E

This abnormal hemoglobin has an extremely high occurrence in individuals from southeast Asian countries. Individuals may inherit the hemoglobin either heterozygously and homozygously. Surprisingly, the homozygous conditions of this abnormal hemoglobin presents no clinical complications. Individuals show a marked microcytic hypochromic picture, with some target cells and slight polychromasia, but are asymptomatic. On alkaline electrophoresis, there is a strong band located in the same position as hemoglobin C, while the heterozygous condition shows 70% hemoglobin A and 30% hemoglobin E. Hemoglobin E is the second most common hemoglobin variant worldwide and is being seen with increasing frequency due to large numbers of southeast Asians emigrating to North America (Fig. 8.9).

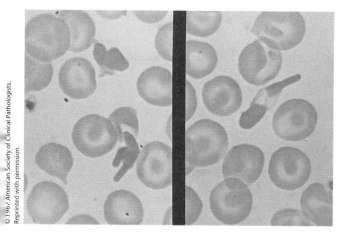

Figure 8.8 Hemoglobin SC. Note the presence of crystals with pointed projections.

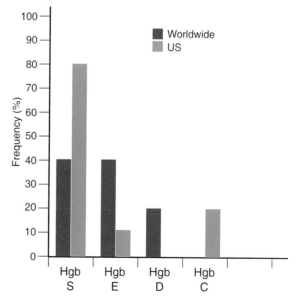

Figure 8.9 Variants of hemoglobin in United States versus worldwide.

Hemoglobin D~Punjab~/Hemoglobin G~phila~

Not often seen, hemoglobin D$_{Punjab}$ is a clinical variant in which both genetic states are asymptomatic. There is a higher incidence of hemoglobin D in Great Britain, and this is thought to reflect the large number of Indian wives brought to England during Great Britain's long occupation of the Punjab region of India and Pakistan. The prevalence of this variant in these regions is 3%.

Although rare, hemoglobin G$_{phila}$ is seen in American blacks. It is an alpha chain variant that migrates in the same position as hemoglobin S at alkaline electrophoresis at pH 8.6. There are no hematological abnormalities, but there is a high incidence in Ghana.

Hemoglobin O~Arab~

An uncommon hemoglobin, hemoglobin O$_{Arab}$ is found in 0.4% of American blacks. Most individuals are asymptomatic, but this hemoglobin must be distinguished from hemoglobin C at alkaline electrophoresis, because it migrates to the same location. Citrate electrophoresis at pH 6.4 will isolate this band for positive identification.

CONDENSED CASE

A 6-year-old Indian girl was brought to the emergency department with a fever, malaise, and joint pain. Lab results were WBC = $13,000 \times 10^9$/L, Hgb = 9.0 g/dL, Hct = 27%, and MCV = 85%. Her peripheral smear revealed a moderate number of target cells, with 2+ polychromasia and moderate oat-shaped cells. **Based on this sketch, what is the first diagnosis that comes to mind?**

Answer
Based on her peripheral smear and the fact that she is anemic with joint pain, sickle cell anemia is a strong possibility. She needs to have this condition confirmed with hemoglobin electrophoresis or IEF. Oat-shaped cells are reversible sickle cells seen in many sickle cell anemia individuals. Obviously her bone marrow is responding because she is exhibiting polychromasia. Splenic function needs to be carefully monitored in individuals of this age group.

Summary Points

- Most hemoglobinopathies are the result of single amino acid substitution in the beta chain.
- In sickle cell disorders, valine is substituted for glutamic acid in the sixth position of the beta chain.
- In hemoglobin C disorders, lysine is substituted for glutamic acid in the sixth position of the beta chain.
- The presence of hemoglobin S affords some protections against malarial infection of red blood cells.
- Cells containing hemoglobin S as the majority hemoglobin are insoluble in areas of the body with low oxygen tension.
- Sickle cells clog small vessels during sickling crisis, causing extensive organ damage and pain.
- Homozygous inheritance of hemoglobin S produces sickle cell anemia (Hgb SS); heterozygous inheritance produces sickle cell trait (Hgb AS).
- Hypoxia, acidosis, dehydration, cold, and fever will predispose the patient to sickling episodes.
- In the African American population, there is an 8% to 10% prevalence of the sickle cell gene.

- Autosplenectomy is a consequence of repeated infarctions to the spleen in young children with sickle cell disease.
- Stroke and acute chest syndrome represent serious complications to sickle cell patients.
- During sickle crisis episodes, patients will show nRBCs, sickle cells, target cells, and polychromasia.
- The white count may need to be corrected due to nRBCs present during sickling episodes.
- Individuals with sickle cell trait are asymptomatic with rare abnormalities in the peripheral smear.
- Newborn screening for hemoglobinopathies is available in the United States through state health laboratories.
- Dithionite solubility is usually the screening procedure used to determine if hemoglobin S is present.
- Acid or alkaline electrophoresis and IEF provide better methods to isolate hemoglobin bands.
- Hemoglobin C disease occurs when hemoglobin C is inherited homozygously; hemoglobin C trait occurs when hemoglobin C is inherited heterozygously.

- Hemoglobin C disease may produce hemoglobin C crystals on Wright's stain.
- Hemoglobin SC is the result of inheriting two abnormal hemoglobins, hemoglobin S and C.
- Hemoglobin SC may produce abnormal crystal formation resembling the Washington Monument or fingers in a glove presentation.

- Hemoglobin S-beta thalassemia may produce conditions as severe as sickle cell disease.
- Hemoglobin E is the third most prevalent hemoglobin variant and is seen with great frequency in the southeast Asian populations.
- Hemoglobin D and hemoglobin G_{phila} migrate with hemoglobin S on alkaline electrophoresis.

Review Questions

1. What is the amino acid substitution in sickle cell anemia patients?
   a. Adenine for thymine
   b. Lysine for valine
   c. Valine for glutamic acid
   d. Cytosine for guanine

2. Which of the following factors contributes to the pathophysiology of sickling?
   a. Increased iron concentration
   b. Hypochromia
   c. Fava beans
   d. Dehydration

3. Which of the following statements pertain to most of the clinically significant hemoglobin variants?
   a. Most are fusion hemoglobins.
   b. Most are singe amino acid substitution.
   c. Most are synthetic defects.
   d. Most are extensions of the amino acid chain.

4. Which of the following hemoglobins ranks second in variant hemoglobins worldwide?
   a. Hgb S
   b. Hbg E

   c. Hgb H
   d. Hgb C

5. Which hemoglobin will show crystals appearing like bars of gold in the peripheral smear?
   a. Hemoglobin CC disease
   b. Hemoglobin DD disease
   c. Hemoglobin EE disease
   d. Hemoglobin SS disease

6. Which one of the following conditions is the leading cause of hospitalization for sickle cell patients?
   a. Acute chest syndrome
   b. Priapism
   c. Painful crisis
   d. Splenic sequestration

7. Which of the following hemoglobin separation methods is used for most newborn hemoglobin screening?
   a. High-performance liquid chromatography
   b. Alkaline electrophoresis
   c. Isoelectric focusing
   d. Acid electrophoresis

CASE STUDY

A 3-year-old boy of Ghanaian ethnicity came to the emergency department acutely ill, with fever, chest pain, and a heavy cough. He was accompanied by his parents, who said that he seemed to have a mild cold and slight fever. However, his condition had become more serious in the last 24 hours. His temperature was 103°F. His parent informed the emergency department staff that he has a diagnosis of **sickle cell anemia**, but they thought that this episode was different from his previous crisis episodes. A CBC was ordered and, because of his cough, he was helped to cough up a sputum sample for culture. He was given ibuprofen for pain and fever. Four hours from the time he was seen in the emergency department, he was admitted and put in the critical care unit, in grave condition. His breathing was compromised and he was placed on mechanical ventilation and lapsed into a coma. He developed disseminated intravascular coagulation (DIC), using 10 units of fresh frozen plasma, 10 units of platelets, and 20 units of packed cells to control the bleeding. Twenty-four hours after admission, he died from overwhelming sepsis. Initial results are as follows (see cover for normal values). **What role does splenic function play in the management of sickle cell patients?**

(continued on following page)

(Continued)

WBC	20.0×10^9/L
RBC	2.82×10^{12}/L
Hgb	11.5 g/dL
Hct	34%
MCV	85 fL
MCH	29.8 pg
MCHC	35.0%
Platelets	160×10^9/L
RDW	18.0%

The differential showed a left shift with heavy toxic granulation and Döhle bodies. The initial coagulation results are:

PT   12.0 seconds (normal value, 11 to 13 seconds)

PTT   26.0 seconds (normal value, <40 seconds)

Insights to the Case Study

This account represents the worst case scenario for a young sickle patient. Patients in this age range who have sickle cell anemia are vulnerable to virulent infections by encapsulated organisms, acute chest syndrome, and dactylitis . When they are admitted to the hospital, coordinated care by a staff knowledgeable about sickle cell complications is increasingly important because time is usually the enemy and the situation can rapidly escalate. In this case, even though the parent mentioned the child's sickle cell diagnosis, he was treated far too casually and not as a young child with special medical needs. *Streptococcus pneumoniae* grew from his sputum culture and a gram positive organism was seen on Gram stain, but he was not treated aggressively when one considers that his spleen was compromised. Functional asplenia is serious and life threatening, especially if the patient becomes infected with an encapsulated organism. Patients such as this merit special attention. This patient died of overwhelming sepsis due to the streptococcal infection, which triggered DIC and uncontrollable bleeding. His platelet count plummeted to 40,000 within 2 hours of admission and he began to bleed from the venipuncture site. He was too young to withstand the numerous assaults on his body system.

⊙ TROUBLESHOOTING

What Is the Proper Procedure If the Automated WBC Does Not Correlate With a Slide Estimate?

A 14-year-old boy presented to the emergency department with a fever of unknown origin. A CBC, blood cultures, and routine chemistries were ordered. The chemistries came back as normal and the blood cultures would be read in 24 hours. The CBC results were as follows:

WBC:	35.0	H
RBC	4.19	L
Hgb	9.3	L
Hct	27.8	L
MCV	66.3	L
MCH	22.3	L
MCHC	33.5	
Platelets	598	H
RDW	21.0	H

The elevated WBC flagged and reflex testing indicated that a manual differential should be performed.

The technologist performed the differential and noted several items:

- The WBC count of 35,000 did not correlate with the slide.
- 100 nRBCs were counted while completing the differential.
- The patient had anisocytosis, probably due to younger polychromatic cells.
- The patient had poikilocytosis including moderate target and moderate sickle cells present.
- The patient had the presence of RBC inclusions: Pappenheimer and Howell-Jolly bodies.

It was obvious to the technologist that this was a sickle cell patient in a crisis with an elevated RDW and the peripheral smear indicative of sickle cell crisis. The presence of 100 nRBCs counted in the differential is a significant finding. nRBCs were most likely being counted as white cells, falsely elevating the white cell count. The Coulter LH750 usually corrects for the presence of nRBCs when the nRBCs are in the low range, but an nRBC count of 100 is fairly high and the instrument calculation has not been reliable in the high range. The instrument reported out a white count of 35,000, but the technologist thought that this count did not agree with the peripheral smear. The technologist needed to manually correct the white count. In order to perform this function, the technologist referred to the raw data function available in the Coulter instrument, to find what the WBC count was prior to correction by the instrument. The number of the WBC was 49,800 and represents the raw number of white cells counted on the initial run of this sample. This number was used to correct for the nRBCs using the formula shown in Figure 8.4.

$$\frac{\text{Uncorrected WBC} \times 100}{100 + 100} = \frac{49.8 \times 100}{200}$$

$$= \frac{4980}{200} = 24,900, \text{ the corrected WBC}$$

The corrected white count was reported to the floor. This case illustrates the value of reflex testing, prompting the performance of a manual differential. A careful observation of the peripheral smear indicated that the instrument correction for nRBCs, 35,000, was not valid (the white count seemed lower) and that the technologist needed to intervene to provide a reliable white count.

WORD KEY

Autosomal • Referring to chromosome, a non–sex-linked chromosome

Embolism • Occlusion of a blood vessel

Infarction • Area of tissue that has been deprived of blood and therefore has lost some of its function

Hypovolemic • Low blood pressure

Placebo • Substance having no medical effect when given to an individual as if a medicine

Viscosity • Thickness

References

1. Ingram VM. Gene mutations in human hemoglobins: The chemical differences between normal and sickle hemoglobins. Nature (Lond) 180:326, 1957.
2. Huisman TH, et al. A Syllabus of Human Hemoglobin Variants, 2nd ed. August, GA: The Sickle Cell Anemia Foundation, 1998.
3. McGhee DB. Structural defects in hemoglobin (hemoglobinopathies). In: Rodak B, ed. Hematology: Clinical Principles and Applications, 2nd ed. Philadelphia: WB Saunders, 2002; 321.
4. Smith-Whitley K. Sickle Cell Disease: Diagnosis and Current Management. Workshop material from the American Society for Clinical Laboratory Sciences National Meeting, Philadelphia, July 2003.
5. Smith JA, Kinney TR (co-chairs). Sickle Cell Disease Guideline Panel: Sickle cell disease guideline and overview. Am J Hematol 47:152–154, 1994.
6. Pawars DR, Chan L, Schroeder WB. B^s– gene cluster haplotypes in sickle cell anemia: Clinical implications. Am J Pediatr Hematol Oncol 12:367–374, 1990.
7. Pawars DR, Weiss JN, Chan LS, et al. Is there a threshold level of fetal hemoglobin that ameliorates morbidity in sickle cell anemia? Blood 63:921–926, 1984.
8. Barnhart MI, Henry RL, Lusher JM. Sickle Cell. A Scope Publication. Kalamazoo, MI: The Upjohn Co., 1976; 12–14. Monograph.
9. Armbruster DA. Neonatal hemoglobinopathy screening. Lab Med 21:816, 1990.
10. Singer K, Motulsky AG, et al. Aplastic crisis in sickle cell anemia. J Lab Clin Med 35:721, 1950.
11. Pearson HA, Cornelius EA, et al. Transfusion reversible functional asplenia in young children with sickle cell anemia. N Engl J Med 283:334, 1970.
12. Gaston MH, Vwerter JL, Woods G, et al. Prophylaxis with oral penicillin in children with sickle cell anemia: A randomized trial. N Engl J Med 314:1593–1599, 1986.
13. Gladwin MT, Sachdev V, Jison ML, et al. Pulmonary hypertension as a risk factor for death in patients with sickle cell disease. N Engl J Med 350:886–895, 2004.
14. Barnhart MI, Henry RL, Lusher JM. Sickle Cell. A Scope Publication. Kalamazoo, MI: The Upjohn Co., 1974; 45. Monograph.
15. Vichinsky EP, Neumaur LD, Earles AN, et al. Causes and outcomes of acute chest syndrome in sickle cell disease. National Acute Chest Syndrome Study Group, 2000.
16. Konotey-Ahulu FI. Sickle cell disease. Arch Intern Med 133:616, 1974.
17. Dampier C, Ely E, Brodecki D, et al. Home management of pain in sickle cell disease: A daily diary study in children and adolescents. J Pediatr Hematol Oncol 24:643–647, 2002.
18. Adeyoju AB, Olujohungbe AB, Morris J, et al. Priapism in sickle cell disease: Incidence, risk factors and complications—An international multicenter study. BJU Int 90:898–902, 2002.
19. Babalola OE, Wambebe CO. When should children and young adults with sickle cell disease be referred for eye assessments? Afr J Med Sci 30:261–263, 2001.
20. Embury SH, et al. Sickle Cell Disease: Basic Principles and Clinical Practice. New York: Raven Press, 1994.

21. Adams RJ, et al. Prevention of a first stroke by transfusion in children with sickle cell anemia and abnormal
results on transcranial Doppler ultrasonography
N Engl J Med 317:781, 1987.

22. Pelehach L. Understanding sickle cell anemia. Lab Med
126:727, 1995.

23. Gaston M, Rosse WF; The Cooperative Group. The
Cooperative Study of Sickle Cell Disease: Review of
study designs and objectives. Am J Pediatr Hematol
Oncol 4:197–201, 1982.

24. Charache S, Terrin ML, Moore RD, et al. Effect of
hydroxyurea on the frequency of painful crisis in sickle
cell anemia. N Engl J Med 332:1317–1322, 1995.

25. Pearson HA. Neonatal testing for sickle cell disease:
A historical and personal view. Pediatrics 83(Suppl):
815–818, 1989.

26. Galacteros F, Kleman K, Caburi-Martin J, et al. Cord
blood screening for hemoglobin abnormalities by thin
layer isoelectric focusing. Blood 56:1068–1071, 1980.

27. Geist A. Hemoglobinopathies: Diagnosis and Care of
Patients with Sickle Cell Disease. Indiana Univeristy
Medical Center, personal correspondence.

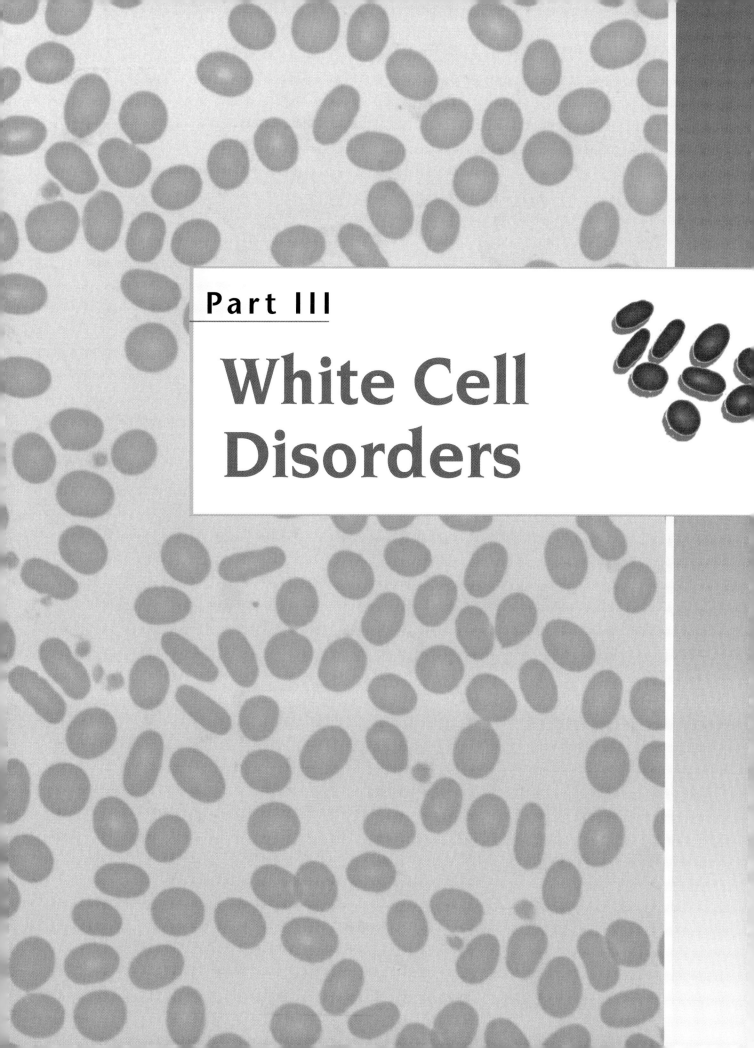

Part III

White Cell Disorders

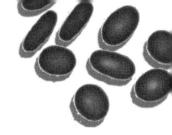

9 Leukopoiesis and Leukopoietic Function

Betty Ciesla

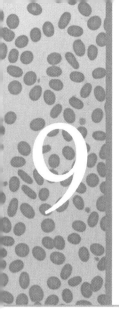

Leukopoiesis

Stages of Leukocyte Maturation

Features of Cell Identification

Myeloblast

Promyelocyte (Progranulocyte)

Myelocyte

Metamyelocyte

Band

Segmented Neutrophil

Eosinophils and Basophils

The Agranular Cell Series

Lymphocyte Origin and Function

Lymphocyte Populations

The Travel Path of Lymphocytes

Lymphocytes and the Development of Immunocompetency

The Response of Lymphocytes to Antigenic Stimulation

Lymphocyte Cell Markers and the Cluster Designation (CD)

Leukocyte Count From the Complete Blood Cell Count to the Differential

Manual Differential Versus Differential Scan

Relative Versus Absolute Values

Objectives

After completing this chapter, the student will be able to:

1. Describe leukopoiesis and the steps leading from immature forms to maturation.

2. List the maturation sequence of the granulocytic series.

3. Name four morphological features that are helpful in differentiating the cells of the granulocytic series.

4. Describe the physiology and function of granulocytes.

5. Describe the features that differentiate the granules of the neutrophilic, eosinophilic, and basophilic cell line.

6. Distinguish between the marginating and circulating pools of leukocytes.

7. Recognize the subtle morphological clues that may distinguish one white cell from another.

8. Describe the lymphatic system and its relationship to lymphocyte production.

9. Describe the role of stimulated and unstimulated lymphocytes.

LEUKOPOIESIS

White cells are a remarkably versatile group of cells whose primary purpose is to defend against bacteria, viruses, fungi, or other foreign substances. To this end, most white cells are granulated and these granules contain enzymes used for digestion and destruction of the invading organisms. In the bone marrow there is a 4:1 ratio, the M:E ratio indicating that four myeloid, or white cells are produced for one erythroid cell. Daily production of white cells is 1.5 billion. Transit from the bone marrow to the peripheral circulation takes place only after white cells have been held in the maturation-storage pool of the bone marrow. For example, segmented neutrophils, the most mature of all of the white cells, are held for 7 to 10 days before their release into the peripheral circulation. Other white cell types have much shorter storage in the maturation pool time.[1] Once released into the circulation, most white cells are short lived before they migrate into tissues. The white cells that are observed in the peripheral circulation are only a snapshot of white cells that are located in three distinct cell compartments: the bone marrow, the circulation, and the tissues.

White blood cells (WBCs) are referred to as leukocytes. For clarity, the word *leukocytic* applies to the white cells of all stages; *granulocytic* applies only to granulated white cells; and *myelocytic* is used in describing a particular white cell condition. The term *myelocytic* may also be used interchangeably for *granulocytic* in conditions such as chronic granulocytic leukemia or chronic myelocytic leukemia. Suffice it to say that these three words—granulocytic, leukocytic, and myelocytic—are all used in denoting some stage of the white cell family. They are not meant to be confusing, but often are, despite good intentions.

WBCs, or leukocytes, have a more complex maturation cycle than erythrocytes. To begin, there is only one mature red cell form as opposed to five mature white cell forms. Red blood cells journey through the circulation for 120 days while white cells spend only *hours* in the circulating blood. Like red cells, white cells originate from the pluripotent stem cell. The pluripotent stem cell gives rise to the myeloid stem cell and the lymphoid stem cell. Through a series of interventions from interleukins (chemical stimulators) and growth factors, a CFU-GEMM is structured to give rise to granulocytes, erythrocytes, monocytes, and macrophages. Curiously, megakaryocytes, eosinophils, and basophils have their own CFU: CGU-Meg and CFU-eosinophil/basophil. Lymphocytes originate not only from the bone marrow but also from the **thymus** and thus, they have a distinctive place on the hematopoietic maturation chart (see Fig. 2.3).

Most of the function of the white cells is performed in the tissues, and it is here that white cells reside for 2 to 5 days. WBCs that appear in the circulation are part of two distinctive cell pools: the marginating pool and the circulating pool. The marginating pool designates those white cells that are located along the vessel endothelium ready to migrate to a site of injury or infection. The circulating pool designates those white cells actually in the bloodstream.[2] At any particular point in the peripheral circulation, the white cells are evenly divided in either pool and there is rapid transfer from pool to pool. An additional site of white cell storage is the spleen, which harbors one fourth of the white cell population.

STAGES OF LEUKOCYTE MATURATION

The white cell series encompasses those cells that are distinguished by their granules and those that are agranular. In all, there are five maturation stages for neutrophils, four for eosinophils and basophils, and three each for monocytes and lymphocytes. Key features in distinguishing immature and mature stages of any of these cells are cell size, nucleus-to-cytoplasm ratio (N:C), chromatin pattern, cytoplasmic quality, and presence of granules. Cell identification is an organized process. Each cell can be identified using the characteristics listed and each student must survey the cell for each characteristic it presents. The stages of maturation for the neutrophilic series from least mature to most mature are:

- Myeloblast
- Promyelocyte or progranulocyte
- Myelocyte
- Metamyelocyte
- Band
- Segmented neutrophil

FEATURES OF CELL IDENTIFICATION

Descriptions for this section represent composite criteria for each cell identification.[3–5] In addition to key distinguishing features, differentiating characteristics are presented for most cells.

Myeloblast

Size: 12 to 20 μm
N:C: 4:1 with round, oval, or slightly indented nucleus

Chromatin: Light red-purple with a fine mesh-like and transparent structure/close-weaved texture; may see two to five nucleoli, which appear as lightened, refractile round structures

Cytoplasm: Moderate blue and usually nongranular

Differentiating characteristic: Nucleus has thin chromatin strands that are distributed throughout the nucleus uniformly; chromatin appears smooth and velvety (Fig. 9.1).

Cluster designation (CD)45, CD38, CD34, CD33, CD13, human leukocyte antigen (HLA)-DR

Promyelocyte (Progranulocyte)

Size: 15 to 21 μm

N:C: 3:1, oval, round, or eccentric flattened nucleus

Chromatin: Light red-purple of medium density, may see single nucleoli

Cytoplasm: Moderate blue color but difficult to observe because fine to large blue-red azurophilic granules are scattered throughout the chromatin pattern; granules are NONSPECIFIC

Differentiating characteristic: Cell is larger than the blast with large prominent nucleoli, nuclear chromatin is slightly coarse (Fig. 9.2).

CD45, CD33, CD13, CD15

Myelocyte

Size: 10 to 18 μm
N:C: 2:1

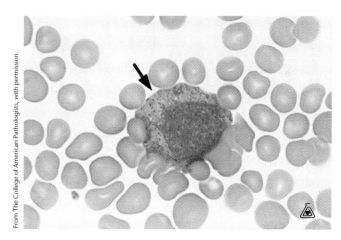

Figure 9.2 Promyelocyte. Prominent nuclei, prominent nonspecific granules, and slightly coarse nuclear chromatin.

Chromatin: Oval indented nucleus, denser, red-purple with slight granular appearance, coarser, clumped appearance

Cytoplasm: Specific granules present, neutrophilic granules are dusty, fine, and red-blue; eosinophilic granules are large red-orange, and singular; basophil granules are large, deep blue-purple

Last stage capable of dividing

Differentiating characteristic: Small pink-purple granules for the neutrophilic myelocyte, nucleus stains deeper color, granular pattern to the chromatin (Fig. 9.3).

CD45, CD33, CD13, CD15, CD11b/11c

Metamyelocyte

Size: 10 to 15 μm
N:C: 1:1

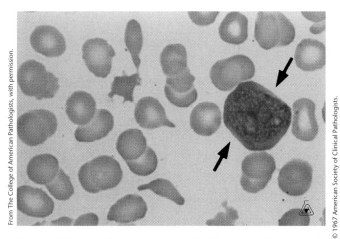

Figure 9.1 Myeloblast. Large cell with high N:C ratio and thin chromatin strands distributed evenly throughout the nucleus; no granules observed.

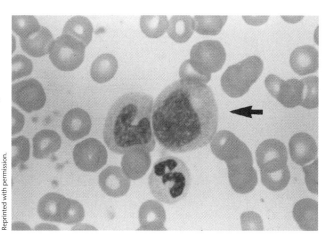

Figure 9.3 Myelocyte. Oval indented nucleus with small, specific granules, granular pattern to the chromatin.

Chromatin: Indented shaped nucleus resembling a kidney bean structure, patches of coarse chromatin in spots

Cytoplasm: Pale blue to pinkish tan with moderate specific granules

Differentiating characteristics: Nuclear indentation and condensed chromatin with no nuclei (Fig. 9.4).

CD markers are the same as for the myelocyte

Band

Size: 9 to 15 μm

Chromatin: Band shaped like a cigar band, C or S shaped, unable to see filament, coarsely clumped almost like leopard spot coarseness

Cytoplasm: Brown-pink, with many fine secondary granules

Differentiating characteristics: No filament, may resemble a metamyelocyte but indentation is more severe and chromatin is more clumped (Fig. 9.5).

CD45, CD13, CD15, CD11b/11c

Segmented Neutrophil

Size: 9 to 15 μm

Chromatin: Two to five lobes of nucleus connected by thin thread-like filaments, cannot observe chromatin pattern in filaments

Cytoplasm: Pale lilac with blue shading and many fine secondary dust-like granules

Distinguishing characteristics: If chromatin can be observed in filament, then the identification is a band; if no constriction is observed in nucleus, then the cell is a band (Fig. 9.6).

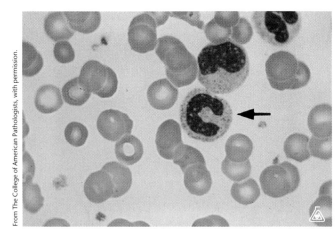

Figure 9.5 Band. No nuclear lobes, no filament, and clumped chromatin.

Eosinophils and Basophils

Eosinophil

Eosinophils can appear at the *myelocytic* stages and move through the maturation sequence.

Size: 10 to 16 μm

N:C: Barely 1:1

Chromatin: Eccentric nucleus, usually bilobed

Cytoplasm: Large, distinctive red-orange SPECIFIC granules with orange-pink cytoplasm, granules are highly metabolic and contain histamine and other substances

Distinguishing characteristics: Granules are uniformly round, large, and individualized; if stain is less than adequate, observe granules carefully for their crystalloid nature (Fig. 9.7).

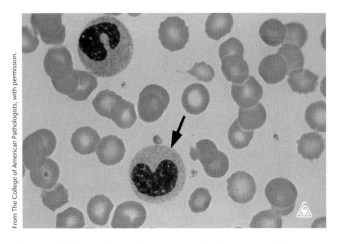

Figure 9.4 Metamyelocyte. Indented nucleus with condensed chromatin, small granules, and no nuclei.

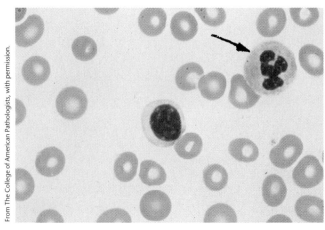

Figure 9.6 Segmented neutrophils. Note two to five lobes in the nucleus with well-distinguished filament, pale dustlike granules.

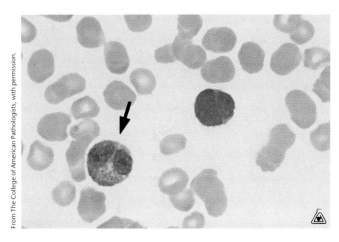

Figure 9.7 Eosinophil. Bilobed nucleus with large uniformly round orange-red granules.

Basophil

Basophils can appear at the *myelocytic* stage and move through the maturation sequence.

Size: 10 to 14 μm

N:C: Difficult to determine

Chromatin: Coarse, clumped bilobed

Cytoplasm: Many large SPECIFIC purple-black granules seem to obscure the large cloverleaf form nucleus, may decolorize during staining leaving pale areas within cell; granules much larger than neutrophilic granules

Distinguishing characteristics: Size and color of granules will obscure the nucleus (Fig. 9.8).

The Agranular Cell Series

The Monocytic Series

Monoblast

See description for myeloblast.

Promonocyte

Size: 12 to 20 μm

N:C: 3:1

Chromatin: Round, flattened nucleus, nucleoli may be present, folding, and creasing, and crimping may be observed

Cytoplasm: Gray-blue, some blobbing may appear, rare granules

Distinguishing characteristics: None noted

Monocyte

Size: 12 to 20 μm

N:C: 1:1

Chromatin: Nuclei take different shapes from brainy convolutions to lobulated and S shaped, chromatin is loose-weaved, lacey, open, and thin

Cytoplasm: Abundant gray-blue with moderate granules, may show area of protrusion or blebbing

Distinguishing characteristic: Nuclear chromatin lacks density, it is open weaved, soft and velvet-like (Fig. 9.9).

CD33, CD13, CD14

The Lymphocytic Series

Outlining CD markers for the lymphocyte cell population is a complex task and beyond the scope of this chapter. Lymphocytes develop subpopulations along the path to maturity, each with a unique CD subset. For this reason, only a modified CD list will be included (Table 9.1).

Lymphoblast

Size: 10 to 20 μm

N:C: 4:1

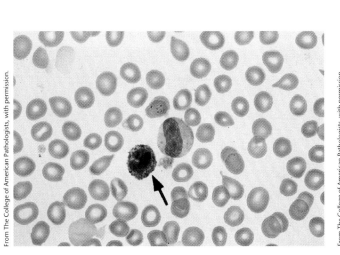

Figure 9.8 Basophil. Indistinguishable nucleus with large, purple-black granules.

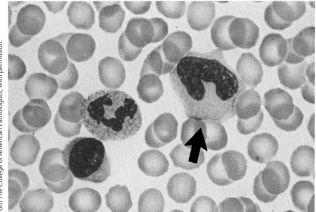

Figure 9.9 Monocyte. Nuclear chromatin is loose-weaved and open, abundant gray-blue cytoplasm.

Table 9.1 ● A Modified List of Antigen Markers of Lymphocytes*

LSC-HLA-DR

CD34, CD45

tDt

Pre-B (most mature)

CD19, CD24, CD45, CD10

tDt

Cyto μ

B cell (mature)

CD19, CD20, CD22, CD45

IgM, IgD

S Ig

T cell (most mature)

CD2, CD3, CD4, CD5, CD7

*List does not represent all possible CD cell designations.

Chromatin: One or two nucleoli with smudgy chromatin

Cytoplasm: Little, deep blue staining at edge

Distinguishing characteristics: Nucleoli is surrounded by dark rim of chromatin

Prolymphocyte

Size: 9 to 18 μm

N:C: 3:1

Chromatin: Nucleoli present, slightly coarsened chromatin

Cytoplasm: Gray-blue, mostly blue at edges

Distinguishing characteristics: None noted

Small Lymphocyte

Size: 7 to 18 μm

N:C: 4:1

Chromatin: Oval nucleus with coarse lumpy chromatin with specific areas of clumping, a compact cell

Cytoplasm: Usually just a thin border, with few azurophilic, red granules

Distinguishing characteristics: Clumping of chromatin around the nuclear membrane may help to distinguish this from a nucleated cell (Fig. 9.10).

Large Lymphocyte

Size: 9 to 12 μm

N:C: 3:1

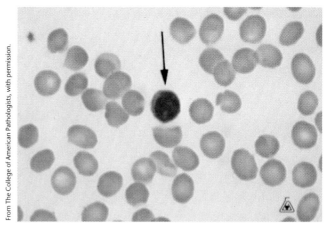

From The College of American Pathologists, with permission.

Figure 9.10 Small lymphocyte. Oval nucleus with coarse, lumpy chromatin.

Chromatin: Looser chromatin pattern, more transparent

Cytoplasm: Larger amount of cytoplasm, lighter in color

Distinguishing characteristic: Cytoplasm is more abundant with tendency for azurophilic granules (Fig. 9.11).

LYMPHOCYTE ORIGIN AND FUNCTION

The lymphocytic series is distinctive in its presentation and function. In contrast to most other white cells, which are derived solely from the bone marrow, lymphocytes are derived from two locations. The primary lymphoid organs are the bone marrow and thymus. The secondary lymphoid organs are the spleen, lymph nodes, Peyer's patches of the gastrointestinal tract, and the tonsils. Additionally, the lymphatic system plays an essential role in lymphocyte development, differentia-

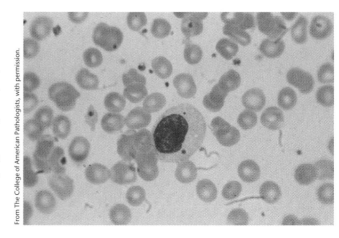

From The College of American Pathologists, with permission.

Figure 9.11 Large lymphocyte. Oval nucleus with looser, more transparent chromatin pattern.

tion, and function. More than 100 lymph nodes form a nexus known as the lymphatic system, which runs from the **cervical** lymph nodes of the neck to the inguinal lymph nodes in the groin area (Fig. 9.12). The lymphatic system plays an important role in blood filtration, fluid balance, antibody generation, and lymphopoiesis.[6] A major part of this system is lymph, a clear, thin fluid derived from plasma that bathes the soft tissues. Once

an injury has occurred and fluid is accumulated through swelling, the lymphatic system moves fluid from the affected area back to the circulation through the capillaries of the lymph nodes. Because the lymphatic system has no pumping mechanism like the heart, it derives its circulatory ability from respiration, muscle movement, and pressure from nearby blood vessels. Excess fluid is transported to two large vessels:

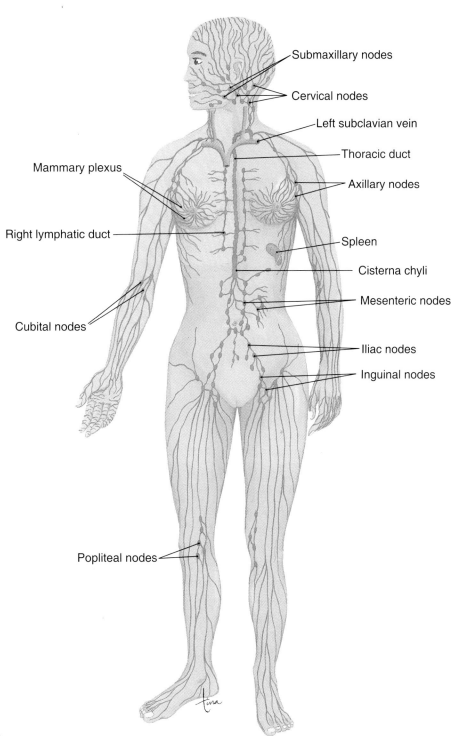

Figure 9.12   The lymphatic system.

the thoracic duct near the left **subclavian** vein and the right thoracic duct near the right subclavian vein.

The primary function of lymphocytes is immunologic: recognizing what is foreign, non-self; forming antibodies; and securing immunity. Non-self or foreign substances may appear as bacteria, cell substances, proteins, or viruses.

Lymphocyte Populations

There are two general subpopulations of lymphocytes—B lymphocytes and T lymphocytes—which appear morphologically similar on peripheral smear. Yet their derivation and function are quite different. B lymphocytes comprise 10% to 20% of the total lymphocyte population, while T lymphocytes comprise 60% to 80%. A third minor population, natural killer (NK) lymphocytes, constitute less than 10% of the total lymphocyte population (Fig. 9.13).

B lymphocytes are derived from bone marrow stem cells. The pluripotent stem cell is activated by interleukin (IL)-1 and IL-6 to differentiate into the lymphocyte stem cell (LSC). In general, the LSC gives rise to the progression of the pre-B cell, the lymphoblast, the B cell, and the terminal cell, the plasma cell. The plasma cell is responsible for antibody production and **humoral** immunity, antibodies to a specific antigen. T cells arise from the LSC, which migrates to the thymus. The thymus, a gland located above the heart, gives rise to the prothymocyte, T lymphoblast, and T cell responsible for cell-mediated immunity. This gland, although highly active in infants and children, is not functional in adults. Determining lymphocyte life span is difficult. Long-lived lymphocytes product cytokines, whereas short-lived lymphocytes produce antibodies. Plasma and tissue environmental influences either promote or delay longevity. There has been speculation that some lymphocytes may live up to 4 years.[7]

T and B cells are dependent on their interaction with their microenvironment: bone marrow versus thymus, versus lymph nodes, versus peripheral blood. Their specific derivation is defined from the surface membrane markers they possess and their stimulation toward a particular immune response. Classification of stages of T and B cells is complex and dominated by which CD markers or surface antigens they possess.

The Travel Path of Lymphocytes

Lymphocytes may originate in the bone marrow, the thymus, and the lymphatic system. Because the lymphatic system is a network of tissues, the travel path of lymphocytes from blood to thymus to lymphatics is less than straightforward. Most white cells proliferate and mature in the bone marrow and are released into peripheral circulation. From the circulation, they may either migrate to tissues or wind their way through circulation until they degenerate. Lymphocytes travel two paths. They either travel between areas of inflammation, or they move from the bone marrow to the thymus and then into secondary lymphoid tissue, the lymphatic system. Mature lymphocytes primarily move back and forth the between the lymphatic system, while imma-

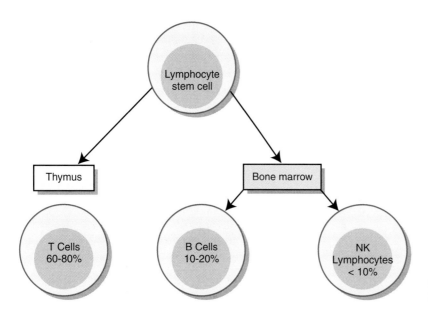

Figure 9.13 Subpopulations of lymphocytes.

ture lymphocytes move from the bone marrow to the thymus and then into the lymphatic system. Because the lymphocyte is a highly mobile cell, it will interact with the endothelial cells of blood vessels as it migrates to tissues. This migration is carefully orchestrated through a series of receptors and cytokines from the endothelial network. Lymphocytes spend far more time in travel through tissues than the marrow or circulation.[8] Extensive transit is meant to increase their opportunities to become exposed to foreign antigenic stimuli and mount an appropriate response.

Lymphocytes and the Development of Immunocompetency

Initially, lymphocytes that are developing and maturing in the bone marrow and thymus are not responsive to provocative antigens. It is only when they reach the lymphatic system that they begin to develop a response to antigenic stimulation and become immunocompetent. Migration through the lymphatic system is carefully orchestrated through a series of receptors, and chemokines on the endothelial network of blood vessels surrounding lymphatic tissue.[8] Immunoblasts are large activated lymphocytes capable of mustering an immune response. Antigenic presentation to lymphocytes may take many forms from altered cells to the body or foreign antigens or proteins. When a foreign antigen is presented to the body, it is usually phagocytized and destroyed by the macrophages of the lymph nodes or tissues. If this mechanism is not complete and some part of the invading mechanism is left behind, then an immune response begins to take place. Lymphocytes become activated and proceed to "battle" foreign antigens with many immune capabilities. Activated lymphocytes take on many roles and proliferate in the first few days after recognition of a foreign antigen or antigenic products. B cells begin to synthesize antibodies to the particular antigen as a primary response. Once the antigen is presented to T cells by macrophages or B cells, then T cells respond by participating in cell-mediated immunity activities. These include:

- Delayed hypersensitivity
- Tumor suppression
- Resistance to intracellular organisms

In addition to each of these responses, T cells release lymphokines, which activate B lymphocytes and assist in humoral immunity and the production of plasma cells. Therefore, T cells play a vital role in cell-mediated and humoral response and are essential to immune development.

The Response of Lymphocytes to Antigenic Stimulation

Once resting lymphocytes respond to antigenic stimulation, they begin to synthesize receptors, signals, or antigenic markers. T cells, which represent 60% to 85% of total lymphocytes, can be subdivided into two populations: T helper (CD4) or T cytotoxic/suppressor (CD8). T helper cells interact with macrocytes and macrophages, secrete cytokines, and promote humoral immunity. T-cytotoxic cells promote memory cells and help to eliminate non-self by promoting enzyme activity, which can significantly alter the cell membrane. B cells, which represent 10% to 20% of total lymphocytes, differentiate into plasma cells. This transformation takes place as T cells recognize antigens and release lymphokines. Lymphokines assist B lymphocytes in transforming into plasma cells, detecting antigens, and producing antibodies. NK cells represent a small subpopulation of lymphocytes with a highly specific function. These cells are non-T or non-B in origin and do not need antigenic stimulation to function. Originating in the bone marrow, they play a role primarily in resisting bacteria, viruses, and fungi.

Lymphocyte Cell Markers and the Cluster Designation (CD)

Before 1980, lymphocytes were demarcated by surface and cytoplasmic immunoglobulins, HLA markers, and terminal deoxynucleotidyl transferase (tDt) antigens. For a listing of CD markers in the unstimulated B and T cells, see Table 9.1. At present, most lymphocyte subpopulations are recognized by their CD markers. CD refers to *cluster designation*, a series of monoclonal antibodies manufactured by public and private companies to identify surface antigens on the many lymphocyte subsets. Lymphocytes can now by identified at successive stages in their maturation by their pattern of reaction to monoclonal antibodies. Most lymphocytes have several CD designations that they may initially possess and then lose or may carry with them throughout their maturation sequence.

LEUKOCYTE COUNT FROM THE COMPLETE BLOOD CELL COUNT TO THE DIFFERENTIAL

White cell counts that are reported on the CBC are directly counted from an automated instrument or by manual method. The age of the patient directly influences whether this number is within or outside of the reference range (Table 9.2). Pediatric reference ranges show more variability than do ranges for adults. Some of the peculiarities of the newborn include highest white counts at 3 months.

The WBC differential is an evaluation of the types of mature white cells in the peripheral circulation. Although only a snapshot of the white cell concentration at a particular moment in time, the differential offers valuable information as to the hematological status of an individual and their response to any circumstances which may alter hematological status. In general terms, the differential is performed on a well-stained, well-distributed peripheral smear.

The peripheral smear is evaluated for distribution at ×10 and then a white cell estimate is performed at ×40 (refer to Chapter 20 for procedures). Following this, a differential count is performed. One hundred white cells are counted and the percentage and identification of each type of white cell is recorded. These percentages are compared to the reference ranges for an individual according to age (Table 9.3). White cell estimates provide important quality control data for the technologist performing the differential. If the white cell estimate fails to agree with the automated count, then perhaps the wrong smear was pulled and an investigation should proceed to correct this error. In most cases, one hundred white cells are carefully counted and identified, but there are circumstances which may warrant counting two hundred white cells. Students will need to refer to the Standard Operating Procedure at each clinical site for recommendations for counting a 200-cell differential. If this is the case, the physician should be aware that a 200-cell count was performed. Table 9.4 lists general conditions when a 200 cell count differential may be desirable. Critical values outside of the reference range have been established for each clinical facility regarding the CBC and the differential. These values are usually flagged by the automated instrument and must be reported to the physician and/or the pathologist in a timely fashion. Laboratory personnel keep careful

records concerning notification of a patient with a critical value. Date, time, and person receiving the information are usually recorded. For a list of sample critical values refer to Table 9.5.

Manual Differential Versus Differential Scan

Most automated hematology instruments have the capacity to perform a differential count. This advance in instrumentation has dramatically shifted work patterns, because less time is spent in reviewing peripheral smears. When a differential is ordered and reported from instrumentation, there are some conditions in which the automated differential count may be questionable. If certain parameters in the differential have been flagged or if a peripheral smear needs to be reviewed as a result of a delta check or reflex testing, the peripheral smear is actually reviewed by a laboratory professional. For these circumstances, there are two levels of technologist review: a manual leukocyte differential count or a differential scan. A manual leukocyte differential count implies that 100 WBCs are counted along with red cell morphology and platelets. A diff scan implies that approximately 50 cells are reviewed to

Table 9.3 ⊙ Manual Differential Reference Ranges for Adults and Infants		
	Adults	**Up to 1 Year**
Segmented neutrophils	50% to 70%	20% to 44%
Bands	2% to 6%	0% to 5%
Lymphocytes	20% to 44%	48% to 78%
Monocytes	2% to 9%	2% to 11%
Eosinophils	0% to 4%	1% to 4%
Basophils	0% to 2%	0% to 2%

Table 9.2 ⊙ Leukocyte Counts at Different Ages*	
Age	**Leukocyte Count**
Birth	4 to 40
4 Years	5 to 15
Adult	4 to 11

*All values × 10⁹/L.

Table 9.4 ⊙ When to Consider Counting More Than 100 Cells on Differential*
• WBC >35.0 × 10⁹/L
• Lymphocytes > 40% or <17 %
• Monocytes >12%
• Blasts (first-time patient)

*These values will vary with every clinical site.

Table 9.5 ○ Sample Critical Values	
WBC	Low 3.0 × 10⁹/L
	High 25.0 × 10⁹/L
Hemoglobin	Low 7.0 g/dL
	High 17.0 g/dL
Platelet	Low 50.0 × 10⁹/L
	High 1.0 × 10¹²/L
Differential	Refer to Standard Operating Procedure for each facility for criteria. *Blasts,* which are reported on a new patient, are always a critical result.

Table 9.6 ○ Absolute Reference Range for Adult Differential*	
• Neutrophils	1.4 to 6.5
• Lymphocytes	1.2 to 3.4
• Monocytes	0.11 to 0.59
• Eosinophils	0.0 to 0.5

*All values ×10⁹/L.

verify the automated result. The criteria for performing either a full differential or a "diff scan," are usually well outlined in the standard operating procedure for each clinical facility. Generally, these criteria include items such as total leukocyte count, lymphocytes, and monocytes above a certain level, an abnormal scatter plot, or thrombocytopenia. Patients whose peripheral smears need review usually represent a pool of individuals who are seriously ill or whose conditions are deteriorating or changing. Needless to say, reviewing peripheral smears on these patients requires a high level of morphological skill from the laboratory professional.

Relative Versus Absolute Values

Relative and absolute counts are terms referring to the white cell differential. The absolute count refers to the count derived from the total white count multiplied by the percentage of any particular white cell. The relative count refers to the percentage of a particular cell counted from the 100 WBC differential. Absolute reference ranges have been compiled for each cell in the white cell differential (Table 9.6). For an example of how to calculate and interpret the relative and absolute count, see below:

If the WBC is 5.0 × 10⁹/L

And the differential reads:

Segmented neutrophils: 40% (Ref. range = 50% to 70%)

Bands: 3% (Ref. range = 2% to 6%)

Lymphocytes: 55% (Ref. range = 20% to 44%)

Monocytes: 2% (Ref. range = 2% to 9%)

Then the absolute count of lymphocytes would be 5000 × 0.55 = 2500.

Reference range for absolute lymphocyte count = 1200 to 3400

In this patient, there is a relative lymphocytosis but not an absolute lymphocytosis.

CONDENSED CASE

A routine CBC was received in the clinical laboratory on a patient who had been receiving daily blood work. On this particular day, the computer flagged (delta checked) a variety of parameters pertaining to the CBC. The parameters that were flagged were: WBC, Hemoglobin, Hematocrit, and MCV. **What are the steps needed to investigate the discrepancy in this patient's results?**

Answer

1. Realize that the delta check is the historical reference on the patient. If the results are flagged, then there is a discrepancy in patient results.
2. Visually inspect the CBC tubes, and peel back the label looking for identification.
3. Check the sample for a clot.
4. Re-run the sample to ensure that there is the proper amount of sample and proper mixing.
5. Check whether there is a transfusion history on the patient.
6. Call the floor and ask how the sample was drawn.

After performing these steps, decide on a course of action.

Summary Points

- The myeloid:erythroid ratio (M:E) is 4:1.

- Segmented neutrophils are held in the marginating pool for 7 to 10 days before release to circulation.

- The white cell series in order of least mature to most mature is myeloblast, promyelocyte, myelocyte, metamyelocyte, band, and segmented neutrophils.

- Cell identification is based on cell size, N:C ratio, presence or absence of granules, presence or absence of nucleoli, chromatin pattern, and texture of cytoplasm.

- The marginating pool designates those white cells located along the vessel endothelium.

- The circulating pool designates those white cells present in the bloodstream.

- Lymphocytes originate not only from the bone marrow but also from the thymus and the lymphatic system.

- The bone marrow and the thymus are the primary lymphoid organs.

- Spleen, lymph nodes, Peyer's patches, and the tonsils are the secondary lymphoid organs.

- The lymphatic system plays an important role in blood filtration, fluid balance, antibody generation, and lymphopoiesis.

- T cells represent 60% to 80% of the total lymphocyte count.

- B cells represent 10% to 20% of the total lymphocyte count.

- T helper and T cytotoxic/suppressor cells are essential in cell-mediated immunity.

- B cells support humoral immunity, which is antibody production by plasma cells.

- Absolute counts are derived from the total white counts multiplied by the relative percentage of a particular cell in the differential.

CASE STUDY

A 45-year-old woman presented to the emergency department with vague complaints of dizziness, right-sided abdominal pain, and intermittent blurred vision. A baseline CBC was drawn with the following results:

WBC	6.5×10^9/L
RBC	4.02×10^{12}/L
Hgb	13.2 g/dL
Hct	37.3%
MCV	86 fL
MCH	24.2 pg
MCHC	30.3×10^9/L
Platelets	30.3×10^9/L

Is this a critical platelet count?

Insights to the Case Study

The patient was admitted to the hospital as a result of the extremely low platelet count. The risk of spontaneous bleeding was a consideration. No further testing was order because it was the weekend and a hematology consult could not be arranged before Monday. The patient had two subsequent CBCs during this time and eventually a peripheral smear was pulled. Once the peripheral smear was stained and reviewed, the technologist noted that most of the platelets were spreading around the neutrophils, a condition known as platelet satellitism (see Fig. 10.18). This condition is a reaction by some patients to the EDTA in the lavender top tubes. Once this was observed, the patient's blood was redrawn in a sodium citrate tube and cycled for a platelet count. The platelet count on this sample was recorded at 230,000. In the usual course of events, a flag on the platelet count would probably not warrant a peripheral smear review. However, this situation may serve as a catalyst for a review of the flagging policy.

Review Questions

1. The primary lymphoid organs are the
   a. liver and spleen.
   b. gallbladder and liver.
   c. bone marrow and thymus.
   d. spleen and tonsils.

2. Which one of these features distinguishes a monocyte from a lymphocyte?
   a. Nucleoli
   b. Abundant gray-blue cytoplasm
   c. Round, flattened nucleus
   d. Large blue-black granules

3. In which stage of neutrophilic maturation are specific granules?
   a. Myeloblast
   b. Metamyelocyte
   c. Myelocyte
   d. Band

4. Which CD marker is specific for monocytes?
   a. CD45
   b. CD19
   c. CD20
   d. CD14

5. Which subpopulation of T cells alters the cell membrane?
   a. T cytotoxic
   b. T helper
   c. NK cells
   d. None of the above

● TROUBLESHOOTING

What Do I Do When Samples Are Sent to the Lab Within Minutes on the Same Patient and the Results Do Not Match?

A 74-year-old patient who was in the critical care unit was having daily hematology blood work performed. The first sample was sent to the laboratory at 2:23 P.M. Hemoglobin and hematocrit were the only analyses requested. The results were verified without delta flags. The second sample was sent 20 minutes later with a request for hemoglobin and hematocrit. Both samples were cycled through the automated instrument and a full CBC was obtained. Only the hemoglobin and hematocrit were reported. The results:

	First Sample at 2:23 P.M.	Second Sample at 2:43 P.M.
WBC	16.9×10^9/L	12.5×10^9/L
Hgb	9.3 g/dL	8.4 g/dL
Hct	26.5%	24.2%
Platelets	104×10^9/L	97×10^9/L

Hemoglobin and hematocrit were the only two tests ordered and both results seem totally verifiable. Since the technologist had access to the complete CBC on the computer screen, she noticed the disparity in white counts. The change in white count, however, is troubling and alerted the technologist to the possible problems with the sample. She considered these possibilities:

1. Is the specimen clotted or contaminated?
2. Did the same patient have blood drawn for specimen 1 and for specimen 2?
3. How was the specimen obtained?

Both samples were checked for clots. After contacting the floor nurse, the following information was obtained. Both samples were drawn through an arterial line, an "A line." Arterial lines are inserted in critically ill patients who have frequent blood draws and receive frequent medications. The procedure when drawing through an A line is to draw off and discard the first 10 mL of blood and then proceed with the blood draw, usually filling tubes directly from the line. In this case, the blood draw for the first sample was difficult and the blood from the A line was not free flowing. The second sample, however, was obtained without difficulty. Proper blood drawing procedure with the A line was followed with both samples. After consultation with the lead technologist and the nurse, it was decided to release the second set of results and remove the first set from the computer. The patient did have a blood bank history and had received units of packed red cells and fresh frozen plasma. This information, however, did not have relevance in this case, considering that the parameter in question was the white count.

WORD KEY

Cervical • Relating to the neck

Inguinal • Relating to the groin area

Subclavian • Situated beneath the clavicle or collarbone

Thoracic • Relating to the chest

Humoral • When relating to immunity it means antibody formation

Thymus • Ductless gland located above the heart that plays a role in immunity

References

1. Turgeon ML. Clinical Hematology: Theory and Procedures. Philadelphia: Lippincott Williams & Wilkins, 1999; 160.
2. Parsons D, Marty J, Strauss R. Cell biology, disorders of neutrophils, infectious mononucleosis and reactive lymphocytes. In: Clinical Hematology and Fundamentals of Hemostasis, 4th ed. Philadelphia: FA Davis, 2002; 252.
3. Heckner F, Lehman P, Kao Y. Practical Microscopic Hematology, 4th ed. Philadelphia: Lea and Febiger, 1994; 14–16.
4. Carr JH, Rodak BF. Clinical Hematology Atlas. Philadelphia: WB Saunders, 1999.
5. O'Connor BH. A Color Atlas and Instructional Manual of Peripheral Blood Cell Morphology. Baltimore: Williams & Wilkins, 1984.
6. Brown B. Hematology: Principles and Procedures, 6th ed. Philadelphia: Lippincott Williams & Wilkins, 2000; 74–79.
7. Rossi MI, Yokota T, Medin KL, et al. B lymphopoiesis is active throughout human life, but there are developmental age related changes. Blood 101:576–584, 2003.
8. Steine-Martin EA, Lotspeich-Steininger CA, Koepke JA. Clinical Hematology: Principles, Procedures, and Correlations, 2nd ed. Philadelphia: Lippincott, 1998; 326–327.

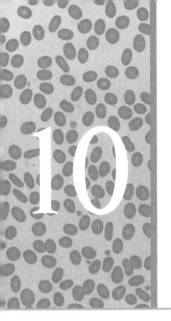

10

Abnormalities of White Cells: Quantitative, Qualitative, and the Lipid Storage Diseases

Betty Ciesla

Introduction to the White Cell Disorders

Quantitative Changes in the White Cells
  Conditions With Increased Neutrophils
  Conditions With Increased Eosinophils
  Conditions With Increased Basophils
  Conditions With Increased Monocytes
  Specific Terminology Relating to Quantitative White Cell Changes

Stages of White Cell Phagocytosis

Qualitative Defects of White Cells
  Toxic Changes in White Cells
  Nuclear Abnormalities: Hypersegmentation

Hereditary White Cell Disorders
  May-Hegglin Anomaly
  Alder's Anomaly (Alder-Reilly Anomaly)
  Pelger-Huët Anomaly
  Chediak-Higashi Syndrome

Reactive Lymphocytosis in Common Disease States
  Other Sources of Reactive Lymphocytosis

The Effect of Human Immunodeficiency Virus/Acquired Immune Deficiency Syndrome on Hematology Parameters

Lipid Storage Diseases (Briefly)
  Common Features of a Few of the Lipid Storage Diseases
  Bone Marrow Cells in Lipid Storage Disorders

Bacteria and Other Unexpected White Cell Changes

Objectives

After completing this chapter, the student will be able to:

1. Recall the physiology and function of granulocytes.

2. Describe the steps involved in phagocytosis.

3. Identify conditions that cause a quantitative increase or decrease in a particular white cell line.

4. Describe the changes observed when white cells respond to infection.

5. Identify the acquired and inherited qualitative changes in the white cell.

6. Identify conditions that lead to hyposegmentation or hypersegmentation of the segmented neutrophils.

7. Define the probable causes for an increased lymphocyte count.

8. Define the differences seen in an adult's versus a child's lymphocyte count.

9. Describe the effects of the human immunodeficiency virus on the complete blood count and the peripheral smear.

10. Recall the reactive symptoms of infectious mononucleosis and cytomegalovirus.

11. Define white cell–related terms such as *leukocytosis, left shift, leukemoid reaction,* and *leukoerythroblastic reaction.*

12. Briefly describe the lipid storage diseases, such as Gaucher's, Niemann-Pick, and Tay-Sachs diseases.

INTRODUCTION TO THE WHITE CELL DISORDERS

Because white cells have such a short time span in the peripheral circulation, alterations either in the quantity of or the quality of a particular cell can be quite dramatic. With the normal differential reference ranges for adults and children as a benchmark, any increase or decrease in a particular type of cell signals the body's unique response to "assaults" of any kind. Infection, inflammation, chronic disease, parasitic infestations, etc., each represents an unexpected occurrence, an opportunity for white cells to mobilize. As white cells respond to infection or other stimuli, changes are seen in the number of and types of a particular cell line. If a cell line is increased, the suffix used to designate an increase is "osis" or "philia," such as "eosinophilia" and "leukocytosis." If a cell line is decreased, the suffix used to designate a decrease is "penia," such as "neutropenia." Changes are observed in the complete blood count (CBC) as well as in the peripheral blood smear. An interesting situation is the role that granules from a particular cell line play in producing symptoms. For example, eosinophilic granules contain histamine. In allergy patients, eosinophils are usually seen in excess. Once histamine is released from eosinophils, this chemical stimulates allergy-related symptoms such as watery, itching eyes and **rhinorrhea.** Interestingly, most allergy medications contain antihistamines, formulated to block allergy symptoms.

In most cases, patients who have newly acquired infections will show an increase in white cells from the reference range. Care must be taken, however, when assessing a patient with an increased white count. Ethnic differences have been suggested in the normal white cell reference range, with blacks having a lower normal white count than whites. A symptomatology that reflects an infection combined with an elevated white count strongly suggests an infectious process.[1]

QUANTITATIVE CHANGES IN THE WHITE CELLS

Various conditions give rise to increases or decreases in a particular cell line. These conditions are usually transient, and once the underlying condition has resolved itself, for the most part the counts return to normal. A partial list of disorders that increase or decrease leukocytes is included. Lymphocytes will be considered under a separate heading.

Conditions With Increased Neutrophils

- Infections
- Inflammatory response
- Stress response
- Malignancies

Conditions With Increased Eosinophils

- Skin disease
- Parasitic disease
- Transplant rejection[2]
- Myeloproliferative disorders

Conditions With Increased Basophils

- Myeloproliferative disorders
- Hypersensitivity reactions
- Ulcerative colitis

Conditions With Increased Monocytes

- Chronic infections like tuberculosis
- Malignancies
- Leukemias with a strong monocytic component
- Bone marrow failure

With regard to a decrease in cell lines, perhaps the most significant finding is neutropenia in which the absolute neutrophil count is less than 2.0×10^9/L. This occurs due to medications, bone marrow assaults due to chemicals, viral infections, or splenic sequestration.[3]

Specific Terminology Relating to Quantitative White Cell Changes

For the most part, four terms are used to describe white cell conditions: *leukocytosis, left shift, leukemoid reaction,* and the *leukoerythroblastic picture.* These terms are usually not used interchangeably, but they are a source of confusion for the student. Leukocytosis simply means that an increase in white cells has occurred; left shift means that the bone marrow is responding to the increased white count by sending out younger cells (metamyelocytes, bands) into the peripheral circulation. Leukemoid reaction is an exaggerated response to infections and inflammation in which the baseline leukocyte count may be between 20 and 50×10^9/L. This count may appear as preleukemic; however, the white cells that are seen in the peripheral smear are slightly immature to mature with no blasts present. The leukoerythroblastic picture is a significant feature of the myeloproliferative disorders and refers to the presence in the peripheral smear of immature white cells, immature red cells (nucleated RBCs [RBCs]), and platelet abnormalities (Table 10.1).

STAGES OF WHITE CELL PHAGOCYTOSIS

The phagocytic process by which bacteria and other infectious agents are recognized and destroyed is a critical function of neutrophils and monocytes. The neutrophil role in phagocytosis is localized and immediate; the monocyte role is related to immune response and more tissue oriented. The process by which bacteria are digested and immobilized can be broken down in several simplified steps (Fig. 10.1).

- Stage 1—CHEMOTAXIS: Foreign body invades tissues; neutrophils, which usually move in random motion through the tissue, are attracted directly to site of invasion through chemical signals sent by foreign body (bacteria). More neutrophils mobilize and rush to site of infection.
- Stage 2—OPSONIZATON: Neutrophilic attachment of the invading foreign body can only take place once the foreign body has been opsonized or prepared to be ingested through interaction with the complement system and other immunoglobulins.
- Stage 3—INGESTION: The opsonized foreign body is ingested by the neutrophil. The foreign body is engulfed by the neutrophilic pseudopod membranes.
- Stage 4—KILLING: The neutrophilic granules release their contents, which contain various lytic elements. The pH of the cell is reduced and hydrogen peroxide is produced by the neutrophil as a result of respiratory burst and released to accelerate the destruction process. The neutrophil is also destroyed in this process.

Bacteremia or sepsis may occur if invading organisms or foreign bodies are not destroyed upon entry into the body. They may locate in secondary sites such as the lymph nodes, where they will rapidly multiply and release toxins.

Phagocytic activity is a complex process involving phagocytic cells, the complement system, cytotoxins, and acute-phase reactants. Each of these systems must have coordinated activities to ensure that pathogens will be destroyed[4] (Table 10.2).

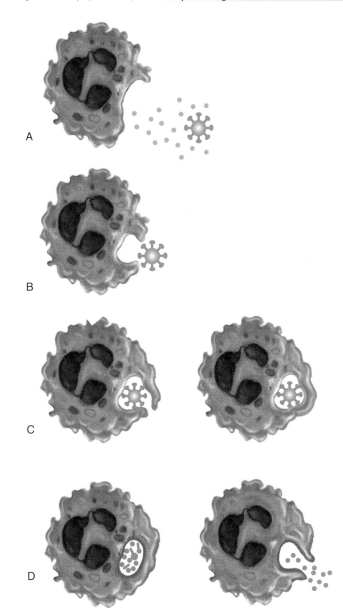

Figure 10.1 Mechanism of phagocytosis. Stages depicted are (*A*) chemotaxis and directed motility, (*B*) opsonization, (*C*) ingestion, (*D*) degranulation and digestion.

QUALITATIVE DEFECTS OF WHITE CELLS

Qualitative changes of the white cell take place either in the cytoplasm or the nucleus. These changes are classified as either inherited or acquired. Acquired defects are seen with much greater frequency than inherited abnormalities. Once a patient has developed an increased white count, toxic changes of the white cells usually occur due to stress during maturation and as a result of activity in the circulation or tissue. A

Table 10.1 ● White Cell Terminology

- **Neutrophilia** Increase in segmented neutrophils
- **Leukocytosis** Increase in white cells
- **Left shift** Increase in bands and metamyelocytes in the peripheral smear; seen in response to infection
- **Leukemoid reaction** Exaggerated response to infection; resulting in high white count and increased numbers of metamyelocytes, bands, and possibly younger cells
- **Leukoerythroblastic picture** Immature white cells, immature red cells, and platelet abnormalities seen in the peripheral smear

careful and patient review of the peripheral smear of these individuals will reveal many of the changes discussed (Fig. 10.2).

Toxic Changes in White Cells

The visible response of white cells to infection or inflammation occurs along two paths. As white cells increase, what is usually seen in the peripheral smear is either an increase in the number of segmented neutrophils giving rise to a neutrophilia or a shift to the left, where younger cells are noted. In either of these cases, toxic changes such as toxic granulation, toxic vacuolization, or the presence of Döhle bodies may be observed and should be carefully sought.

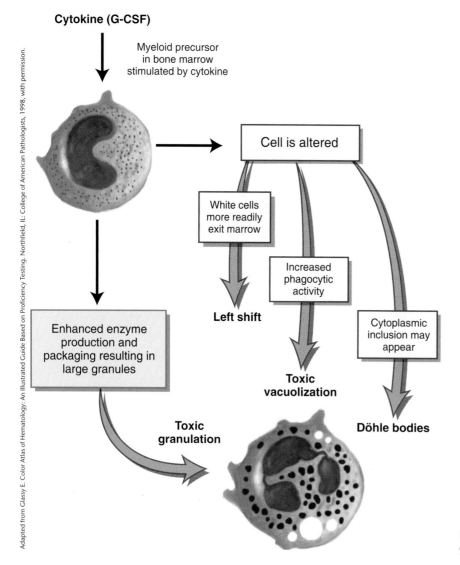

Cytokine (G-CSF)

Myeloid precursor in bone marrow stimulated by cytokine

Cell is altered

White cells more readily exit marrow

Left shift

Increased phagocytic activity

Toxic vacuolization

Cytoplasmic inclusion may appear

Döhle bodies

Enhanced enzyme production and packaging resulting in large granules

Toxic granulation

Figure 10.2 The evolution of toxic granulation.

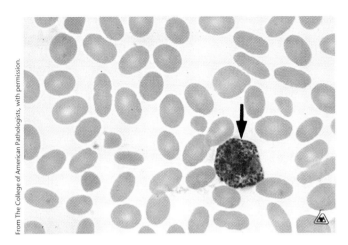

Figure 10.3   Toxic granulation. Note heavier granulation throughout the cytoplasm.

Toxic Granulation

Normal granulation in the segmented neutrophils shows a dustlike appearance, with the red and blue granules being difficult to observe. Toxic granulation is excessive granulation in amount and intensity, with more prominent granules in segmented neutrophils in direct response to enhanced lysosome enzyme production. These granules are more frequent and have much more vivid blue-black coloration (Fig. 10.3). Cluster of toxic granules usually appear in neutrophils. At times the granulation is so heavy as to resemble basophilic granules.

Toxic Vacuolization

This change occurs in segmented neutrophils. Vacuoles appear in the cytoplasm of this cell and may be small or large (Fig. 10.4). Prolonged exposure of blood to drugs

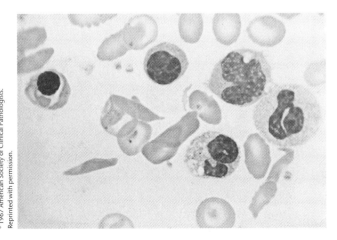

Figure 10.4   Toxic vacuolization. Note large vacuoles located in the cytoplasm.

Table 10.2 ● Essential Elements Leading to Phagocytosis

Cells
- Neutrophils: Attracted to pathogen, are activated by endothelial cell surface receptors, will recruit more neutrophils to infection site through cell surface receptors
- Monocytes: Cells in transit between marrow, tissues circulating blood, will move to area of stimuli and possess lytic enzymes
- Basophils, eosinophils: React in concert with complement and hormones to suppress inflammation

Complements
- C5a: Coats the pathogen, making it "tasty" to phagocytic cells
- C3b: Causes increase in vascular permeability

Cytokines
- Tumor necrosis factor
- Interleukins 1, 8, and 10

such as sulfonamides or chloroquine or prolonged storage may lead to phagocytosis of granules or cytoplasmic contents.[5] Additionally, small uniformly placed vacuoles may be seen in peripheral smear made from blood that has held for long periods of time. In cases where the creation of peripheral smears has been delayed, pseudo-vacuolization will be recognized. This phenomenon must be distinguished from the pathogenic variety. Larger vacuoles unevenly distributed throughout the cytoplasm usually signal serious infections and possible **sepsis.** Studies have shown that when 10% of neutrophils are affected by vacuoles in a fresh sample, this ranks as a serious and significant **prognostic indicator**[6] (Table 10.3).

Table 10.3 ● Significant Alterations in Neutrophils in Peripheral Smears

- Döhle bodies
- Toxic granulation
- Toxic vacuolization
- Hyposegmentation
- Hypersegmentation
- Bacteria (intracellular or extracellular)
- Platelet satellitism
- Chediak-Higashi granules

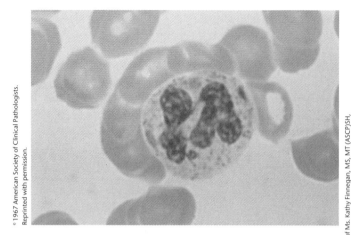

Figure 10.5   Döhle bodies are inclusions that are pale, peripherally located in the cytoplasm, and rodlike.

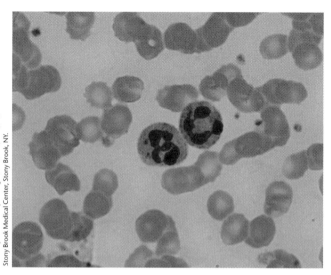

Figure 10.6   Human ehrlichiosis.

Dohle Bodies

These cytoplasmic inclusions consist of ribosomal RNA. They range from 1 to 5 μm in size, are located near the cytoplasmic membrane, and appear as a rod-shaped pale bluish-gray structure (Fig. 10.5). These transient inclusions are frequently observed in neutrophils but may be seen in monocytes and bands. Dohle bodies are difficult to observe under light microscopy, and peripheral smears must be carefully scrutinized for their presence. Dohle bodies may also be seen in nonpathological conditions such as pregnancy.

Human Ehrlichiosis

Named for the noted microbiologist, Paul Ehrlich, human ehrlichiosis infections are a fairly new group of tick-borne diseases, which show a notable white cell inclusion in some cases. There are two varieties: human monocytic ehrlichiosis (HME), caused by the *Rickettsia*-like bacteria *Ehrlichia chafeensis*, and human granulocytic ehrlichiosis (HE), caused by the *Rickettsia*-like bacteria *Ehrlichia phagocytophilia*. These diseases are difficult to diagnose because patients show vague symptomatology that is often mistaken for other infectious diseases. HME cases are usually located in the southeastern and mid-Atlantic United States[9] and show in initial flu-like presentation. Patients with HE, who are usually located in the midwestern United States, show an acute onset of high fever, chills, and headache.[10] Common to both illnesses is low white count, extremely elevated liver enzymes, and thrombocytopenia. Inclusions may be seen in the granulocytes or monocytes from the bone marrow, and these morula, mulberry-like, inclusions are large, 1 to 3 μm, and resemble berries in appearance

(Fig. 10.6). These inclusions, if identified, are specific for these diseases but are difficult to observe and are not seen in every case. However, peripheral smears and bone marrow smears should be carefully reviewed for identification of these inclusion bodies.

Nuclear Abnormalities: Hypersegmentation

Normal segmented neutrophils will have between three and five lobes in the nucleus. Hypersegmentation is defined as a segmented neutrophilic nucleus having more than five lobes (Fig. 10.7). This condition is usually seen in the megaloblastic processes such as folic acid, pernicious anemia, or vitamin B_{12} deficiency and is usually accompanied by oval macrocytes.

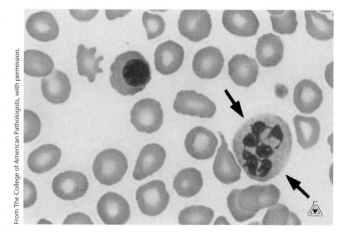

Figure 10.7   Hypersegmented neutrophil.

HEREDITARY WHITE CELL DISORDERS

May-Hegglin Anomaly

This inherited disorder is associated with thrombocytopenia and giant platelets. Abnormal bleeding may be seen in a small number of affected individuals. Döhle bodies are seen in the cytoplasm of neutrophils and are larger than the Dohle bodies seen in neutrophils responding to infections or inflammation.

Alder's Anomaly (Alder-Reilly Anomaly)

This rare genetic disorder is associated with the presence of coarse dark granules in neutrophils, lymphocytes, monocytes, eosinophils, and basophils (Fig. 10.8). This granulation is thought to consist of lipid depositions in the cytoplasm as a result of decreased mucopolysaccharide production.[7] Prominent deposition of granules in *every* cell line is a differentiating feature between this condition and toxic granulation, which appears in clusters only in neutrophils and monocytes.

Pelger-Huët Anomaly

This fairly common inherited disorder shows hyposegmentation of the nucleus of segmented neutrophils. In heterozygotes, the nucleus is seen as peanut shaped, dumb-bell shaped, or pince-nez shaped (Fig. 10.9). In homozygotes, the nucleus is spherical with no lobes and prominent nuclear clumping. Initially, when observing cells with the Pelger-Huët anomaly, they may appear as bands or metamyelocytes. When considering these cells in a peripheral smear, it is important

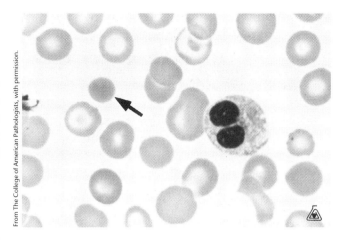

Figure 10.9   Pelger-Huët. Note spherocyte (at *arrow*) and the typical bilobed appearance of Pelger-Huët cells.

to make two judgments. Is the hyposegmentation seen in the majority of neutrophils? Is the nuclear content mature? Even experienced morphologists have misidentified these cells as bands or metamyelocytes, greatly skewing the peripheral smear results. In a true Pelger-Huët anomaly, almost 70% to 95% of the neutrophils will show hyposegmentation. The cells, however, will be functional neutrophils. There are a number of conditions in which the neutrophils may present with a pseudo–Pelger-Huët look, such as leukemias, myeloproliferative disorders, and severe infections.

Chediak-Higashi Syndrome

This is a rare autosomal disorder of neutrophilic granules. Neutrophils in these individuals show giant gray-green cytoplasmic granules (Fig. 10.10). Lymphocytes

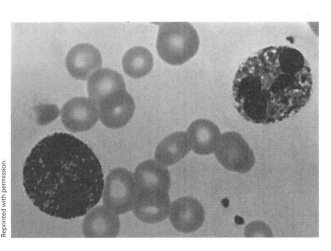

Figure 10.8   Alder's anomaly. Note deep granulation.

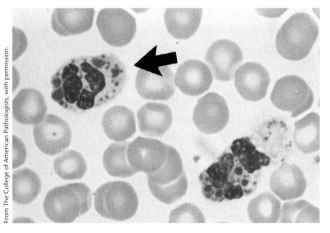

Figure 10.10   Chediak-Higashi anomaly. Note large gray-green granules in the cytoplasm.

and monocytes show a single red granule in the cytoplasm. Current studies suggest that there is a defective fusion protein in these individuals, which is crucial to lysosomal secretion.[8] White cells in patients with Chediak-Higashi syndrome are not fully functioning and show reduced chemotaxis and bactericidal killing function. Affected children show neutropenia, **albinism,** and photophobia and develop recurrent infections with *Staphylococcus aureus*. Hepatosplenomegaly and liver failure may develop. Platelet function is affected with abnormal bleeding times and small vessel bleeding. The prognosis is poor in most children, who usually die young due to complications of infections.

REACTIVE LYMPHOCYTOSIS IN COMMON DISEASE STATES

It is normal for young children between the ages of 1 and 4 to have a relative lymphocytosis. The white cell differential in this age group will show a reversal in the number of lymphocytes to segmented neutrophils from the adult reference range. The lymphocytes, however, will have normal morphology (Fig. 10.11). By far the most common disease entity displaying variation in lymphocytes is infectious mononucleosis. This is viral illness caused by the Epstein-Barr virus (EBV), a member of the human herpes virus family, type 4. Although young children may become infected with EBV, the virus has a peak incidence at around 20 years of age. Most adults have been exposed to EBV by midlife, and this is recognized by demonstratable antibody production whether or not they have had an active case of infectious mononucleosis. The virus is found in body fluids, especially saliva, and is frequently passed through exchanges such as kissing, sharing food utensils, or drinking cups. The virus, which incubates for 3 to 4 weeks, enters through the oral passages and infects B lymphocytes. Normal lymphocytes become infected and are transformed into "reactive" (old terminology, "atypical") lymphocytes. Symptoms include sore throat, fatigue, anorexia, fever, and headache. The lymph nodes are usually always enlarged and there may be hepatosplenomegaly. Most individuals have a self-limited course of disease, which is uncomfortable but uncomplicated. Autoimmune hemolytic anemia and elevated liver enzymes may be a complication in less than 1% of patients.

Differential diagnosis includes careful examination of the peripheral smear, the results of rapid agglutination tests, and more sophisticated procedures such as ELISA or indirect immunofluorescence, which track

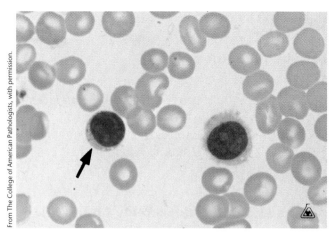

From The College of American Pathologists, with permission.

Figure 10.11   Normal lymphocyte.

EBV antigen positivity and measure IgG titers in **convalescence.** The peripheral smear is particularly impressive and usually shows a reactive lymphocytosis, with between 10% and 60% reactive lymphocytes (Fig. 10.12). Morphologically, these lymphocytes are larger than the normal large lymphocytes with an abundant royal blue cytoplasm, sometimes scalloping the red cells. They are easily identified with clumped chromatin material and must be recorded separately (on the differential counter) from the other nonreactive normal lymphocytes seen in the smear (Table 10.4). At times, the diagnosis of infectious mononucleosis is difficult to make in the event that the rapid agglutination test is negative, which it is in 10% of cases.[11] The clinician should rely on symptoms, peripheral smear, and professional experience in pronouncing the disease. Molecular diagnostics is highly accurate but is expensive and a specialized procedure. There is no treatment for infectious mononucleosis except for bed rest and treatment of additional symptoms or possible subsequent infections.

Other Sources of Reactive Lymphocytosis

In most cases, viral disorders affect the CBC in a similar pattern. Most have an increased white count with a depressed number of segmented neutrophils and an increased lymphocyte count. Conditions such as cytomegalovirus and hepatitis A, B, and C viruses may show reactive lymphocytes of a morphology similar to infectious mononucleosis. Cytomegalovirus (CMV) is a virus that is endemic worldwide. A member of the herpes family, this virus discovered in 1957 is similar to EBV. The virus has been isolated from respiratory secretions, urine, semen, and cervical secretions, but it also found in transplanted organs and donor blood. Indeed,

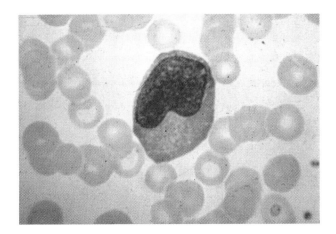

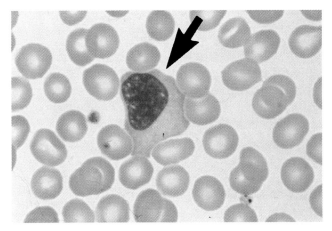

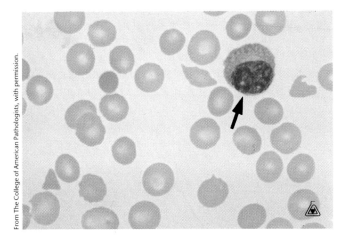

From The College of American Pathologists, with permission.

Figure 10.12 Reactive lymphocytes. Note large cells with abundant basophilic cytoplasm.

	Table 10.4 ⊙ Lymphocyte Morphologies	
	Reactive Lymphocyte	**Resting Small Lymphocyte**
Size	Large (9 to 30 μm)	Small (8 to 12 μm)
N:C ratio	Low to moderate	High to moderate
Cytoplasm	Abundant, color-less to dark blue	Scant, colorless to light blue
Nucleus	Round to irregular	Round
Chromatin	Coarse to moder-ately fine	Coarse
Nucleoli	Absent to distinct	Absent
Typing	Polyclonal	Polyclonal

individuals and the other vulnerable populations, CMV disease can be severe and potentially fatal. Congenital CMV occurs when the mother develops an active CMV infection or when her latent CMV becomes reactivated due to pregnancy. It is the leading congenital viral disease. Affected infants may show low birth weight, jaundice, and enlarged spleen and the disease may predispose to psychomotor defects or deafness. Often, affected mothers are not even aware that they are infected. Donor blood administered to premature infants, multiply transfused populations, or immunocompromised patients must be CMV negative.

THE EFFECT OF HUMAN IMMUNODEFICIENCY VIRUS/ ACQUIRED IMMUNE DEFICIENCY SYNDROME ON HEMATOLOGY PARAMETERS

The HIV is the causative agent of acquired immunodeficiency syndrome (AIDS). In this disease, immune function is eventually obliterated and patients frequently die of opportunistic infections such as *Pneumocystis carinii* or *Mycobacterium avium* or the neoplasm Kaposi's sarcoma. Lymphocytes are primarily involved in this disease process, particularly CD4 helper, inducer cells and CD8 suppressor, cytotoxic cells. The normal ratio of CD4 to CD8 is 2:1. In HIV infection, the level of CD4 is drastically reduced, with the ratio being reversed, leading to a decline in immune capabilities. The CBC shows a pancytopenia with neutropenia, anemia, and a thrombocytopenia. The lymphocytes will show reactive changes such as extremely basophilic cytoplasm or possibly clefting and vacuolization.

40% to 90% of all blood donors show anti-CMV titers, indicating that they have been exposed and have mounted an antibody response. Most individuals have a subclinical infection and do not even realize that they have had a viral infection. Some individuals have a mononucleosis-like syndrome with low-grade fever and flu-like symptoms. But to immunocompromised

Table 10.5 ⊙ Enzyme Deficiencies in Specific Lipid Storage Diseases	
Disease	**Missing Enzyme**
Gaucher's disease	β-Glucocerebrosidase
Niemann-Pick disease	Sphingomyelinase
Tay-Sachs disease	Hexosaminidase A

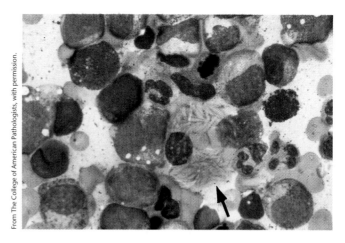

Figure 10.13 Gaucher's cells (BM). Note the crinkled tissue paper appearance of the cytoplasm.

LIPID STORAGE DISEASES (BRIEFLY)

The lipid storage diseases are a group of diseases in which a strategic metabolic enzyme is missing or inactive, usually as a result of a single gene deletion (see Table 10.5). Because of this missing enzyme, undigested metabolic products accumulate in cells and cell integrity is affected. Cells of the reticuloendothelial system (RES) are most often affected. The RES is a network of cells seen throughout the circulation and tissues that provide the phagocytic defense system. Histiocytes, monocytes, macrophages, and the cells of the bone marrow, liver, spleen, and lymph nodes comprise this network. Consequently, large, easily identifiable cells specific to each disease are located in the bone marrow and are part of the diagnostic picture of many of these disorders. For this reason, these disorders are not frequently observed in the clinical laboratory.

Common Features of a Few of the Lipid Storage Diseases

Gaucher's, Tay-Sachs, and Niemann-Pick are the three most common lipid storage diseases, and they have many common features. All are autosomal recessive disorders as a result of a single-gene mutation. Abnormal facial features and liver enlargement are seen in all but Tay-Sachs. Although there is a wide range of clinical presentation, from infant onset to adult onset, those individuals with infant onset have a more severe clinical presentation and a shorter life span. Many of these diseases have a high incidence in the northeast European Jewish population (the Ashkenazi), and for this reason prenatal counseling and genetic screening are highly recommended in affected or extended families. Central nervous system involvement is often a feature of infantile forms of the disease, especially Tay-Sachs, and short life spans usually prevail.[12] There is no cure for the lipid storage diseases, and for the most severe manifestations,

supportive therapy is all that can be offered. Enzyme replacement therapy using biosynthetic enzyme material is available in limited qualities.[13] Bone marrow transplantation is also available, yet the risks and benefits of this procedure in young children must be carefully considered.

Bone Marrow Cells in Lipid Storage Disorders

Gaucher's and Niemann-Pick diseases each have specific bone marrow cells that are representative of the particular disorder. For Gaucher's disease, the cell is large, 20 to 100 μm, with rod-shaped inclusions that appear like crinkled tissue paper in the bone marrow (Fig. 10.13). For Niemann-Pick, the cell is equally large but appears round with evenly sized lipid accumulations (Fig. 10.14). In their own right, each of these cells is

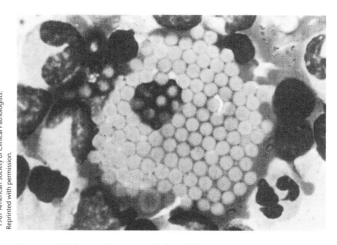

Figure 10.14 Niemann-Pick cell (BM). Cytoplasm shows lipid accumulation.

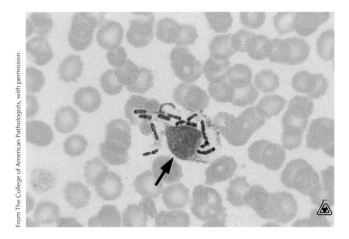

Figure 10.15   Intracellular bacteria in a segmented neutrophil.

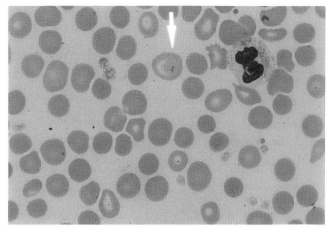

Figure 10.17   Precipitated stain, not bacteria.

striking on bone marrow examination because they are infrequently observed. In Tay-Sachs disease, there is no large identifiable bone marrow cell, yet most of these individuals have a deficiency of hexosamindadase A, which can be tested for prenatally.[14] The lymphocytes in each of these disorders may show vacuolization, and although it is a common finding, it is not specific for the lipid storage disorders.

BACTERIA AND OTHER UNEXPECTED WHITE CELL CHANGES

The presence of bacteria in a peripheral smear indicates bacteremia or sepsis, a condition that may have severe consequence to the patient. Blood is a sterile environment such that the presence of gram-positive or -negative bacteria, fungi, etc., is an unwanted event. Bacteria may be seen intracellularly or extracellularly as either

cocci or rods. In either case, bacteria must be recognized and the significant medical caretakers must be alerted (Figs. 10.15 and 10.16). Precipitated stain may at times resemble bacteria; therefore, it is important to be positive in your identification of bacteria, as artifacts may be confusing (Fig. 10.17).

Platelet satellitism has been discussed in a case study in a previous chapter. However, it represents a phenomenon that must be recognized as an unexpected event in a peripheral smear. The blood of some patients will react with EDTA, causing platelets to form a ring around neutrophils. This is described as platelet satellitism (Fig. 10.18). This event will produce a falsely low platelet count and can be corrected only once the patient sample is collected in a sodium citrate tube for an accurate platelet count (Fig. 10.19). An additional peripheral cell change that may occur in segmented neutrophils is **pyknosis,** or pyknotic changes. This is

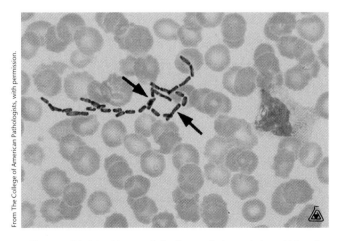

Figure 10.16   Extracellular bacteria in peripheral blood.

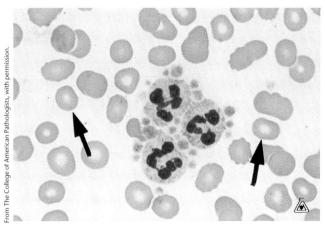

Figure 10.18   Platelet satellitism.

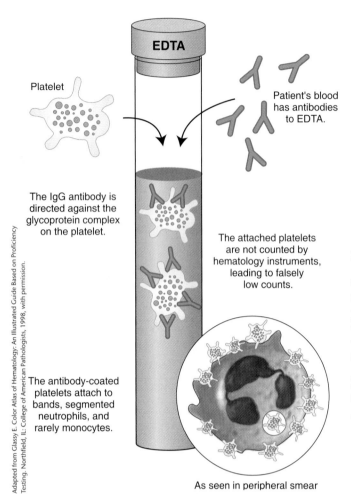

The antibody-coated platelets attach to bands, segmented neutrophils, and rarely monocytes.

Platelet

Patient's blood has antibodies to EDTA.

The IgG antibody is directed against the glycoprotein complex on the platelet.

The attached platelets are not counted by hematology instruments, leading to falsely low counts.

As seen in peripheral smear

Adapted from Glassy E. Color Atlas of Hematology: An Illustrated Guide Based on Proficiency Testing. Northfield, IL: College of American Pathologists, 1998, with permission.

Figure 10.19   Platelet satellitism formation. An unexpected reaction of the patient to the EDTA causes the platelets to ring around segmented neutrophils.

seen in degenerated neutrophils as the segmented nucleus becomes an amorphous, smooth blob-like structure with no clear segmented structure. These cells are not counted in the white cell differential.

Student Challenge

Observe Figure 10.20. Is the cell at the arrow a lymphocyte or an nRBC? Why or why not?

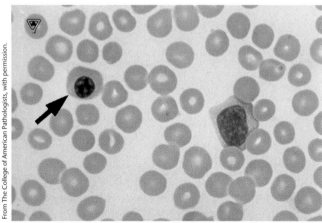

From The College of American Pathologists, with permission.

Figure 10.20   Is this a lymphocyte or an nRBC?

CONDENSED CASE

A hemoglobin and hematocrit were ordered on a patient for a surgical floor. The test was performed on the Coulter LH 750, and the hemoglobin and hematocrit were compatible with previous results. However, the instrument routinely reports the complete CBC, and while observing the entire nine parameters, the operator noticed that the platelet count was only 23,000, a critical value. The delta check on the patient from the previous day showed that the platelet count was 257,000, a significant difference. Corrective action needed to be taken. The operator decided to check the tube that she has just cycled through the instrument for clots, and a small clot was found. **How many times should a purple top tube be inverted once drawn to prevent clotting?**

Answer

The specimen that was sent from the floor was an improper sample that had probably not been properly collected. When drawing blood into a purple top tube, the tube must be inverted five to seven times for proper mixing of the anticoagulant and blood. Once the technologist noticed a small clot, corrective action needed to be taken. The technologist now had the responsibility of notifying the nurse of the erroneous results and asking for a redraw. Additionally, the erroneous results needed to be removed from the computer and the documentation of the situation and corrective action needed to be recorded. The sharp eye of the technologist/technician in this case made it possible for reliable results to eventually be obtained.

Summary Points

- Infections and inflammation will increase the number of neutrophils in the peripheral smear.

- Leukocytosis means an increase in white count.

- Eosinophils will be increased in skin diseases, parasitic infections, and transplant rejection.

- A left shift signifies that younger white cells will appear in the peripheral smear such as occasional metamyelocytes, many bands, and segmented neutrophils.

- Leukemoid reaction is an exaggerated response to infection or inflammation.

- In the leukoerythroblastic picture, young white cells, young red cells, and abnormal platelets will be seen.

- Phagocytosis is a process by which bacteria and other infectious agents are recognized and destroyed by neutrophils and monocytes.

- Toxic changes in white cells are observed as toxic granulation, toxic vacuolization, and Döhle bodies.

- Hereditary white cell disorders include May-Hegglin anomaly, Pelger-Huët anomaly, and Chediak-Higashi syndrome.

- Pelger-Huët anomaly is a hyposegmentation disorder in which the lobes of the segmented neutrophils are peanut shaped or bilobed.

- A hypersegmented nucleus, five lobes or more, is seen in megaloblastic disorders.

- Chediak-Higashi syndrome is a rare autosomal disorder of neutrophilic granules.

- Human ehrlichiosis represents a group of tick-borne diseases caused by *Rickettsia Ehrlichia chafeensis* and *Ehrlichia phagocytophilia*. Inclusions may be seen in the granulocytes and monocytes in the bone marrow.

- Reactive lymphocytes are lymphocytes transformed by viral infections or other disorders.

- Reactive lymphocytes are characterized by abundant basophilic cytoplasm, a lower N:C ratio, and clumped chromatin material.

- Infectious mononucleosis is caused by the Epstein-Barr virus, and patients show low-grade fever, sore throat, swollen glands, anorexia, and headache.

- Individuals with AIDS show a pancytopenia and a reversal in CD4 and CD8.

- Bacteria may appear intracellularly in neutrophils or may appear within the peripheral smear.

- Lipid storage diseases represent a group of inherited disorders in which a key metabolic enzyme is missing or inactive.

- Gaucher's disease and Niemann-Pick disease are lipid storage disorders showing large histiocytic-like cells in the bone marrow.

CASE STUDY

A 60-year-old woman was sent for preoperative blood testing before her elective gallbladder surgery. Her surgeon ordered a complete blood count, a chemistry panel, and a coagulation profile. Her chemistry panel and coagulation profile were normal. Her CBC, however, showed a large number of band forms, which were flagged on the automated differential. This was an unexpected result, and the surgeon called for a repeat sample. Because her differential was flagged, a slide was pulled and observed for a slide review. **Which conditions may show a high number of bands?**

Insights to the Case Study

The CBC on this individual showed all normal parameters except for the band count in the automated differential. The automated differential in this patient reported 50% bands, clearly unexpected results. Reflex testing was ordered and a peripheral smear was reviewed. The smear showed large numbers of segmented neutrophils with bilobed or peanut-shaped nuclear material, suggestive of Pelger-Huët anomaly. Pelger-Huët anomaly, discovered in 1928, is an inherited abnormality of the segmented neutrophils in which there is hyposegmentation of the nuclear material. In most cases, it is a heterozygous disorder and the white cells still function normally showing active phagocytic ability and normal leukocyte function. When the disorder presents homozygously, a single round nucleus is seen. It is essential to differentiate Pelger-Huët anomaly from true band cells because the reporting of 50% bands could lead the physician to suspect septicemia or other serious infectious conditions, which would warrant a left shift. In this case, the surgeon was notified and the surgery was completed as scheduled.

Review Questions

1. Which of the following inclusions are usually only seen in the bone marrow?
   a. Toxic granulation
   b. Chediak-Higashi granules
   c. The morulas from *Ehrlichia* infections
   d. Bacteria

2. In which of the following conditions will monocytes be increased?
   a. Tuberculosis
   b. Parasitic infections
   c. Ulcerative colitis
   d. Skin diseases

3. Which is the causative agent in infectious mononucleosis?
   a. HIV
   b. EBV
   c. CMV
   d. CBC

4. The process of ingesting, digesting, and killing bacteria is termed:
   a. opsonization.
   b. phagocytosis.
   c. neutrophilia.
   d. mobilization.

5. Qualitative changes in the white cell include all except which of the following:
   a. Toxic granulation
   b. Toxic vacuolization
   c. Gaucher's cells
   d. Döhle bodies

● TROUBLESHOOTING

Is It Precipitated Stain or Is It Bacteria?

A 24-year-old man presented to the emergency department with a fever of unknown origin. A CBC, blood cultures, and routine chemistries were ordered. The chemistries came back as normal and the blood cultures would be read in 24 hours. The CBC results were as follows:

WBC	35.0×10^9/L	H
RBC	3.23×10^{12}/L	L
Hgb	9.3 g/dL	L
Hct	27.8%	L
MCV	86.0 fL	L
MCH	28.7 pg	L
MCHC	33.5 %	
Platelets	598×10^9/L	H
RDW	21.0	H

The elevated WBC was flagged, and reflex testing required that a manual differential be completed. The technologist, upon reviewing the peripheral smear, noted several items:

   The 35.0×10^9/L WBC count correlated with the slide.

   Many band forms were seen.

   Toxic granulation was noted.

   The patient's peripheral smear seemed to show the presence of bacteria intracellularly and extracellularly; however, the technologist was fairly new to the hospital facility, and because this was such an important finding, he needed assistance in making a definite identification.

Differentiating precipitated stain from bacteria is often difficult, yet there are some distinct characteristics that can make the identification easier. Microorganisms or bacteria are uniform in size and shape and are usually dispersed throughout the slide. They may be found randomly throughout the peripheral smear, and in most cases, they are lucky to be visualized at all. Precipitated stain, on the other hand, tends to appear in aggregates, which are localized and plentiful. Additionally, precipitated stain tends to lack an organized morphology and looks smudgy or clumpy. In the case of our patient, the technologist consulted several of his peers. Through consensus, it was agreed the inclusions were bacteria. The pathologist was notified and the floor was contacted. The blood cultures were positive, and the patient was started on high-dose antibiotics and made a complete recovery.

WORD KEY

Albinism • Partial or total absence of pigment in the hair, skin, and eyes

Convalescence • Period of recovery after a disease or surgery

Photophobia • Unusual intolerance of light

Prognostic • Prediction of the chance for recovery

Pyknosis • Shrinkage of cells through degeneration

Rhinorrhea • Excessive watery discharge from nose

Sepsis • Systemic inflammatory response to infection that includes symptoms such as fever, hypothermia, tachycardia, and others

References

1. Van Assendelft OW. Reference values for the total and differential leukocyte count. Blood Cells 11:77–96, 1985.
2. Barnes EJ, Abdel-Rehim MM, Goulis Y, et al. Application and limitation of blood eosinophilia for the diagnosis of acute cellular rejection in liver transplantation. Am J Transplant 3:432–438, 2003.
3. Wiseman BK. A newly recognized granulopenic syndrome caused by excessive splenic leukolysis and successfully treated by splenectomy. J Clin Invest 18:473, 1939.
4. Turgeon ML. Clinical Hematology: Theory and Procedures, 4th ed. Baltimore: Lippincott Williams & Wilkins, 2005; 196–200.
5. Ponder E, Ponder RV. The cytology of the polymorphonuclear leukocyte in toxic conditions. J Lab Clin Med 28:316, 1942.
6. Malcolm ID, Flegel KM, Katz M. Vacuolation of the neutrophil in bacteremia. Arch Intern Med 139:675, 1979.
7. Foley A. Nonmalignant hereditary disorders of leukocyte. In: Steine-Martin EA, Lotspeich-Steininger CA, Koepke JA. Clinical Hematology: Principles, Procedures, Correlations, 2nd ed. Philadelphia: Lippincott, 1998; 365.
8. Baetz K, Isaaz S, Griffith SG. Loss of cytotoxic T lymphocyte function in Chediak-Higashi syndrome arises from a secretory defect that prevents granule exocytosis. J Immunol 154:6122, 1995.
9. Eng TR, Harkess JR, Fishbein DB, et al. Epidemiological clinical and laboratory findings of human ehrlichiosis in the U.S. in 1988. JAMA 264;2252–2258, 1990.
10. Bakken JS. Ask the experts: Differentiating human ehrlichiosis from other tick borne illnesses. Infect Dis News September:14–15, 1995.
11. James E. Unmasking infectious mononucleosis. ADVANCE for Medical Laboratory Professionals. March 22, 2004.
12. Kolodney EH, Tenembaum AL. Storage diseases of the reticuloendothelial system. In: Nathan and Oski's Hematology of Infancy and Childhood, 4th ed. Philadelphia: WB Saunders, 1992; 1453–1464.
13. Graubowski GA, Pastores GM. Enzyme replacement therapy in type I Gaucher disease. Gaucher Clin Perspect 1:8, 1993.
14. Harmening DM, Spier CM. Lipid (lysosomal) storage disease and histiocytosis. In: Harmening DM, ed. Clinical Hematology and Fundamentals of Hemostasis, 4th ed. Philadelphia: FA Davis, 2002; 633.

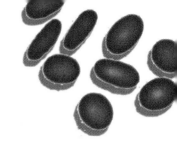

11

Acute Leukemias

Barbara Caldwell

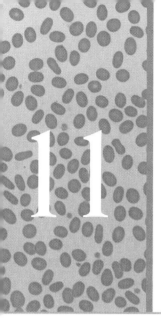

Definition of Leukemia

Comparing Acute and Chronic Leukemia

Leukemia History

Acute Myeloid Leukemia
Epidemiology
Clinical Features
Laboratory Features
Classifications

Acute Lymphoblastic Leukemia
Epidemiology
Clinical Features
Classifications
Prognosis in Acute Lymphoblastic Leukemia

Objectives

After completing this chapter, the student will be able to:

1. Compare and contrast acute versus chronic leukemia with respect to age of onset, presenting symptoms, and organ involvement.

2. Describe acute leukemia with emphasis on symptoms, peripheral smear finding, and bone marrow findings.

3. Classify the acute nonlymphocytic leukemias according to the French-American-British classification system.

4. Describe how cytochemical staining can aid in the diagnosis of the acute leukemias.

5. Briefly describe the World Health Organization classification for acute leukemias.

6. Identify the most consistent cytogenetic abnormalities in the acute leukemias.

7. Describe acute lymphocytic leukemia with emphasis on age of onset, symptoms at presentation, prognosis, and laboratory findings.

8. Describe the most pertinent CD markers for the acute lymphocytic leukemias.

9. Describe the factors that may influence the prognosis in acute lymphocytic leukemias.

10. Characterize the T-cell acute lymphoblastic leukemias.

DEFINITION OF LEUKEMIA

Leukemia is caused by the mutation of the bone marrow pluripotent or most primitive stem cells. This neoplastic expansion results in abnormal, leukemic cells and impaired production of normal red blood cells, neutrophils, and platelets. As the mutant cell line takes hold and normal hematopoiesis is inhibited, the leukemic cells spill into the peripheral blood and invade the reticuloendothelial tissue, specifically the spleen, liver, lymph nodes, and, at times, central nervous system. The leukemic stem cells have atypical growth and maturation capability. The mutant clone may demonstrate unique morphologic, cytogenetic, and immunophenotypic features that can be used to aid in the classification of the particular type of leukemia. Many of the leukemias have similar clinical features, but regardless of the subtype, the disease is fatal if left untreated.

COMPARING ACUTE AND CHRONIC LEUKEMIA

The initial evaluation of leukemia is initially made by:

1. Noting the onset of symptoms
2. Analyzing the complete blood count (CBC) results
3. Observing the *type* of cell that predominates (cell **lineage**)
4. Assessing the *maturity* of cells that predominate

Because leukemia is a disease of the bone marrow that causes normal bone marrow cell production to be crowded out as the abnormal, neoplastic cells take over, the CBC results will commonly show a decreased red cell count or anemia, as well as a decrease in platelets or thrombocytopenia. The level of anemia and thrombocytopenia tends to be more severe in acute leukemia. Leukocytosis is a hallmark feature of chronic leukemia, and because the spleen also becomes a site of extramedullary (outside of the bone marrow) hematopoiesis, prominent hepatosplenomegaly is most often associated with chronic leukemia.

The type of cell that predominates in the peripheral blood and the bone marrow is defined according to *cell lineage* as either myeloid or lymphoid. The myeloid stem cell gives birth to granulocytes, monocytes, megakaryocytes, and erythrocytes (see Fig. 2.3). Therefore, as will be described in the various sections of this chapter, the myeloid leukemias can involve proliferation of any stage of these four cell lines. By contrast, the lymphoid stem cell gives rise solely to lymphocytic lineage cells.

Cell maturity can be used to separate the initial diagnosis between acute and chronic leukemias. When blasts or other immature cells predominate, the leukemia is classified as *acute,* versus the predominance of more mature cell types being associated with *chronic* leukemia.

The onset of acute versus chronic leukemia is distinctly different. Acute leukemia has a quick onset, whereas chronic leukemia has a slow, insidious course and may even be discovered on routine physical examination. Age is another factor that is often consistent in the different leukemic variants. Although acute leukemia may occur at any age, chronic leukemia is usually a disease seen in adults (Table 11.1).

To summarize, using both the cell lineage and the maturity of cells that predominate, leukemias can be categorized into four broad groups:

1. Acute myeloid leukemias
2. Acute lymphoblastic leukemias
3. Chronic myelocytic leukemias (see Chapter 12)
4. Chronic lymphocytic leukemias (see Chapter 13)

LEUKEMIA HISTORY

It is important to give credit to those early scientists who were able to recognize and define leukemia in an age when little technology existed save a crude microscope and who had the ability to make astute clinical observa-

Table 11.1 ● Comparison of Characteristics of Acute and Chronic Leukemia

Characteristic	Acute Leukemia	Chronic Leukemia
Onset	Abrupt	Subtle
Morbidity	Months	Years
Age	All	Adults
WBC	Variable	Elevated
Predominant cells	Blasts and other immature white cells	Mature
Anemia, thrombocytopenia	Present	Variable
Neutropenia	Present	Variable
Organomegaly	Mild	Marked

tions and perform postmortem analysis. A brief discussion of the pertinent discoveries that occurred more than 100 years ago gives one a great appreciation of just how far the science of hematology has progressed in such a short time. Two scientists in separate countries made early descriptions of leukemia in 1845. Bennett in Scotland and Virchow in Germany both studied a series of autopsy findings from individuals who died with very enlarged spleens and livers (hepatosplenomegaly).[1,2] Virchow is credited with assigning the term *weisses blut* (meaning "white blood"), which is translated into Greek as *leukemia*. Both Bennett and Virchow came to believe that leukemia is caused by a cancerous overgrowth of the white cells. Virchow was able to demonstrate by further studies that one could classify the cases into two groups: those with mostly large spleens and those with predominantly enlarged lymph nodes.[3] We now know that these groups represent a distinction between chronic myelocytic leukemia (CML) and chronic lymphocytic leukemia (CLL).

The next conceptual proposal came in 1878 from Neumann, who suggested that the origin of blood cells was the bone marrow, and hence leukemia was a disease of the bone marrow. He used the term *myelogene*, which is the origin of the later term "myelogenous leukemia."[4] Epstein in 1889 was the first to assign the term *acute leukemia*, designating cases wherein the patients died from the disease in a matter of months from manifestation of first symptoms. He noted that these patients had very purulent blood and surmised by this gross observation of white blood that there was an incredible increase in white cells. He was eventually able to lead the hematology forefathers of his day to recognize a separation between what we now call acute myelogenous leukemia (AML) and a more chronic, slow onset that we now recognize at CML.[5]

Proof of the early scientist's ingenuity is the fact that until Ehrlich developed a polychromatic stain in 1877 that allowed blood cells to be distinguished, scientists were only able to observe colorless cells under the microscope[6]! Once the use of his stains became widespread around the turn of the century, scientists were able to show that acute leukemia was associated with early blast cells, and chronic leukemia with more mature cells. Thus, in 1900 the description of a myeloblast and a myelocyte were documented by Naegeli,[7] and several years later the existence of monoblastic leukemia was first described by Schilling. Hirschfield's important contribution was that he made the connection that red cells and white cells share a common cell of origin.[8] The combined discoveries of these scientists laid the foundation for our current understanding of leukemia. As new research and application of new techniques continue to refine the classification of leukemia, changes in treatment protocols lead to improved survival statistics.

ACUTE MYELOID LEUKEMIA

AML is malignant, clonal disease that involves proliferation of blasts in bone marrow, blood, or other tissue. The blasts most often show myeloid or monocytic differentiation. Almost 80% of patients with AML will demonstrate chromosome abnormalities, usually a mutation resulting from a chromosomal translocation (the transfer of one portion of the chromosome to another).[9] The translocation causes abnormal **oncogene** or tumor suppression gene expression, and this results in unregulated cellular proliferation.[10] Genetic syndromes and toxic exposure contribute to the pathogenesis in some patients.

Although the diseases grouped into the acute myelogenous leukemia categories have similar clinical manifestations, the morphology, immunophenotyping, and cytogenetic features are distinct. Cytochemical stains are used along with morphology to help identify the lineage of the blast population. Electron microscopy may also be used to subclassify the various leukemias. When morphology and/or **cytochemistry** evidence of lineage is absent, flow cytometry is used to specifically tag the myeloid or lymphoid antigens and thus classify the acute leukemias.

Epidemiology

The incidence of AML increases with age, accounting for 80% of acute leukemias in adults and for 15% to 20% of acute leukemias in children. Of note, however, is that when congenital leukemia (occurring during the neonatal period) does rarely occur, it is paradoxically AML rather than ALL and is often monocytic. The rate of AML is somewhat higher in males than females, and there is an increased incidence in developed, more industrialized countries. Eastern European Jews have an increased risk of developing AML, whereas Oriental populations have a decreased risk.[11]

Table 11.2 lists the conditions that have been documented as predisposing to development of AML. The high incidence of individuals having congenital defects such as Down syndrome and bone marrow failure syndromes such as Fanconi's anemia has demonstrated that these factors are often implicated in the pathogenesis of

Table 11.2 ⊙ Conditions and Disorders With Increased Risk for Development of Acute Leukemia		
Congenital Defects	**Acquired Diseases**	**Environmental Factors**
Down syndrome	Aplastic anemia	Ionizing radiation
Klinefelter syndrome	Myeloma	Alkalating agents
Turner syndrome	Sideroblastic anemia	Cytotoxic drugs
Monosomy 7 syndrome	Acquired genetic changes	Pesticide exposure
Fanconi's anemia	Translocations	Solvents
Wiskott-Aldrich syndrome	Inversions	
Neurofibromatosis	Deletions	
Familial aplastic anemia	Point mutations	
Fraternal twins and nonidentical siblings	Paroxysmal nocturnal hemoglobinuria	
Combined immunodeficiency syndrome	Transition from other hematopoietic diseases (myeloproliferative disorders)	
Blackfan-Diamond syndrome		

AML. It has also been well documented that leukemia is associated with exposure to ionizing radiation, as this was most notably reported with the increase in leukemia that occurred following the release of atomic bombs over Hiroshima and Nagasaki in 1945. The fallout from atomic bombs and exposure to nuclear reactor plants has caused much well-founded public apprehension, fear, and concern over the past 50 years.[12,13] A wide variety of chemicals and drugs have been linked to AML. In a study involving factories in China, the risk of developing leukemia was five to six times higher in workers with recurrent exposure to benzene than in the general population.[14] Many drugs, in particular, therapy-related alkylating drugs, are associated with AML emerging after the treatment. All of the chronic myeloproliferative disorders (chronic myelocytic leukemia [CML], idiopathic myelofibrosis [IMF], polycythemia vera [PV], essential thrombocythemia [ET]) have an increased propensity for terminating in AML, with 60% to 70% of CML cases undergoing a transition to AML.

Clinical Features

All of the signs and symptoms that present so abruptly in patients with AML are caused by the infiltration of the bone marrow with leukemic cells and the resulting failure of normal hematopoiesis. These criminal leukemic cells that invade the bone marrow are dysfunctional, and without the normal hematopoietic elements, the patient is at risk for developing life-threatening complications of anemia, infection due to functional neutropenia, and hemorrhage due to thrombocytopenia (Table 11.3).

Fatigue and weakness are the most common complaints that reflect the development of anemia. Pallor, **dyspnea** on exertion, heart palpitations, and a general loss of well-being has been described.[15] Fever is present is about 15% to 20% of patients and may be the result of bacterial, fungal, and, less frequently, viral infections, or from the leukemic burden of cells on tissues and organs. Easy bruising, petechiae, and mucosal bleeding may be found due to thrombocytopenia. Other more severe symptoms related to decreased platelet counts that occur less commonly are gastrointestinal or genitourinary tract and central nervous system (CNS) bleeding. CNS infiltration with high numbers of leukemic cells has been reported in 5% to 20% of children and approximately 15% of adults with AML.[16,17] Headache, blindness, and other neurological complications are indications of meningeal involvement. Leukemic blast cells circulate through the peripheral blood and may invade any tissue. Extramedullary hematopoiesis is common in monocytic or myelomonocytic leukemias. Organs that were active in fetal hematopoiesis may be reactivated to again produce cells when stressed by the poor performance of the overburdened leukemic bone marrow. Hepatosplenomegaly or lymphadenopathy may occur but is not as prominent as that seen in the chronic leukemias. Skin infiltration is very characteristic in monocytic leukemias, particularly gum infiltration, which is termed **gingival hyperplasia.** When

Table 11.3 ● Clinical Findings in Acute Leukemia

Pathogenesis	Signs and Symptoms
Bone Marrow Infiltration	
Neutropenia	Fever, infection
Anemia	Pallor, dyspnea, lethargy
Thrombocytopenia	Bleeding, petechiae, ecchymosis, intracranial hematoma and gastrointestinal or conjunctival hemorrhage (rare)
Medullary Infiltration	
Marrow	Bone pain and tenderness, limp, arthralgia
Extramedullary Infiltration	
Liver, spleen, lymph nodes, thymus	Organomegaly
Central nervous system	Neurological complications including dizziness, headache, vomiting, alteration of mental function
Gums, mouth	Gingival bleeding and hypertrophy
Skin	Lesions or granulocytic sarcoma

leukemic cells crowd the bone marrow of the long bones, joint pain may be produced.

Laboratory Features

Peripheral Blood and Bone Marrow Findings

The CBC and examination of peripheral blood smear are the first step in the laboratory diagnosis of leukemia. Blood cell counts are variable in patients with AML. The WBC may be normal, increased, or decreased. It is markedly elevated, over 100×10^9/L cells in less than 20% of cases. Conversely, the WBC is less than 5.0×10^9/L with an absolute neutrophil count of less than 1.0×10^9/L in about half the patients at the time of diagnosis.[18] Blasts are usually seen on the peripheral smear examination, but in leukopenic patients, the numbers may be few and require a diligent search to uncover. Cytoplasmic inclusions known as **Auer rods** often present in a small percentage of the myeloblasts, monoblasts, or promyelocytes present in the various subtypes of AML. Auer rods are elliptical, spindle-like inclusions composed of azurophilic granules. Nucleated red blood cells may be present, as well as myelodysplastic features, including pseudo-hyposegmentation (pseudo Pelger-Huët cells) or hypersegmentation of the neutrophils, and hypogranulation.

Anemia is a very common feature due to inadequate production of normal red cells. The reticulocyte count is usually normal or decreased. Red cell anisopoikilocytosis is mildly abnormal, with few poikilocytes present. Thrombocytopenia, which can be severe, is almost always a feature at diagnosis. Giant platelets and agranular platelets may be seen. Disseminated intravascular coagulation (DIC) is most commonly associated with one of the types of AMLs known as acute promyelocytic leukemia. The DIC is caused by the release of tissue factor–like procoagulants from the azurophilic granules of the neoplastic promyelocytes, which in turn activate coagulation and further consume platelets, leading to dangerous bleeding diathesis.

Before treatment, serum uric acid and lactic dehydrogenase (LDH) levels often are mild or moderately increased.

The hallmark feature of acute leukemia is always a hypercellular bone marrow, with 20% to 90% leukemic blasts at diagnosis or during relapse. The blast population grows indiscriminately as these cells have only limited differentiation capability and are frozen in the earliest stage of development. The lineage of blasts that predominate depends on the specific type of acute leukemia. The most current classification for hematological and lymphoid tumors published by the World Health Organization (WHO) recommends that the requisite blast percentage for a diagnosis of acute myeloid leukemia be greater than or equal to 20% myeloblasts in the blood or marrow.[19] When performing a peripheral blood smear on a patient with a suspected diagnosis of leukemia, at least 200 WBCs should be classified. It is recommended that the blast percentage in the bone marrow be derived from a 500-cell differential count. If the WBC is less than 2.0×10^9/L, buffy coat smears should be prepared for differential counting.

Myeloblasts may be distinguished from lymphoblasts by three distinct ways: presence of Auer rods, reactivity with cytochemical stains, or reactivity with cell surface markers (for example, clusters of differentiation [CD] groups CD13, CD33) on blasts with specific monoclonal antibodies. The morphology of blasts can often be determined by an experienced morphologist; however, other supporting tests are always needed to confirm the initial designation. The features that can be used to differentiate a myeloblast from a lymphoblast are outlined in Figure 11-1. The chromatin material of a myeloblast is usually much finer than that of a lymphoblast. A myeloblast often has more cytoplasm than a lymphoblast. Both size of the blast and number of nucleoli may not be helpful characteristics. Although a myeloblast is usually larger than a lymphoblast, sufficient variations are seen that this is not the best factor to consider. Along the same lines, the number of nucleoli that can be seen in a myeloblast is one to four, and a lymphoblast one or two, so when deciding lineage on a blast with two obvious nucleoli, either choice would be acceptable. Therefore, of the characteristic features listed in Figure 11.1, the most helpful is usually the chromatin staining pattern. As mentioned previously, other methods besides morphological examination must be used to confirm the type of blasts present, and often to quantify the number of blasts, particularly when two blast populations coexist in significant amounts in the leukemic bone marrow.

Other studies that can be used to diagnose the acute leukemias include chromosome analysis, molecular genetic studies, DNA flow cytometry, and electron microscopy.

From 5% to 10% of the AMLs have a preleukemic presentation termed "myelodysplastic syndrome." These patients are usually over the age of 50 and have anemia, thrombocytopenia, and monocytosis but with bone marrow blast percentages of less than 20% (see Chapter 14).

Cytochemical Stains

Cytochemical stains are very helpful in the diagnosis and classification of acute leukemias (Table 11.4). These stains are usually performed on bone marrow smears but may also be done on peripheral smears or bone marrow touch preps. The special stains are used to identify enzymes or lipids within the *blast* population of cells—hence, the reaction in mature cells is not of importance. The positive reactions that occur will be associated with a particular lineage, and with some of the stains (e.g., myeloperoxidase [MPO] and Sudan Black B [SBB]), the fine or coarse staining intensity is an indication of the lineage of blast cells. All of the cytochemical stains described below are negative in lymphoid cells (with rare exceptions), so a positive result with any of these will most often rule out acute lymphoblastic leukemia.

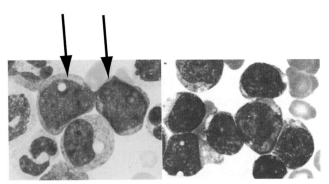

	Myeloblast	*Lymphoblast*
Size	15-20 μm	10-15 μm
Chromatin	Fine	Moderately condensed
Nucleoli	1-4, prominent	1-2, often inconspicuous
Cytoplasm	Moderate, basophilic	Scant
Auer rods	May be present	Absent

Figure 11.1 Comparison of myeloblast and lymphoblast morphology.

Table 11.4 ● Cytochemical Reactions in Acute Leukemia

Cytochemical Reaction	Cellular Element Stained	Blasts Identified
Myeloperoxidase (MPO)	Neutrophil primary granules	Myeloblasts strong positive; monoblasts faint positive
Sudan Black B (SBB)	Phospholipids	Myeloblasts strong positive; monoblasts faint positive
Specific esterase	Cellular enzyme	Myeloblasts strong positive
Nonspecific esterase (NSE)	Cellular enzyme	Monoblasts strong positive
Terminal deoxynucleotidyl transferase (TdT)	Intranuclear enzyme	Lymphoblasts positive
Periodic acid-Schiff	Glycogen	Variable, coarse or block-like positivity often seen in lymphoblasts and pronormoblasts, myeloblasts usually negative although faint diffuse reaction may occasionally be seen

Myeloperoxidase

Primary granules of myeloid cells contain peroxidase. The granules are found in the late myeloblast and exist throughout all the myeloid maturation stages. Because primary granules are absent in myeloblasts, there is limited MPO activity in early myeloblasts; however, those blasts that are closer to maturing to the promyelocyte stage will stain positive. Promyelocytes, myelocytes, metamyelocytes, and band and segmented neutrophils will stain strongly positive, indicated by the presence of blue-black granules. Monocytic granules stain faintly positive. Because lymphoid cells, nucleated red cells, and megakaryoblasts lack this enzyme, they will stain negative. This negative reaction is useful in initially differentiating ALL from AML. Eosinophils will also stain positive for MPO. Auer rods are strongly positive for peroxidase. The enzymatic activity in blood smears will fade over time, so slides should not be held for staining for longer than 3 weeks. The MPO stain will be positive in acute myeloid leukemia (>3% positive), acute promyelocytic leukemia (90% to 100% positive), acute myelomonocytic leukemia (including AMML with abnormal eosinophils, AMML Eo [variable, >3% positive]), acute monoblastic and monocytic leukemia (variable), and in the myeloblasts present in acute erythroid leukemia (myeloblasts, >3% positive).

Sudan Black B

Phospholipids and other intracellular lipids are stained by SBB. Phospholipids are found in the primary (nonspecific) and secondary (specific) granules of neutrophilic cells and eosinophils, and in smaller quantities in monocytes and macrophages. The stain will be negative in lymphocytes, although rarely the azurophilic granules of lymphoblasts may demonstrate positivity. The SBB pattern of staining mimics the MPO stain in that it is very sensitive for granulocyte precursors, increases in staining intensity with the later stages of granulocytic maturation, and stains weakly positive with monocytic cells. Thus, this stain can also be used to differentiate AML from ALL. A distinct advantage of the SBB over the MPO stain is that the SBB-stained slides are stable for a longer period of time.

Specific Esterase (Naphthol AS-D Chloracetate Esterase)

The specific esterase enzyme is present in the primary granules of myeloid cells. Accordingly, myeloblasts and other neutrophilic cells in AML will stain positive. This stain will also be positive in basophils and mast cells but is negative in eosinophils, monocytes, and lymphocytes. The specific esterase enzymatic reaction is stable in paraffin-embedded tissue sections, making this an extremely useful stain for identifying cells of myeloid lineage in extramedullary myeloid tumors.[20]

Nonspecific Esterase (Alpha-Naphthyl Butyrate or Alpha-Naphthyl Acetate Esterase)

These stains are used to identify monocytic cells and will stain negative with granulocytes. Different substrates are available, with alpha-naphthyl butyrate stain considered more specific and alpha-naphthyl acetate stain being more sensitive. Many cells in addition to monocytes will stain positive (macrophages, histiocytes, megakaryoblasts, and some carcinomas), so the sodium fluoride inhibition step is used to differentiate the positivity. With this step, following initial staining, the NSE activity of monocytes and macrophages is inhibited (reaction was positive, then reaction is negative), whereas the activity of the other cells remains positive. Mature T lymphocytes will stain a coarse dot-like pattern. The NSE stain is used to identify the monoblast and promonocyte populations in acute monoblastic leukemia and acute myelomonocytic leukemia. However, in 10% to 20% of cases of acute monoblastic leukemia, the NSE stain is weakly positive or negative. In these cases, immunophenotyping may be used to confirm monocytic differentiation.[19]

Terminal Deoxynucleotidyl Transferase

Terminal deoxynucleotidyl transferase (TdT) is an intranuclear enzyme found in stem cells and immature lymphoid cells within the bone marrow, but not in mature B lymphocytes. It is present in 90% of acute lymphoblastic leukemias and in only 5% to 10% of acute myeloblastic leukemias.[21] It has also been demonstrated in one-third of cases of the blast crisis stage of chronic myelogenous leukemia and is a good prognostic indicator in these patients.[22,23]

Immunophenotype

Immunophenotyping can help to classify the clone of leukemic blasts by using monoclonal antibodies directed against cell surface markers. The specific lineage and stage of maturation can be tagged, and this information then is used to indicate appropriate therapy and can be correlated to prognosis. Immunophenotyping can be done by flow cytometry or by immunohistochemistry methods. Multiple antigens can be detected simultaneously on a single cell using flow cytometry. A selected panel of monoclonal antibodies is presented in Table 11.5.

The assignment of the particular nomenclature for the type of leukemia is based on the combined morphologic, immunophenotypic, and cytochemical information, as well as any unique clinical presentation. The information is used to suggest the best approximation of the subtype of leukemia, recognizing that our knowledge is sometimes imperfect and that changes in these classifications may again take place in the future as our understanding of the science of leukemia improves.

Classifications

The morphological variants of acute myeloid leukemia may occur as a primary presentation or may be the result of a clonal evolution from other disorders such as the myeloproliferative disorders of chronic myelogenous leukemia, idiopathic myelofibrosis, or essential

Table 11.5 ● Immunophenotypic Classification	
Lineage	**Marker**
Hematopoietic precursor	CD117 (HLA-DR), CD34
Myeloid	CD11b, CD13, CD33, CD15
T-lineage	CD1, CD2, CD3, CD4, CD5, CD7, CD8, TdT
B-lineage	CD10, CD19, CD20, CD21A, CD22, CD23, CD24, CD79a, TdT
Erythroid	Glycophorin A
Monocytic	CD14, CD4, CD11b, CD11c, CD36, CD64
Megakaryocytic	CD41, CD42, CD61

thrombocythemia. The acute leukemias are categorized according to the cell line and stage of maturation that predominate. In order to classify the acute leukemias consistently, in 1976 the French-American-British (FAB) group developed a system of nomenclature that separated the acute myeloid from acute lymphoid leukemias. The classification scheme, as it evolved over the years, designates multiple subtypes for the various acute myeloid leukemias, M0 to M7, and three subtypes, L1 to L3, for the lymphoid leukemias (Table 11.6). The classification was initially based solely on morphology of the cells present; however, later results of cytochemistry staining reactions were incorporated into the classification. The requisite blast percentage derived from bone marrow examination using the FAB classification is greater than 30%.

The FAB classification has been problematic for several reasons. Immunophenotyping and cytogenic and molecular analyses are not well defined for the individual subtypes. Also, the FAB classification does not clearly separate groups of patients who have positive clinical outcomes. Because of these limitations, and due to the discovery of a number of genetic lesions that can predict clinical outcomes much better than just a morphology-based delineation, the group of hematopathologists convened by WHO in 1997 proposed a new classification for the acute myeloid leukemias (Table 11.7). The resulting scheme proposed by the WHO group incorporated specific genetic data into the classification of hematopoietic and lymphopoietic tumors[24] (Table 11-8). They also included a sepa-

Table 11.6 ● FAB Classification of Acute Leukemia

Designation	Descriptive Name
M0	Acute myeloblastic leukemia, minimally differentiated
M1	Acute myeloblastic leukemia without maturation
M2	Acute myeloblastic leukemia with maturation
M3	Acute promyelocytic leukemia, hypergranular
M3v	Acute promyelocytic leukemia, microgranular
M4	Acute myelomonocytic leukemia
M4Eo	Acute myelomonocytic leukemia with eosinophilia
M5a	Acute monoblastic leukemia, poorly differentiated
M5b	Acute monoblastic leukemia, with differentiation
M6	Erythroleukemia
M7	Acute megakaryoblastic leukemia
L1*	Acute lymphoblastic leukemia
L2*	Acute lymphoblastic leukemia
L3*	Acute lymphoblastic leukemia, leukemic phase of Burkitt's lymphoma

*Based on blast morphology.

Table 11.7 ● World Health Organization Classification of Acute Myeloid Leukemias

Acute myeloid leukemia with recurrent genetic abnormalities
- Acute myeloid leukemia with t(8;21)(q22;q22)
- Acute myeloid leukemia with abnormal bone marrow eosinophils
  - inv(16)(p13q22) or t(16;16)(p13;q22)
- Acute promyelocytic leukemia (AML with t(15;17)(q22;q12)
- Acute myeloid leukemia with 11q23

Acute myeloid leukemia with multilineage dysplasia

Acute myeloid leukemia and myelodysplastic syndromes, therapy-related

Acute myeloid leukemia not otherwise categorized
- Acute myeloid leukemia minimally differentiated
- Acute myeloid leukemia without maturation
- Acute myeloid leukemia with maturation
- Acute myelomonocytic leukemia
- Acute monoblastic and monocytic leukemia
- Acute erythroid leukemia
- Acute megakaryoblastic leukemia
- Acute basophilic leukemia
- Acute panmyelosis with myelofibrosis
- Myeloid sarcoma

Acute leukemia of ambiguous lineage
- Undifferentiated acute leukemia
- Bilineal acute leukemia
- Biphenotypic acute leukemia

rate designation for the acute leukemias that arise from a previous myelodysplastic syndrome (preleukemia/myelodysplastic syndrome, see Chapter 14) or those occurring as a result of transition from a myeloproliferative disorder (see Chapter 12). In addition, they recognized two other categories of AML as distinct: therapy-related AMLs and those not otherwise categorized. Therefore, the four main WHO groups are:

I. AML with recurrent cytogenetic abnormalities
II. AML with myelodysplasia
III. Therapy-related AML and myelodysplastic syndrome
IV. AML not otherwise categorized

It is noteworthy that the most significant change from the FAB classification is that the required blast percentage for a diagnosis of AML using the WHO criteria is greater than or equal to **20%** myeloblasts in the blood or marrow compared to the FAB blast percentage criteria of **30%** that has been used for many years.[19]

Because the WHO is the most current classification, each of these groups is discussed. However, as technology of genetic and molecular analysis is moving so rapidly, it is likely that modifications to this classification scheme will be necessary in the near future.

I. Acute Myeloid Leukemia With Recurrent Genetic Abnormalities

The most important features of this group are the recurrent genetic abnormality and favorable prognosis. The abnormalities that are commonly identified involve reciprocal translocations. Four subtypes are described here. The reader is referred to other hematology refer-

Table 11.8 ⊙ Chromosomal Alterations*	
Chromosome Abnormality	**Clinical Correlation**
AML	t(8;21)(q22;q22)
	11q23
	Trisomy 7, 8, 13
AML with abnormal bone marrow eosinophils	inv(16)(p13q22)
	t(16;16)(p13;q22)
APL	t(15;17)(q22;q12)
AMML	t(8;16)(p11;p13)
AMonoL	t(9;11)(p22;q23)
B-ALL	Hyperdiploid >50
	t(1;19)(q23;p13.3)
	t(12;21)(p13;q22)
T-ALL	t(1;14)(p32;q11.2)
	t(1;7)(q32;q35)

*These are example of chromosome abnormalities; the list is not intended to be comprehensive.

ence texts for an in-depth discussion of immunophenotypes and genetics that are characteristic for each disorder.

Acute Myeloid Leukemia With t(8;21)(q22;q22)

This leukemia occurs most often in children or young adults and represents 5% to 12% of AML cases.[25] The translocation t(8;21)(q22;q22) is the hallmark feature of this subtype. The morphology associated with this AML include the presence of myeloblasts having abundant cytoplasm, often containing azurophilic granules and sometimes containing large, pseudo–Chediak-Higashi granules. Auer rods are common, and maturation in the neutrophil lineage (promyelocytes, myelocytes, neutrophils) is seen. Dysplastic neutrophilic features that may be seen include pseudo–Pelger-Huët hyposegmentation and hypogranulation. Eosinophils are often increased, and monocyte percentages are usually decreased (Fig. 11.2).

AML with t(8;21) is associated with good response to chemotherapy and long-term survival rates.

Acute Myeloid Leukemia With inv(16)(p13q22) or t(16;16)(p13;q22)

This acute myeloid leukemia occurs in all ages but most often in younger patients. The inv(16)(p13q22) is found in approximately 10% to 12% of all AML cases.[19] This leukemia was previously referred to using the FAB classification as acute myelomonocytic leukemia with eosinophilia (AMML Eo). Various stages of monocytic,

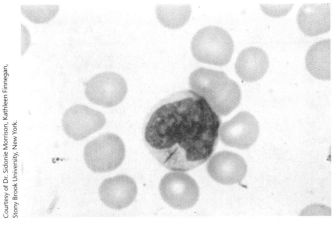

Courtesy of Dr. Sidonie Morrison, Kathleen Finnegan, Stony Brook University, New York.

Figure 11.2 Acute myeloid leukemia with t(8;21)(q22;q22). Note Auer rod in myeloblast.

granulocytic, and eosinophilic maturation are present, as well as abnormal granulations in the immature eosinophils (Fig. 11.3). Rarely, cases of inv(16)(p13q22) lack the eosinophilia.[26] The monoblasts and promonocytes will stain positive for nonspecific esterase (NSE) stain, and the myeloblasts and monoblasts show greater than 3% positivity.

AMML with inv16 and t(16;16) also show high complete remission rates.

Acute Promyelocytic Leukemia [AML With t(15;17)(q22;q12)]

Acute promyelocytic leukemia (APL) accounts for 5% to 8% of AML and can occur in any age but most often

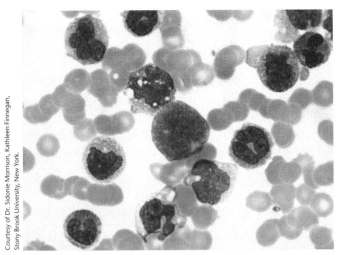

Courtesy of Dr. Sidonie Morrison, Kathleen Finnegan, Stony Brook University, New York.

Figure 11.3 Acute myeloid leukemia with inv(16)(p13q22). Numerous monoblasts, promonocytes, and monocytes are present. Also note few eosinophils that are often characteristically increased in AML with this cytogenetic abnormality.

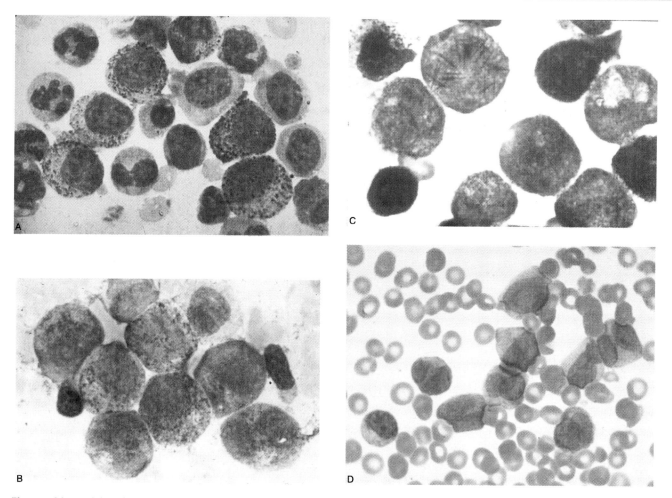

Figure 11.4 *(A)* and *(B),* Hypergranular acute promyelocytic leukemia, promyelocytes with prominent azurophilic granules. *(C)* Hypergranular APL with multiple Auer rods. *(D)* Microgranular APLv. These abnormal promyelocytes have lobulated nuclei and absent or fine azurophilic granules.

in middle-aged patients.[27] Abnormal, hypergranular promyelocytes predominate in the bone marrow in APL with t(15;17)(q22;q12). Numerous Auer rods (fused azurophilic granules) are present in the myeloblasts and promyelocytes, and bundles of Auer rods ("faggot cells") may be seen (Fig. 11.4, C). The azurophilic granules from leukemic promyelocytes have procoagulant activity and predispose the patient to a bleeding diathesis as a result of DIC. The MPO reaction is strongly positive in the promyelocytes. In about 20% of APL cases, a variant type of APL referred to as *microgranular* APL is found. These cases are characterized by cells with convoluted or lobulated nuclei that mimic promonocytes (Fig. 11.4D). These leukemic promyelocytes contain such small azurophilic granules that they are not visible by light microscopy. These cells may cause confusion with acute monocytic leukemia; however, the strong positive MPO reaction (weak in AMonoL) and the bundles of Auer rods are clear clues pointing to a diagnosis of microgranular APL. In addition, the WBC

is often markedly elevated in the microgranular variety of APL.

The prognosis in APL patients with t(15;17) (q22;q12), as with the other leukemias grouped in this category, is also very good.

Acute Myeloid Leukemia With 11q23

This 11q23 deletion/translocation cytogenetic abnormality is found in 5% to 6% of AML cases. It occurs in more often in children but can occur at any age. Monoblasts and promonocytes predominate in the bone marrow and peripheral blood. The monoblasts have abundant cytoplasm, often showing pseudopodia, and fine nuclear chromatin with one or more nuclei. Azurophilic granules are often seen in the monoblasts, and cytoplasmic vacuoles may be present in monoblasts and promonocytes (Fig. 11.5). The NSE reaction is strongly positive in the monoblasts and promonocytes, and the MPO reaction is often negative. The prognosis in AML with 11q23 abnormalities is intermediate.

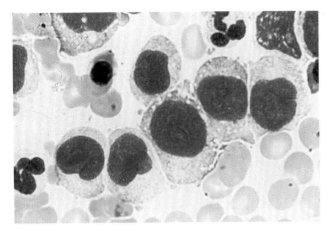

Figure 11.5 Acute myeloid leukemia with 11q23. Note monoblastic leukemia features; monoblasts have abundant cytoplasm, often showing pseudopodia, and fine nuclear chromatin, with one or more nucleoli.

II. Acute Myeloid Leukemia With Myelodysplasia

AML with **myelodysplasia** is seen primarily in adults.[28] The blast percentage in blood or bone marrow is 20% or greater, with abnormal characteristics, called **dysplasia,** observed in at least two cell lines. Some of the dysplastic features that can be observed in neutrophils are hypogranulation, hyposegmentation or pseudo-Pelgeroid neutrophils, and/or bizarre segmented nuclei. In the erythroid cell line, the dyserythropoiesis may present as nucleated red cells with nuclear fragments or multinucleated cells, megaloblastic features, cytoplasmic vacuoles, or karyorrhexis. Ringed sideroblasts may also be seen. The platelet cell line may also be dysplastic, as micromegakaryocytes with one lobe instead of multiple lobes are often present. It is important to be able to recognize these dwarf megakaryocytes because they may be seen by a technologist performing a peripheral smear examination and can be confused with other cells having a round nucleus, for example, mimicking the appearance of a myelocyte. The dysplasia must be present in at least two cell lines to fit the criteria for this category of AML. AML with myelodysplasia may follow a myelodysplastic syndrome (see Chapter 14). Patients with this disorder often present with a decrease in WBC, RBC, and platelet counts, termed pancytopenia. The prognosis of patients with AML with myelodysplasia is poor.[29]

III. Therapy-Related Acute Myeloid Leukemia and Myelodysplastic Syndrome

Treatment with cytotoxic chemotherapy and/or radiation therapy has been associated with the development of AML and myelodysplastic syndrome. The two major agents implicated are alkylating agents/radiation and topoisomerase II inhibitors.[30] These therapy-related leukemias have different epidemiologies, as the alkylating agent/radiation induced disorders usually occur 5 to 6 years after exposure, whereas the topoisomerase II inhibitor disorders occur after an average of 2 to 3 years after exposure.[31] The alkylating agent–related AMLs usually start with a myelodysplastic presentation, with the blast percentage less than 5%, and having the typical myelodysplastic features. Nuclear hypolobulation, cytoplasmic hypogranulation, dyserythropoiesis, and an increase in ringed sideroblasts are characteristic features seen. This may progress into an AML or more pronounced myelodysplastic syndrome. There is a generally poor prognosis associated with alkylating agent/radiation therapy–related AML.

Topoisomerase II inhibitor–related AML does not usually have a preleukemic or myelodysplastic syndrome phase. This type of therapy-related AML often has morphology consistent with that seen in acute monoblastic or myelomonocytic leukemia, although cases showing involvement of other cell lineages have also been described. The prognosis is similar to that of patients with the corresponding morphologically classified AML.

IV. Acute Myeloid Leukemia (Not Otherwise Categorized)

Leukemias with features that do not fit into the previously described categories fall into this grouping. These leukemias are primarily classified according to morphology and cytochemistry reactions. As with the other AMLs, the presence of at least 20% blasts is a hallmark characteristic.

Acute Myeloid Leukemia, Minimally Differentiated

There is little evidence of maturation beyond the blast stage in AML, minimally differentiated, and the marrow is replaced by a homogeneous population of blasts (Fig. 11.6). The myeloid lineage of the blasts is defined by immunophenotyping with a positive expression of CD13, CD33, CD34, and CD117. The MPO and SBB cytochemical stains are usually negative (<3% blasts reacting) and Auer rods are absent. This phenotype comprises approximately 5% of the AML cases and is associated with a poor prognosis.

Acute Myeloid Leukemia Without Maturation

Similar to AML, minimally differentiated, the category of AML without maturation also involves cases where at least 90% of the nonerythroid cells in the bone marrow are myeloblasts (Fig. 11.7). However, at least 5% of the

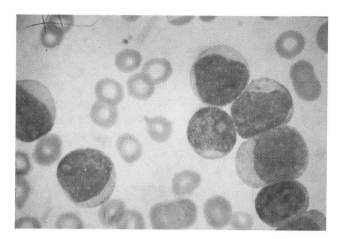

Figure 11.6   Acute myeloid leukemia, minimally differentiated.

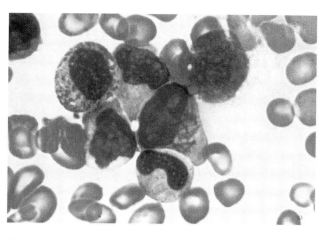

Figure 11.8   Acute myeloid leukemia, with maturation. Note myeloblast with multiple Auer rods.

blasts, and usually a much higher percentage, have a positive reaction with MPO or SBB and Auer rods may be present. AML without maturation constitutes about 10% of AML cases. The blasts in this AML variant express CD13, CD33, CD34, and CD117. AML without maturation appears to have a poor prognosis, especially in patients with a markedly increased WBC.[19]

Acute Myeloid Leukemia With Maturation

AML with maturation is a common leukemia, comprising approximately 30% to 45% of all AML cases. Again, following the definition for acute leukemia, blasts will constitute at least 20% of all nucleated cells in the bone marrow. However, in this variant, greater than 10% of neutrophils with maturation beyond the promyelocyte stage are observed. Additionally, the monocytic component will comprise less than 20% of nonerythroid cells.

Blasts frequently demonstrate Auer rods and variable degrees of dysplasia may be seen (Fig. 11.8). More than 50% of the blasts and maturing cells are MPO and SBB positive. The morphology of the previously described AML with t(8;21)(q22;q22) is usually that of AML with maturation. This phenotype responds variably to chemotherapy, with the t(8;21) cases having a favorable prognosis.

Acute Myelomonocytic Leukemia

A mixture of malignant cells with both myelocytic and monocytic features are found in the blood and bone marrow of patients with acute myelomonocytic leukemia (AMML). The bone marrow has greater than 20% blasts, with both myeloid cells and monocytic cells each comprising greater than 20% of all marrow cells. The monoblasts are large cells with abundant, basophilic cytoplasm with fine azurophilic granules and often pseudopod cytoplasmic extensions; the nucleus has a lacy chromatin and one to four nucleoli. Promonocytes have a more convoluted nucleus with a somewhat more condensed, mature chromatin pattern and may have cytoplasmic vacuoles (Fig. 11.9). Interestingly, the monocytic component may be more prominent in the peripheral blood than in the bone marrow. The NSE reaction is usually strongly positive in AMML, and at least 3% of the blasts are MPO positive. The naphthol ASD chloracetate esterase (specific esterase) reaction is also positive. The leukemic cells variably express myeloid antigens of CD13 and CD33 and usually demonstrate one or more of the monocytic-associated antigens such as CD14, CD4, CD11c, CD64, and CD36.[19] Cases of AML with inv(16) that display AMML with eosinophilia are discussed under AML with recurrent genetic abnormalities. This particular variant

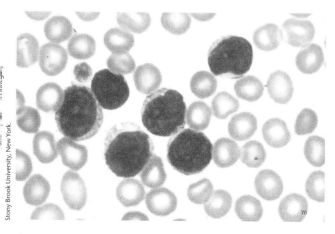

Figure 11.7   Acute myeloid leukemia, without maturation.

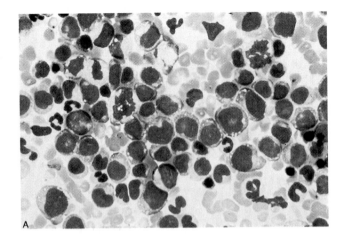

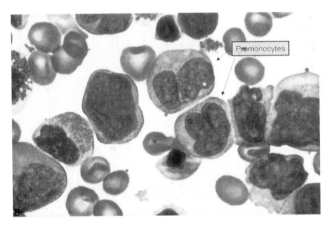

Figure 11.9 Acute myelomonocytic leukemia. *(A)* AMML with prominent monoblasts, promonocytes, and spectrum of myeloid/monocytic cells. *(B)* AMML with promonoblast, promonocytes, and eosinophil on edge of frame at *arrow* (AMMLe)

is associated with favorable prognosis, whereas survival rates for the other AMMLs vary.

Acute Monoblastic and Acute Monocytic Leukemia

Acute monoblastic leukemia accounts for 5% to 8% of AMLs, whereas acute monocytic leukemia comprises 3% to 6% of cases.[27] The bone marrow in both of these leukemias shows greater than 20% blasts, with greater than 80% of the cells having monocytic origin, including monoblasts, promonocytes, and monocytes. The distinction between monoblastic and monocytic leukemia subtypes depends on the proportions of monoblasts and promonocytes present in the bone marrow. Acute monoblastic leukemia has a predominance of monoblasts, which are large cells with moderate to intensely basophilic, abundant cytoplasm, and prominent round nuclei with fine chromatin. A spectrum of monocytic cells is seen in acute monocytic leukemia, with the majority of cells being promonocytes. The

nuclear chromatin of promonocytes is more condensed and they often have a convoluted or cerebriform configuration. The cytoplasm of promonocytes contain azurophilic granules and may be vacuolated. Less than 20% of the cells are of granulocytic origin. Auer rods are usually absent in acute monoblastic leukemia but are frequently seen in the promonocytes of acute monocytic leukemia (Fig. 11.10). In most cases, monoblasts

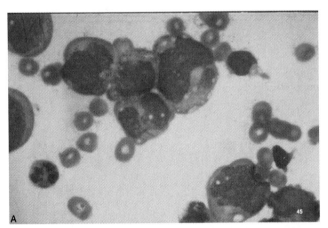

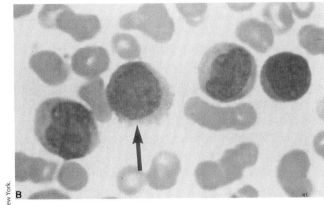

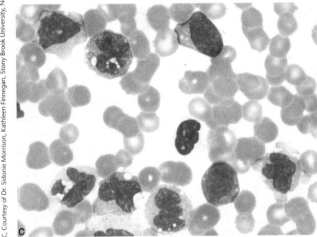

C, Courtesy of Dr. Sidonie Morrison, Kathleen Finnegan, Stony Brook University, New York.

Figure 11.10 *(A)* Acute monoblastic leukemia with Auer rods. *(B)* Acute monocytic leukemia, one monoblast, three promonocytes. *(C)* Acute monocytic leukemia, monoblast, several promonocytes, and monocytes are present.

and promonocytes will stain intensely positive with NSE. Monoblasts are typically MPO or SBB negative; promonocytes may be very weakly positive with these staining reactions. The characteristic immunoreactivity of the monocytic leukemic cells for lysozyme is also a common finding.

Acute monoblastic leukemia may occur at any age, but the majority of patients tend to be younger, have increased blast percentages in the peripheral blood, and have a poor prognosis.[32] Acute monocytic leukemia is more common in adults, with the median age being 49 years. A hallmark clinical feature of the monocytic leukemias is extramedullary disease, with the most predominant finding being the cutaneous and gum infiltration that results in gingival hypertrophy. Other clinical features include bleeding disorders due to DIC, as well as a high incidence of CNS or meningeal disease either at the time of diagnosis or as a manifestation of relapse during remission.[33] A high WBC count is another common finding reported in 10% to 30% of patients.

Characteristic immunophenotypic markers for cells of monocytic differentiation include CD14, CD4, CD11b, CD11c, CD 36, CD64, and CD68. The strong association between the acute monoblastic leukemia and deletions/translocations involving chromosome 11q23 have been previously described under AML with recurrent genetic abnormalities. In general, both acute monoblastic and acute monocytic leukemias have an unfavorable prognosis due to shorter duration of treatment response and poor prognostic factors.

Acute Erythroid Leukemia

Acute erythroid leukemias are predominantly characterized by abnormal proliferation of erythroid precursors. The additional presence or absence of a myeloid element defines the two subtypes, erythroleukemia and pure erythroid leukemia. More than 50% of the bone marrow cells are erythroid precursors and at least 30% are myeloblasts in erythroleukemia (erythroid/myeloid) (Fig. 11.11). Pure erythroid leukemia is defined by the majority of marrow cells (>80%) being comprised of erythroid precursors, without a myeloid proliferation.[19]

Erythroleukemia is usually found in patients 50 years of age or older and accounts for approximately 5%

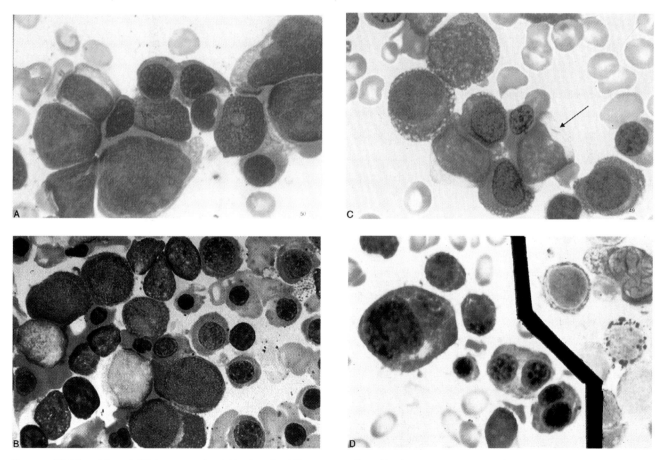

Figure 11.11   *(A)* and *(B)* Acute erythroid leukemia. *(C)* Acute erythroid leukemia, note Auer rod in myeloblast. *(D)* Acute erythroid leukemia, left frame shows binucleated pronormoblasts and dysplastic features, right frame shows PAS block positivity in a ring around the nucleus.

to 6% of AML cases. Characteristics that are commonly seen in the abundant erythroid precursors include dysplastic features such as bizarre multinucleation, cytoplasmic vacuolization, and megaloblastic nuclear changes. The differential diagnosis includes megaloblastic anemia; however, patients with vitamin B$_{12}$ or folic acid deficiency will respond to treatment with these vitamins, and the dysplastic features are not as pronounced as those seen in cases of erythroleukemia.

Myeloblasts containing Auer rods may be observed in up to two-thirds of patients with erythroleukemia.[34] Abnormal megakaryocytes may also be noted. Anemia is often markedly severe in patients with erythroleukemia, and indeed may be more profound that the degree seen in other AML subtypes. The peripheral blood may contain a striking amount of nucleated red cells. However, it is interesting to note that the crowding of the normal elements of the bone marrow by the leukemic cell population results in ineffective erythropoiesis, which actually leads to reticulocytopenia. The bone marrow iron stain often demonstrates ringed sideroblasts, and the PAS stain may be positive in the classic "block" or coarse positivity in the pronormoblasts. The myeloblasts will stain MPO and SBB positive.

Pure erythroid leukemia is the more rare subtype of the two acute erythroid leukemias and may be seen in any age. The stem cells in this leukemia give rise predominantly to erythroid lineage; therefore, any myeloid cell markers will be negative. The pronormoblasts can be identified by immunohistochemical reactivity with antibody to hemoglobin A and expression of glycophorin A, a red cell membrane protein.[19]

Erythromyeloleukemia may evolve to an acute myeloblastic leukemia, with similar prognostic results as other subtypes in patients of similar ages.[35] Pure erythroid leukemia is usually associated with an aggressive clinical course.

Acute Megakaryoblastic Leukemia

Acute megakaryoblastic leukemia (AMegL) is the most rare form of the AMLs, comprising approximately 3% to 5% of cases. This diagnosis is made if at least 20% of blasts in the bone marrow are megakaryoblasts. This leukemia occurs in both children and adults.

Megakaryoblasts are small, medium to large in size, often found as heterogeneous mix in the same patient in regard to size, with some blasts being of small or medium size with scant basophilic cytoplasm and others much larger with more abundant cytoplasm and distinct blebbing pseudopod formation. The nucleus is round or slightly indented with delicate chromatin and one to three prominent nucleoli. Although megakary-

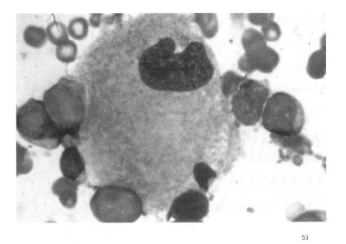

Figure 11.12   Acute megakaryoblastic leukemia.

oblasts may be difficult if not impossible to identify by light microscopy, the presence of blasts with cytoplasmic blebbing may provide a hallmark clue as to the lineage of the blasts. Megakaryoblastic fragments or micromegakaryocytes, along with giant, hypogranular platelets, are sometimes present (Fig. 11.12).

The diagnosis of AMegL is usually made based on immunophenotyping results because megakaryoblasts will express one or more of the platelet glycoproteins: CD41 (glycoprotein IIb/IIIa), CD61 (glycoprotein IIIa), and, less frequently, CD42 (glycoprotein Ib). Cytochemical stains are not as useful, as the MPO, SBB, and TdT are negative, whereas the alpha-naphthyl acetate esterase reaction is usually positive with a negative alpha-naphthyl butyrate esterase reaction (both types of NSE would be positive in acute monocytic leukemia). Megakaryoblasts manifest platelet peroxidase activity that can be identified by electron microscopy cytochemistry.

Although adult patients usually present with the typical acute leukemia symptoms related to cytopenias of pallor, weakness, and excessive bleeding, unlike other leukemias, organomegaly is uncommon at diagnosis. Thrombocytosis may rarely occur and dysplastic features of platelets and neutrophils may be seen. The AMegL that occurs in children has been associated with t(1;22), and these individuals may present with significant abdominal masses[36] and lytic bone lesions.[37] Children with Down syndrome who develop an acute transient leukemia often have AMegL as the predominant morphological subtype. Patients with this rare form of AMegL associated with Down syndrome may undergo spontaneous remission, in contrast with the poor prognosis that is typical of most cases of AMegL, especially in infants with the t(1;22).[38]

Other Acute Leukemias

Several other acute leukemias account for less than 5% of cases of acute leukemia. *Acute basophilic leukemia* is a very rare leukemia that may occur "de novo" or more commonly may arise as a blastic transformation in patients with a preceding CML. The predominant circulating cell appears blast-like with one to three nucleoli and prominent, but variable number of, coarse basophilic granules. The cells will stain positive with the metachromatic stain tolidine blue. Additionally, the blasts will stain positive with acid phosphatase and show block positivity with PAS but are negative with MPO, SBB, and NSE stains. The blasts usually are positive for myeloid markers CD13, CD33, and CD34, and also will show reactivity with CD9. The special stains and immunophenotyping will distinguish acute basophilic leukemia from acute promyelocytic leukemia, as the early basophilic myelocytes may be confused with promyelocytes.

Acute myelofibrosis is another rare leukemia characterized by marked peripheral blood pancytopenia and marrow hyperplasia of the erythroid, granulocytic, and megakaryocytic components, combined with a variable degree of fibrosis. Differential diagnosis from chronic idiopathic myelofibrosis (IMF) can be made since more immature cells are seen in the acute process and the splenomegaly that is a hallmark feature of IMF is absent in acute myelofibrosis.

There are several types of acute leukemias that the WHO group has combined into "acute leukemia of ambiguous lineage." These include leukemias where the morphologic, immunophenotypic, and/or cytochemical findings are not helpful in the classification of a particular type of myeloid or lymphoid process or, conversely, where the features indicate a combination of different lines.[39–41] *Undifferentiated acute leukemias* lack markers consistent with a specific lineage, *bilineal acute leukemias* contain different populations of cells that express both myeloid and lymphoid markers, and *biphenotypic acute leukemias* are typified by cells that have both myeloid- and T or B lineage–specific antigens on the same blast population.[19]

ACUTE LYMPHOBLASTIC LEUKEMIA

Acute lymphoblastic leukemia (ALL) is a malignant disease that evolves as a result of mutation of lymphoid precursor cells that have their origin in the marrow or thymus, at a particular stage of maturation. The immunophenotype reflects the antigen expression of the stage of differentiation of the dominant clone. The leukemic cells persistently accumulate in intramedullary and extramedullary sites, constantly competing with normal hematopoietic cell production and function. This results in anemia, thrombocytopenia, and neutropenia, as well as an overpopulation of lymphoblasts in the tissues such as liver, spleen, lymph nodes, meninges, and gonads.

Epidemiology

ALL is predominantly a disease of children, with highest incidence in children between the ages of 2 and 6. It accounts for 76% of all leukemias diagnosed in children younger than age 15.[42] According to National Cancer Institute statistics, there is an increased incidence of ALL seen in all age groups in males compared to females of European or African descent.[43] The exception is a slight female predominance in infancy.[44] Although more uncommon in adults, ALL occurs in all ages, and rising incidence rates are seen with increasing age, with a second peak incidence in the elderly population.

The etiology of ALL is unknown in the vast majority of cases. Environmental agents, such as ionizing radiation and chemical mutagens, have been implicated, and there is evidence to suggest a genetic factor in some patients. Children with Down syndrome have an increased risk of leukemia, particularly precursor B lymphoblastic leukemia. There is a higher frequency of childhood ALL in industrialized countries compared with in developing countries. It has also been postulated that some cases of childhood leukemia stem from an adverse cellular response to common infections that occur at a later time than was typically experienced in past centuries.[45,46] These "delayed" exposures are believed to increase the risk of genetic mutations in the lymphoid precursors, leading to the development of leukemia.

Clinical Features

Clinical presentation is variable; symptoms may be subtle and develop over months or they may be acute and quite severe. The presenting symptoms are directly related to the degree of bone marrow failure or extramedullary involvement (see Table 11.3). Symptoms that are seen in about half of the patients include fever that stems from the leukemic process itself (tumor burden) and from the neutropenia and pallor and fatigue that are caused by the anemia. Bleeding, purpura, and bone and joint pain are other common presenting complaints. Children often present with a limp or the inability to walk due to the pain caused by the leukemic infiltration of the periosteum (bone covering) or due to the actual bone itself causing osteoporosis or bone erosion. Hepatosplenomegaly and lymphadenopathy may be prominent symptoms. Uncommon symptoms include cough, dyspnea, cyanosis, and syncope related to a bulky mediastinal mass that can compress blood vessels or the trachea.[47]

Classifications

The FAB classification defined three morphological subtypes—L1, L2, and L3—based on the appearance of the blasts that predominate. L1 lymphoblasts are small with scant cytoplasm, are uniform in size, and have indistinct nucleoli. L2 blasts are larger and more pleomorphic, often containing abundant cytoplasm and prominent nucleoli (Table 11.9). Both LI and L2 blasts cannot be determined from morphology alone as they may be easily confused with myeloblasts seen in AML. L3 lymphoblasts are characterized by intensely basophilic cytoplasm that has many vacuoles. Because of the differences in prognosis based on immunophenotype and cytogenetics, the WHO has recognized just two groups of acute lymphoblastic leukemias, precursor B-cell and precursor T-cell lymphoblastic leukemia/lymphoma.

Precursor B Lymphoblastic Leukemia/ Lymphoblastic Lymphoma

Precursor B lymphoblastic leukemia (B-ALL)/lymphoblastic lymphoma (B-LBL) is a malignancy where B-lineage lymphoblasts predominate in the bone marrow (B lymphoblastic leukemia). Sometimes there is primary involvement of lymph nodes or extranodal sites (B lymphoblastic lymphoma). Greater than 25% of bone marrow cells must be identified as lymphoblasts to meet the WHO definition of acute lymphoblastic leukemia; however, the bone marrow aspirate typically consists of almost entirely lymphoblasts at diagnosis. When the leukemic process is limited to a mass lesion and 25% or fewer lymphoblasts are seen in the marrow, the designation **lymphoma** is used.[19] B-ALL comprises approximately 85% of all childhood ALL, whereas B-LBL is a rare type of lymphoma and constitutes approximately 10% of lymphoblastic lymphoma cases.[48] B-ALL may also develop in adults, and the prognosis is generally much poorer in adults.

The bone marrow and blood will manifest blasts in all cases of B-ALL. Extramedullary sites of hematopoiesis cause hepatosplenomegaly, and there is a predilection for CNS (**meningeal leukemia**), lymph nodes, and gonad involvement. Bone pain from marrow hyperplasia is also a frequent clinical symptom.

Laboratory Features

The WBC is variable in B-ALL—it may be markedly elevated, normal, or decreased. As with all other acute leukemias, anemia and thrombocytopenia are apparent at diagnosis. The blood and bone marrow contains lymphoblasts with L1 or L2 morphology (Fig. 11.13). Coarse azurophilic granules may be present in the lymphoblasts in up to 10% of cases. Lymphoblasts with pseudopod projections, termed "hand-mirror cells," are occasionally found. Although not as important as the immunophenotypic characterization, cytochemistries may be helpful until further studies can be performed to help separate the preliminary diagnosis of lymphoid from myeloid leukemia. The myeloid stains SBB and MPO will be negative or very weakly positive as compared to the intensely positive stain seen in myeloblasts. The NSE reaction is generally negative. By contrast, the PAS stain is positive in over 70% of ALL cases, with the nuclei often giving the appearance of being rimmed with a punctate PAS-positive string of beads.

Immunophenotype

As previously noted, the immunological classification should be performed in all cases as it allows for more

---

Table 11.9 ⊙ FAB Morphological Classification of Acute Lymphoblastic Leukemia

Feature	L1	L2	L3
Cell size	Small, regular	Large, mixed sizes	Large
Nuclear chromatin	Fine or condensed	Fine or condensed	Fine
Nuclear shape	Regular, cleft or indentation possible	Irregular, cleft or indentation more common	Regular, round or oval
Nucleoli	Indistinct	1 to 2, prominent	1 to 2, prominent
Cytoplasm	Scant	Variable, often moderately abundant	Deeply basophilic, vacuolated

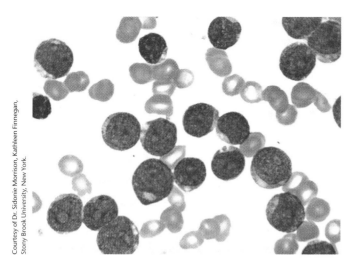

Figure 11.13   Precursor B lymphoblastic leukemia.

differentiation (CD) groups is done. Because no one surface marker is 100% specific, a panel is needed to establish the diagnosis and sort the leukemia into the appropriate subtype. To be able to interpret the CD information, it is important to have a basic understanding of lymphocyte ontogeny.

Each of the two lineages of lymphocytes (B and T cells) can be subclassified into several maturational stages by the expression of their surface antigens. Accordingly, ALLs are divided by immunophenotype, first into B- or T-cell lineages. In leukemia, the lymphoblasts are "frozen" at a specific stage of maturation, and these blasts can then be further categorized by using CD markers into the particular stage of differentiation, that is, precursor B, pre-B, and mature B-ALL.

The lymphoblasts in B-ALL/LBL are uniformly TdT positive and HLA-DR positive. The flow cytometric immunophenotype in most cases is positive for CD 10, CD19, CD20, CD24, cytoplasmic CD22, and CD79a (Fig. 11.14).

precise diagnosis and important prognostic correlations. In order to define a particular population of lymphoblasts in leukemia, evaluation of the results of a panel of antibodies used to distinguish the clusters of

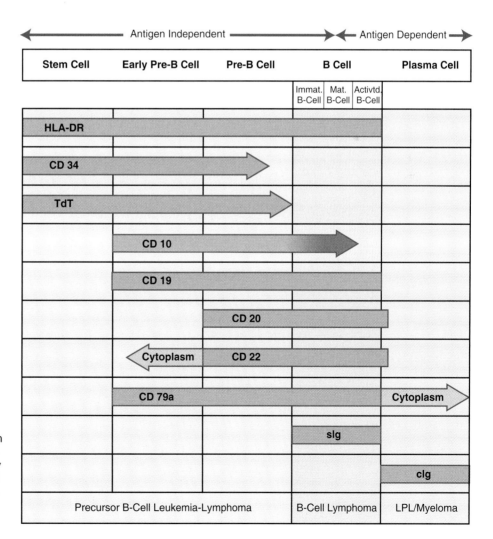

Figure 11.14   B-lineage antigen expression. Stages of B-cell differentiation can be demonstrated by antigen expression. TdT, terminal deoxynucleotidyl transferase; sIg, surface immunoglobulin; cIg, cytoplasmic immunoglobulin.

Cytogenetic Findings

In addition to immunophenotype, certain chromosomal alterations have been identified in B-ALL that are considered prognostically important (see Table 11-8). While these abnormalities are not as consistently associated as the Philadelphia chromosome seen in CML, they do provide additional information that can help to refine the treatment regimen. Two abnormalities that have been associated with a good prognosis are (1) hyperploidy greater than 50 and (2) t(12;21)(p13;q22). Other cytogenetic findings have been linked to a poor prognostic outcome (Table 11.10).

Precursor T Lymphoblastic Leukemia/ Lymphoblastic Lymphoma

Precursor T lymphoblastic leukemia/lymphoma is a malignancy of lymphoblasts with pre-T markers predominating in the bone marrow (T-ALL). When there is primary involvement of lymph nodes or extranodal sites, it is termed T lymphoblastic lymphoma. As in B-ALL, greater than 25% of bone marrow cells must be identified as lymphoblasts to meet the WHO definition of acute lymphoblastic leukemia; however, the bone marrow aspirate typically consists of almost entirely lymphoblasts at diagnosis. When the leukemic process is limited to a mass lesion and at least 25% lymphoblasts are seen in the marrow, the designation *lymphoma* is used.[19]

T-ALL represents approximately 15% to 20% of all childhood ALL, is more prevalent in adolescents than young children, and is seen more frequently in males than females. T-ALL accounts for 25% of adult cases. T-lymphoblastic lymphoma (T-LBL) is the subtype of 85% to 90% of lymphoblastic lymphomas[19] and is seen more frequently in males.

The bone marrow and blood will manifest blasts in all cases of T-ALL. Both T-ALL and T-LBL patients often present with large mediastinal or other tissue masses; other sites of involvement include lymph nodes, liver, spleen, skin, CNS, and gonads.

Laboratory Features

The leukocyte count may be quite high in precursor T-ALL ($>100 \times 10^9$/L). The lymphoblasts often have L2 morphology, medium-size blasts with a moderate amount of cytoplasm and prominent nucleoli, occasional nuclear clefting; or, less frequently, have L1 morphology with smaller blasts, a high nucleus-to-cytoplasm ratio, scant cytoplasm, and indistinct cytoplasm. Sometimes, a mixture of both L1 and L2 morphology is observed in the same case (see Table 11.9 and Fig. 11.15). The number of mitotic blast cells is usually higher in T-ALL than in B-ALL.

Immunophenotype

Most precursor T-ALL malignancies have an immunophenotype that corresponds to an immature thymocyte

---

Table 11.10 ● Prognostic Factors in Acute Lymphoblastic Leukemia

Risk Factors	Favorable	Unfavorable
WBC Count	$<10 \times 10^9$/L	$>50 \times 10^9$/L
Hemoglobin	<10 g/dL	>7 g/dL
Age	2 to 9 years	<2 and >10 years
Race	White	Black
Sex	Female	Male
Response to treatment	<14 days	>28 days
CNS leukemia	Absent	Present
Immunophenotype	Precursor B-cell	Precursor T-cell or mixed lineage
Cytogenetic	Hyperploidy >50	Hypoploidy
	t(12;21)(p13;q22)	Translocations, especially
		t(9;22)(q34;q11.2)
		t(1;19)(q23;p13.3)
		t(4;11)(q21;q23)

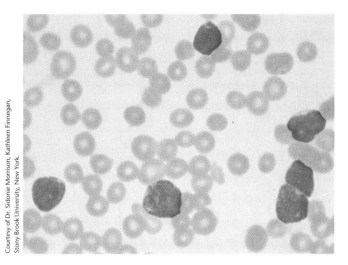

Courtesy of Dr. Sidonie Morrison, Kathleen Finnegan, Stony Brook University, New York.

Figure 11.15   Precursor T lymphoblastic leukemia.

(prothymocyte) stage, originating in the bone marrow. The B-LBL or lymphoma phenotypes correspond to the more mature state of differentiation.[49] The lymphoblasts in T-ALL are TdT, cytoplasmic CD3 and CD7 positive, and variably express CD1, CD2, CD4, CD5, CD8, and CD10. Of interest is the fact that the myeloid-associated antigens CD13 and CD34 are often present,

and this may still be consistent with the diagnosis of T-ALL/LBL (Fig. 11.16).

Cytogenetic Findings

Reciprocal translocations of the T-cell receptor loci have been detected in about one-third of patients with T-ALL/LBL.[19] These translocations arise from mistakes in the normal recombination mechanisms that generate antigen receptor genes. These cellular rearrangements that occur in T-ALL cases affect the proteins that have vital functions in cell proliferation, differentiation, or survival.[50] The association of clinical findings, specific lymphoblast phenotype with particular chromosomal abnormalities has been shown to have prognostic significance. For a detailed discussion of the genes affected by chromosomal translocations in B-ALL and T-ALL, the reader is referred to Williams Hematology, 6th ed. Chapter 97, New York: McGraw-Hill, 2001.

Prognosis in Acute Lymphoblastic Leukemia

In the pediatric age group, children with ALL have an overall complete remission rate of close to 95%; however, the disease-free, long-term response rate is about

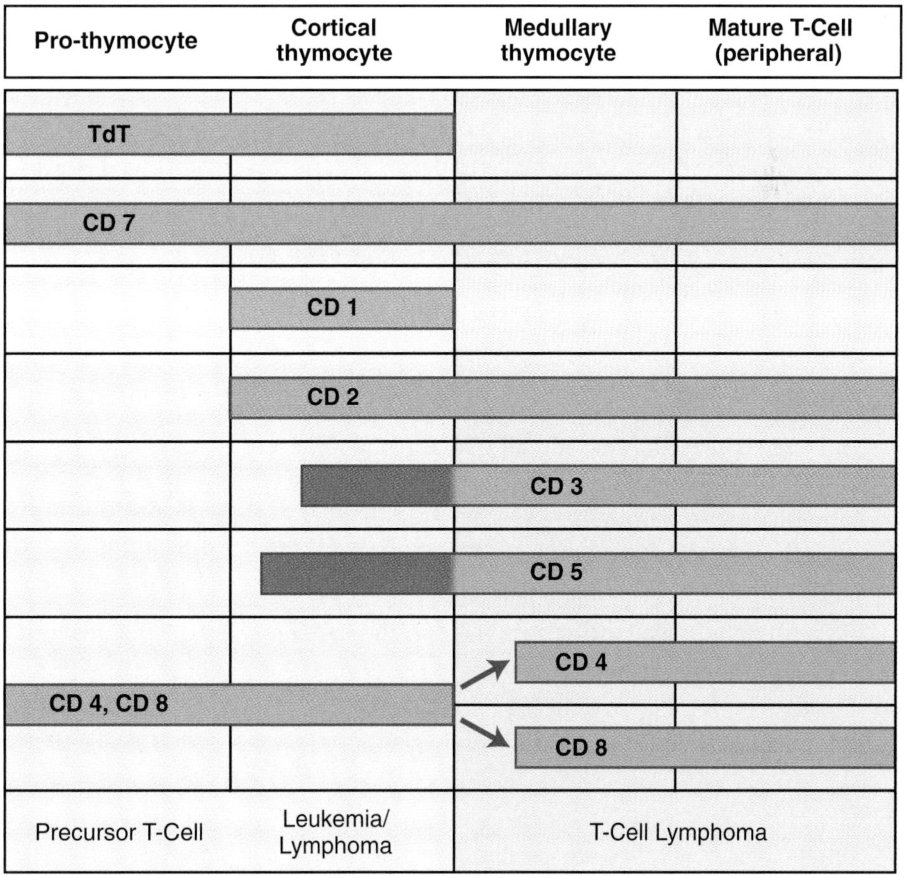

Pro-thymocyte	Cortical thymocyte	Medullary thymocyte	Mature T-Cell (peripheral)
TdT	TdT		
CD 7	CD 7	CD 7	CD 7
	CD 1		
	CD 2	CD 2	CD 2
	CD 3	CD 3	CD 3
	CD 5	CD 5	CD 5
		CD 4 →	CD 4
CD 4, CD 8	CD 4, CD 8	CD 8 →	CD 8
Precursor T-Cell	Leukemia/Lymphoma	T-Cell Lymphoma	T-Cell Lymphoma

Figure 11.16   T-lineage antigen expression. T-cell development originates with prothymocytes in the bone marrow. Further development takes place after these cells migrate to the thymus, where the maturation of the thymocyte can be classified, using specific CD markers, according to the various membrane antigens that are expressed.

70% to 80%.[51,52] The cure rate in adults is somewhat more variable at 60% to 85%.[19] Prognostic indicators in ALL are listed in Table 11.10.

Although the FAB morphology classification has been used for more than a quarter of a century, the discovery of genetic markers that can help predict clinical outcome prompted the WHO to redefine the classification scheme. For a given case, the initial therapy for treating an acute leukemia based on morphological or cytochemical findings may be amended when the cytogenetic and immunophenotypic testing is completed.

Age and WBC count are used for risk assessment in all pediatric clinical trials, with WBC less than 50 × 10⁹/L as the minimal criteria for low-risk ALL.[53] Other prognostic factors used to determine outcome are sex,

immunophenotypic and cytogenetic profiles, and response to treatment. The two most important tests with the greatest prognostic prediction power when the sample of hematopoietic material is limited are flow cytometry and cytogenetics.

The combination of conventional clinical, morphological, and cytochemistry findings with the newer immunophenotypic, cytogenetic, and molecular testing now available affords the pathologist and oncologist the most valuable and comprehensive information to "get to know" each disease entity and its characteristics. It is now even more imperative that there is good communication between the clinician, the laboratory staff, and the pathologist in gathering the important prognostic data so that the most specific diagnosis and treatment can be applied.

CONDENSED CASE

A 10-year-old girl was taken to an outpatient clinic with a complaint of sore throat and a lump in her neck. Upon examination she was observed to have a tonsillar abscess, swollen glands, and widespread bruising in the extremities. She also had a low-grade fever. She was treated with antibiotics and released, but she failed to progress in the next 2 days. Her blood work revealed a white count of 8.0 × 10⁹/L, an hematocrit of 28%, and a platelet count of 10,000. Her parents were contacted and she was immediately admitted to the hospital. A bone marrow examination was performed and revealed an infiltration of blast cells in the marrow. **Why are her other cell counts depressed?**

Answer
Although this is an unusual presentation of an acute leukemia, all of the elements related to symptoms are in place. The depressed hematocrit and platelet count are indicative of the blast burden in the bone marrow crowding out all of the normal elements and causing low counts. This young girl will be transferred to an oncology facility and will most likely be treated aggressively for her leukemia after it is classified. **What is the presumptive diagnosis based upon this information?**

　　1 Monocyte
　　83 Blasts

Summary Points

- Leukemia is caused by the mutation of the bone marrow pluripotent stem cells.

- Individuals with acute leukemia will present with variable white counts, anemia, and platelet counts.

- When blasts cells accumulate in the bone marrow and peripheral smear, the leukemia is classified as acute.

- Hepatosplenomegaly or lymphadenopathy is more prominent in chronic leukemias than in acute leukemias.

- According to the WHO, the peripheral smear must contain 20% myeloblasts or greater for a diagnosis of acute leukemia.

- Skin infiltration is characteristic of monocytic leukemias; extramedullary hematopoiesis is common in monocytic or myelomonocytic leukemias.

- Headache, blindness, and other neurological complications are indicative of blast cells crossing the blood-brain barrier.

- Cytochemical staining can assist in the diagnosis of acute leukemias based on staining patterns.

- Auer rods are composed of fused primary granules and may be present in myeloblasts.

- Immunophenotyping can help to classify the clone of leukemic cells by using monoclonal antibodies in flow cytometry or immunohistochemistry procedures.

- Cytogenetic abnormalities such as translocation and deletion are an important prognostic feature of many acute leukemias.
- Acute promyelocytic leukemia is associated with disseminated intravascular coagulation.
- Treatment with cytotoxic chemotherapy and/or radiation therapy is associated with the development of acute leukemia and myelodysplastic syndrome.
- Acute myelocytic leukemia with maturation of the most common acute myelocytic leukemias.
- Acute lymphoblastic leukemia is the leukemia of childhood with highest incidence between the ages of 2 and 6 years.
- Acute lymphoblastic leukemia accounts for 76% of all leukemias diagnosed in children younger than 13 years.
- Children with Down syndrome have an increased risk of leukemia.
- Lymphoblasts will frequently cross the blood-brain barrier, causing neurological involvement.
- In the pediatric age group, children with acute lymphoblastic leukemia have an overall complete remission rate of close to 95%.

CASE STUDY

A 6-year-old girl presented to her pediatrician with symptoms of fatigue, pallor, bruising, and a pronounced limp. Physical examination revealed moderate splenomegaly, mild lymphadenopathy, and a fever of 101°F. CBC results were as follows:

WBC	60.6×10^9/L	LDH	725 (Nl 277-610 IU/L)
RBC	2.90×10^{12}/L	Reticulocytes	0.7%
Hgb	7.9 g/dL	PT/aPTT	Normal
Hct	24.1%		
MCV	82 fL		
MCH	27.2 pg		
MCHC	32.8 g/dL		
RDW	17.0%		
Platelets	23×10^9/L		
Differential:	2 band neutrophils		
	4 segmented neutrophils		
	10 lymphocytes		
	1 monocyte		
	83 balsts		

Insights to the Case Study

Considering the patient's age and the fact that she has 83% blasts in her peripheral smear, a diagnosis of acute leukemia is highly likely. There is also evidence of hemolysis since the LDH is extremely elevated. The reticulocyte count is low and not representative of a regenerative bone marrow. This is probably due to the crowding out of the normal elements of the bone marrow. A bone marrow biopsy was ordered and showed sheets of small blasts with scanty cytoplasm and indistinct nucleoli. The cytochemical stains were SBB negative and NSE negative. The PAS was positive. Immunophenotyping results showed TdT positive and cells positive for CD10, CD19, CD20, CD24, and CD34. These findings suggest a pre-B acute lymphoblastic leukemia.

Review Questions

1. Which of the following is most often associated with acute leukemia?
   a. Erythrocytosis and thrombocytosis
   b. Neutropenia and thrombosis
   c. Anemia and thrombocytopenia
   d. Lymphocytosis and thrombocythemia

2. What is the requisite blast percentage for the diagnosis of acute leukemia recommended by the World Health Organization (WHO)?
   a. 10%
   b. 20%
   c. 30%
   d. 40%

3. Auer rods may be seen in which of the following cells?
   a. Myeloblasts
   b. Myelocytes
   c. Lymphoblasts
   d. Megakaryoblasts

4. The myeloperoxidase stain will be strongly positive in:
   a. acute lymphoblastic leukemia.
   b. acute monocytic leukemia.
   c. acute megakaryoblastic leukemia.
   d. acute myeloblastic leukemia.

5. Acute promyelocytic leukemia has a high incidence of which of the following cytogenetic abnormalities?
   a. t(8;21)(q22;q22)
   b. inv(16)(p13q22)
   c. t(15;17)(q22;q12)
   d. t(9;11)(p22;q23)

6. Which cytochemical reaction is most helpful in identifying the blasts in acute monoblastic leukemia?
   a. Nonspecific esterase
   b. TdT
   c. PAS
   d. SBB

7. The monoclonal marker that is often positive in precursor B lymphoblastic leukemia/lymphoma is:
   a. CD1.
   b. CD7.
   c. CD10.
   d. CD41.

⊙ TROUBLESHOOTING

What Do I Do to Correct the CBC When the White Count Is Out of Linearity Range?

CBC results

WBC	194.1×10^9/L	
RBC	3.89×10^{12}/L	
Hgb	11.3 g/dL	
Hct	34.0%	
MCV	91.0 fL	
MCH	29.1 pg	
MCHC	32.0 g/dL	
RDW	17.2%	
Platelets	41×10^9/L	
WBC diff:	NE, LY, MO, EO, BA all have R flags	

Flags

+++WBC beyond reportable range, upper linearity limit is 99.9×10^9/L
RL, R, RH, flags
on entire CBC

The entire CBC and differential was "flagged" and considered nonreportable.

1. Which of these CBC results are unacceptable to report out to the clinician without further workup?
   ALL: *WBC out-of-range, inaccurate RBC/HCT/RBC indices, questionable inaccurate platelets*

2. What are the next steps that should be taken to provide accurate results?

Resolution steps

- Dilute blood 1:10 with diluent, re-run
- Calculate to get accurate WBC
- Subtract RBC from WBC, i.e., RBC − WBC = accurate RBC
- Perform microhematocrit (spun HCT)
- Report only WBC, RBC, platelets
- Perform manual WBC differential, verify platelet count (or perform manually)

Example:

1. 1:10 dilution of blood—WBC result was 24.9×10^9/L

   - Calculate to get **accurate WBC**:

     WBC 24.9×10^9/L

     24.9×10 (dilution factor) = 249×10^9/L = *accurate WBC count*

2. Subtract WBC from original RBC, as WBCs are included in original count, to obtain **accurate RBC**

     3.89 (original RBC) − 0.249 (WBC count expressed in millions unit of measure) = 3.64×10^{12}/L = *accurate RBC count*

3. Microhematocrit = 33.5%

   - Be careful to exclude the buffy coat when reading the microhematocrit

4. Perform manual WBC differential and platelet estimate

WORD KEY

Auer rods • Elliptical, spindle-like inclusions composed of fused azurophilic granules that may be present in myeloblasts, monoblasts, or promyelocytes in the various AMLs

Cytochemistry • Special stains usually performed on bone marrow samples that are examined microscopically to identify enzymes, lipids, or other chemical constituents within the blast population of cells in acute leukemia

Dyspnea • Shortness of breath

Dysplasia • Abnormal maturation of cells in the bone marrow

Gingival hyperplasia • Swelling of the gingival tissues (gums); in leukemia, this is due to infiltration of the gum tissues with leukemic cells

Immunophenotyping • Process of using monoclonal antibodies directed against cell surface markers to identify antigens unique to the specific lineage and stage of maturation

Lineage • Referring to one specific cell line

Lymphoma • Neoplasm involving abnormal proliferation of cells arising in the lymph nodes; these tumor cells may also metastasize to involve extranodal sites

Meningeal leukemia • Leukemic cells proliferating in the central nervous system

Myelodysplasia • Abnormal maturation and/or differentiation of granulocytes, erythrocytes, monocytes, and platelets

Oncogene • Gene that is responsible for the development of cancer

References

1. Virchow R. Weisses Blut Froiep's Notizen 36:151, 1845.
2. Bennett JH. Two cases of disease and enlargement of the spleen in which death took place from the presence of purulent matter in the blood. Edinburgh Med Surg J 64:413, 1845.
3. Virchow R. Die farblosen Blutkorperchen. In: Gesammelte Abhandlungen sur Wissen schaftlichen Medizin. Frankfurt: Meidinger, 1856.
4. Neumann E. Ueber myelogene leukäemie. Berl Klin Wochenchr 15:69, 1878.
5. Ebstein W. Ueber die acute Leukämie und Pseudo-leukämie. Dtsch Arch Klin Med 44:343, 1889.
6. Erlich P. Farbenanolytische Untersuchungen zur Histologie und Klinik des Blutes. Berlin: Hirschwald, 1891.
7. Naegeli O. Ueber rothes Knochenmark und Myeloblasten. Dtsch Med Wochenschr 26:287, 1900.
8. Hirschfield H. Zur Kenntnis der Histogenese der granulirten Knochenmarkzellen. Arch Pathol Anat 153:335, 1898.
9. Look AT. Oncogene transcription factors in human acute leukemias. Science 278:1059, 1997.
10. Harmening DH. Clinical Hematology and Fundamentals of Hemostasis, 4th ed. Philadelphia: FA Davis, 2002.
11. Sandler DP, Ross JA. Epidemiology of acute leukemia in children and adults. Semin Oncol 24:3–16, 1997.
12. Caldwell GG, Kelley D, Zack M, et al. Mortality and cancer frequency among military nuclear test (SMOKY) participants 1957 through 1979. JAMA 250:620–624, 1983.
13. United Nations Scientific Committee on the Effects of Atomic Radiation. Sources and Effects of Ionizing Radiation. Publication E.94.IX.2, New York: United Nations, 1972.
14. Sullivan AK. Classification, pathogenesis, and etiology of neoplastic diseases of the hematopoietic system. In: Lee GR, Bithell TC, Foerster J, et al, eds. Wintrobe's Clinical Hematology, 9th ed. Philadelphia: Lea and Febiger, 1993: 1725–1791.
15. Chang JC. How to differentiate neoplastic fever from infectious fever in patients with cancer. Usefulness of naproxen test. Heart Lung 16:122, 1987.
16. Golub TR, Weinstein HJ, Grier HE. Acute myelogenous leukemia. In: Pizzo P, Poplack D, eds. Principles and

Practice of Pediatric Oncology, 3rd ed. Philadelphia: JB Lippincott, 1997: 463–482.

17. Rohatiner A, Lister TA. The general management of the patient with leukemia. In: Henderson ES, Lister TA, Greaves MF, eds. Leukemia, 6th ed. Philadelphia: WB Saunders, 1996: 247–255.

18. Burns CP, Armitage JO, Frey AL, et al. Analysis of presenting features of adult leukemia. Dancer 47:2460, 1981.

19. Jaffe ES, Harris NL, Stein H, et al. World Health Organization Classification of Tumours; Pathology and Genetics of Tumours of Haematopoietic and Lymphoid Tissues. Lyon: IARC Press, 2001.

20. Traweek ST, Arber DA, Rappoport H, et al. Extramedullary myeloid tumors. An immunohistochemical and morphologic study of 28 cases. Am J Surg Pathol 17:1011–1019, 1993.

21. Chilosi M, Pizzolo G. Review of terminal deoxynucleotidyl transferase. Biologic aspects, methods of detection, and selected diagnostic application. Appl Immunohistochem 3:209–221, 1995.

22. Kung PC, Long JC, McCaffrey RP, et al. Tdt in the diagnosis of leukemia and malignant lymphoma. Am J Med 64:788, 1978.

23. Marks SM, Baltimore D, McCafffrey R. Terminal transferase as a predictor of initial responsiveness to vincristine and prednisone in blastic chronic myelogenous leukemia. A cooperative study. N Engl J Med 298:812, 1978.

24. Harris NL, Jaffe ES, Diebold J, et al. World Health Organization classification of neoplastic diseases of the hematopoietic and lymphoid tissues: Report of the Clinical Advisory Committee meeting-Airlie House, Virginia, November, 1997. J Clin Oncol 17:3835–3849, 1999.

25. Caligiuri MA, Strout MP, Gilliland DG. Molecular biology of acute myeloid leukemia. Semin Oncol 24:32–34, 1997.

26. Stark B, Resnitzky P, Jeison M, et al. A distinct subtype of M4/M5 acute myeloblastic leukemia (AML) associated with t(8:16)(p11:13), in a patient with the variant t(8:19)(p11:q13) – case report and review of the literature. Leuk Res 19:367–379, 1995.

27. Stanley M, McKenna RW, Ellinger G, et al. Classification of 358 Cases of Acute Myeloid Leukemia by FAB Criteria; Analysis of Clinical and Morphologic Findings in Chronic and Acute Leukemias in Adults. Boston: Martin Nijhoff Publishers, 1985.

28. Head DR. Revised classification of acute myeloid leukemia. Leukemia 10:1826–1831, 1996.

29. Leith CP, Kopecky KJ, Godwin J, et al. Acute myeloid leukemia in the elderly: Assessment of multidrug resistance (MDR1) and cytogenetics distinguishes biologic subgroups with remarkably distinct responses to standard chemotherapy. A Southwest Oncology Group study. Blood 89:3323–3329, 1997.

30. Pui CH, Relling MV, Rivera GK, et al. Epipodophyllotoxin-related acute myeloid leukemia: A study of 35 cases. Leukemia 9:1990–1996, 1995.

31. Ellis M, Ravid M, Lishner M. A comparative analysis of alkylating agent and epipodophyllotoxin-related leukemias. Leuk Lymphoma 11:9–13, 1993.

32. Scott CS, Stark AN, Limbert HJ, et al. Diagnostic and prognostic factors in acute monocytic leukemia: An analysis of 51 cases. Br J Haematol 69:247–252, 1988.

33. Finaux P, Vanhaesbroucke C, Estienne MH, et al. Acute monocytic leukaemia in adults: Treatment and prognosis in 99 cases. Br J Haematol 75:41, 1990.

34. Brunning RD, McKenna RW. Acute leukemias. In: Atlas of Tumor Pathology. Tumors of the Bone Marrow. Washington, DC: Armed Forces Institute of Pathology, 1994: 19–142.

35. Davey FR, Abraham N Jr, Bronetto VL, et al. Morphologic characteristics of erythroleukemia (acute myeloid leukemia; FAB-M6): A CALGB study. Am J Hematol 49:29, 1995.

36. Bernstein J, Dastugue N, Haas OA, et al. Nineteen cases of the t(1;22)(p13;q13) acute megakaryoblastic leukaemia of infants/children and a review of 39 cases: Report from a t(1;22) study group. Leukemia 14:216–218, 2000.

37. Nichols CR, Roth BJ, Heerema N, et al. Hematologic neoplasms associated with primary mediastinal germ-cell tumors. N Engl J Med 322:1425–1429, 1990.

38. Bowman WP, Melvin SL, Aur RJ, et al. A clinical perspective on cell markers in acute lymphocytic leukemia. Cancer Res 41:4752–4766, 1981.

39. Hanson CA, Abaza M, Sheldon S, et al. Acute biphenotypic leukaemia: Immunophenotypic and cytogenetic analysis. Br J Haematol 84:49–60, 1993.

40. Legrand O, Perrot JY, Simonin G, et al. Adult biphenotypic acute leukaemia: An entity with poor prognosis which is related to unfavorable cytogenetics and P-glycoprotein over-expression. Br J Haematol 100: 147–155, 1998.

41. Matutes E, Morilla R, Farahat N, et al. Definition of acute biphenotypic leukaemia. Haematologica 82: 64–66, 1997.

42. Gurney JG, Davis S, Serverson RK, et al. Trends in cancer incidence among children in the U.S. Cancer 78:532, 1996.

43. SEER Cancer Statistics Review, 1973-1995. Bethesda, MD: National Cancer Institute, 1998.

44. Reaman GH, Sposto R, Sensel MG, et al. Treatment outcome and prognostic factors for infants with acute lymphoblastic leukemia treated on two consecutive trials of the Children's Cancer Group. J Clin Oncol 17:445, 1999.

45. Greaves MF. Aetiology of acute leukaemia. Lancet 349:344, 1997.

46. Kinlen LJ. High-contact paternal occupation, infection and childhood leukaemia: Five studies of unusual population mixing of adults. Br J Cancer 76:1539, 1997.

47. Ingram L, Rivera GK, Shapiro DN. Superior vena cava syndrome associated with childhood malignancy: Analysis of 24 cases. Med Pediatr Oncol 18:476, 1990.

48. Borowitz MJ, Croker BP, Metzgar RS. Lymphoblastic lymphoma with the phenotype of common acute lymphoblastic leukemia. Am J Clin Pathol 79:387–391, 1983.

49. Weiss LM, Bindl JM, Picozzi VJ, et al. Lymphoblastic lymphoma: An immunophenotype study of 26 cases with comparison to T cell acute lymphoblastic leukemia. Blood 67:474–478, 1986.

50. Look AT. Oncogenic transcription factors in the human acute leukemias. Science 278:1059, 1997.

51. Reiter A, Schrappe M, Tiemann M, et al. Improved treatment results in childhood B-cell neoplasms with tailored intensification of therapy: A report of the Berlin-Frankfurt-Münster group trial NHL-BFM90. Blood 94:3294, 1999.

52. Bowman W, Shuster JJ, Cook B, et al. Improved survival for children with B-cell acute lymphoblastic leukemia and stage IV small noncleaved-cell lymphoma: A Pediatric Oncology Group study. J Clin Oncol 14:1252, 1996.

53. Smith M, Arthur D, Camita B, et al. Uniform approach to risk classification and treatment assignment for children with acute lymphoblastic leukemia. J Clin Oncol 14:18, 1996.

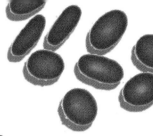

12 Chronic Myeloproliferative Disorders

Kathy Finnegan

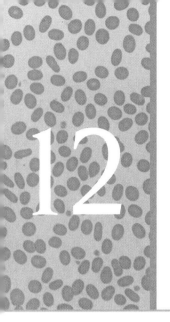

Chronic Myelogeneous Leukemia
 Disease Overview
 Pathophysiology
 Clinical Features and Symptoms
 Peripheral Blood and Bone Marrow
 Diagnosis
 Treatment
 Prognosis

Chronic Neutrophilic Leukemia

Chronic Eosinophilic Leukemia

Polycythemia Vera
 Disease Overview
 Pathophysiology
 Clinical Features and Symptoms
 Peripheral Blood and Bone Marrow Findings
 Diagnosis
 Treatment
 Prognosis

Myelofibrosis With Myeloid Metaplasia
 Disease Overview
 Pathophysiology
 Clinical Features and Symptoms
 Peripheral Blood and Bone Marrow Findings
 Diagnosis
 Treatment
 Prognosis

Essential Thrombocythemia
 Disease Overview
 Pathophysiology
 Clinical Features and Symptoms
 Peripheral Blood and Bone Marrow Findings
 Diagnosis
 Treatment
 Prognosis

Objectives

After completing this chapter, the student will be able to:

1. Define the *myeloproliferative disorders*.

2. List and discuss classification of the myeloproliferative disorders.

3. Identify the major cell lines involved with the myeloproliferative disorders.

4. Discuss the pathogenesis of the myeloproliferative disorders.

5. Identify and differentiate clinical features and signs associated with the chronic myeloproliferative disorders.

6. Identify and describe the peripheral and bone marrow abnormalities associated with the chronic myeloproliferative disorders.

7. Compare and contrast the clinical and laboratory features of the chronic myeloproliferative disorders.

8. Identify the diagnostic criteria for the chronic myeloproliferative disorders.

9. Discuss the treatment of and prognosis for the chronic myeloproliferative disorders.

10. Discuss the cytogenetic abnormalities associated with the chronic myeloproliferative disorders.

The chronic **myeloproliferative** disorders (CMPDs) are a group of disorders that are considered **clonal** malignancies of the hematopoietic stem cell.[1] These disorders include chronic myelogenous leukemia (CML), myelofibrosis with myeloid metaplasia (MMM), polycythemia vera (PV), and essential thrombocythemia (ET). Significant changes have evolved in the last decade with regard to terminology of leukemias and associated disorders. The World Health Organization (WHO) in conjunction with the Society for Hematopathology and the European Association of Hematopathology published a new classification for myeloid and lymphoid neoplasms.[1,2] The WHO based their classification on morphology, genetic, immunophenotypic, biological, and clinical features. For lymphoid disorders, the WHO classification uses the Revised European-American Lymphoma (REAL) Classification. The myeloid disorders include the criteria of the French-American-British (FAB) classification and the guidelines of the Polycythemia Vera Study Group (PVSG).[3,4] The WHO classification of the chronic myeloproliferative diseases recognizes seven entities.[2,3] Table 12.1 lists these entities.[1] These disorders are unified but independent. Each disease has overlapping clinical features but different etiologies. The CMPDs are characterized by proliferation of one or more cell lines and are predominantly mature in cell morphology. The bone marrow shows varying degrees of abnormal proliferation of myeloid, erythroid, and megakaryocytic elements. In the peripheral blood, the red blood cell (RBC), white blood cell (WBC), and platelet counts vary, and each disorder is identified by the predominant cell that is present. Table 12.2 summarizes the characteristics of the CMPDs.

Table 12.1 ◉ WHO Classification of Chronic Myeloproliferative Diseases
Chronic myelogenous leukemia [Ph chromosome, t(9;22) (q34;q11). *BCR-ABL* positive]
Chronic neutrophilic leukemia
Chronic eosinophilic leukemia (hypereosinophilic syndrome)
Polycythemia vera
Chronic idiopathic myelofibrosis
Essential thrombocythemia
Chronic myeloproliferative disease unclassifiable

Adapted from: Jaffee ES, Harris NL, Stein H, Vardiman JW, eds. World Health Organization Classification of Tumors: Pathology and Genetics of Tumors of Haematopoietic Lymphoid Tissues. Lyon: IARC Press; 2001.

Other common features shared by these disorders are splenomegaly, hepatomegaly, increased leukocytosis, thrombocytosis, and erythrocytosis. There may be various degrees of bone marrow fibrosis. All the CMPDs have interrelationships between the disorders. Transitions are common between disorders and many finally terminate into an acute myelogenous leukemia (AML).[1] Review Figure 12.1 for these interrelationships. A very small percentage of CMPDs can terminate into an acute lymphoblastic leukemia (ALL). An increase in the percentage of blasts in the peripheral blood and bone marrow indicates the onset of an accelerated stage or transformation to an acute process.

The CMPDs are primarily diseases of adults. The peak onset is in the fifth to the seventh decades of life.[1] The major clinical and pathological findings are the unregulated proliferation of cells in the bone marrow. This results in the increased numbers of mature cells in peripheral blood. The increase is found in the granulocytes, usually the neutrophils, platelets, or RBCs. These disorders typically manifest a normocytic, normochromic anemia with all three cell lines involved. The dysfunction in the CMPDs is a loss of regulatory signals that control the production of the mature cells. One of the important bone marrow findings that overlap the various CMPDs is marrow fibrosis. *Fibrosis* is defined as the replacement of normal bone marrow elements with connective tissue. Classification of these diseases is based on the lineage of the predominant cell present, marrow fibrosis, and clinical and pathological findings.

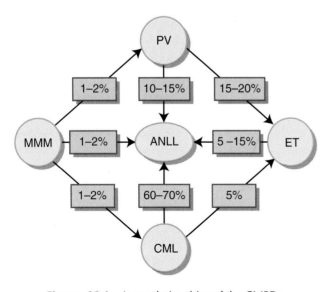

Figure 12.1 Interrelationships of the CMPDs.

Table 12.2 ● Characteristics of Chronic Myeloproliferative Disorders

CMPD	Cell Line	WBC	Bone Marrow Fibrosis	Philadelphia Chromosome (Ph[1])	Organ Involvement
Chronic myelogenous leukemia (CML)	Myeloid	Increased	Variable	Present	Splenomegaly Hepatomegaly
Polycythemia vera (PV)	Erythroid, myeloid megakaryocyte	Increased	None	Absent	Splenomegaly Hepatomegaly
Myelofibrosis with myeloid metaplasia (MMM)	Teardrop, erythrocytes Fibroblasts	Variable	Increased	Absent	Splenomegaly Hepatomegaly
Essential thrombocythemia (ET)	Megakaryocyte	Normal	None	Absent	Splenomegaly

CHRONIC MYELOGENOUS LEUKEMIA

Disease Overview

CML is a hematopoietic proliferative disorder associated with a specific gene defect and a very characteristic blood picture.[5] Synonyms for this disorder include chronic granulocytic leukemia and chronic myelocytic leukemia. There is a marked neutrophil leukocytosis with some circulation of immature neutrophils and an increase in basophils. The gene defect is the translocation of genetic material between chromosome 9 and chromosome 22 (t9:22), which is positive in 90% to 95% of the cases.[6,7] This gene mutation is called the Philadelphia chromosome, or Ph1. This translocation leads to a formation of a hybrid gene called *BCR-ABL*. This fusion gene mutation affects maturation and differentiation of the hematopoietic cells.

This disorder is usually diagnosed in the chronic phase of the disorder. The peripheral blood picture shows an extremely high WBC with the whole spectrum of neutrophilic cell development seen. As the disease evolves, the chronic phase will deteriorate to an aggressive or accelerated phase and terminate in an acute phase or blast crisis. CML is one of the most common forms of chronic leukemia.[1] See Table 12.3 for a summary of key facts for CML.

Pathophysiology

CML is a clonal proliferative disorder. The hallmark of the initial phase is the excess of mature neutrophils in the peripheral blood. The expansion of the myeloid cell results in an alteration of self-renewal and differentiation. There now is an increase in cells. The formation of the Philadelphia chromosome plays a significant role in the understanding of the pathogenesis of CML.

The main portion of the long arm of chromosome 22 is deleted and translocated to the distal end of the long arm of chromosome 9. This results in an elongated chromosome 9 or 9q+. A small part of chromosome 9 is then reciprocally translocated to the broken end of 22 or 22−. This now forms the *BCR-ABL* hybrid gene, which codes for a 210-kDa protein, or p210, which has increased tyrosine kinase activity.[5,8] Tyrosine kinase activity provides an important mediator to regulate metabolic pathways causing abnormal cell cycling. The activation of tyrosine kinase activity may suppress apoptosis (natural cell death) in hematopoietic cells and provide the mechanism for excess cell production.[6,9]

Clinical Features and Symptoms

Most patients are diagnosed in the chronic phase. Many patients are asymptomatic and are diagnosed when an elevated white count is found on a routine complete blood count (CBC). Common findings include fatigue,

Table 12.3 ● Key Facts of CML

- Clonal stem cell disorder
- Marked leukocytosis with all stages of granulocyte maturation
- Hepatosplenomegaly
- Thrombocytosis is common in chronic phase
- Three phases: chronic, accelerated, blast
- Philadelphia chromosome
- *BCR-ABL* fusion gene
- LAP score <10

weight loss, low-grade fever, normocytic, normochromic anemia, night sweats, and splenomegaly. The chronic phase can last for months to years. CML is characterized by a chronic phase, an accelerated phase, and a blast phase. As the disease progresses, the features worsen.

The accelerated phase has a rising peripheral blood count, appearance of peripheral blasts and promyelocytes, increase in splenomegaly, bone pain, thrombocytopenia, and a worsening anemia.

The acute phase or blast crisis is similar to an acute leukemia. Bone marrow and peripheral blood blasts counts are greater than 30%.[1] Excessive bleeding, infection, petechiae, ecchymosis, and bruising are seen more in the later stage due to bone marrow failure.

Peripheral Blood and Bone Marrow

The peripheral blood smear shows the presence of a severe leukocytosis with the entire spectrum of the myeloid cell development. A mild normocytic, normochromic anemia with nucleated red blood cells (nRBCs) is a common finding. Eosinophils and basophils also are increased in number. In the chronic phase, thrombocytosis is present. Figure 12.2 illustrates the spectrum of neutrophilic maturation seen in CML. As the disease progresses, the anemia worsens, and thrombocytopenia and younger and younger cells are

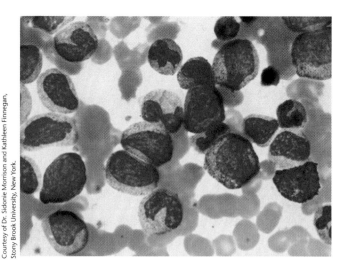

Courtesy of Dr. Sidonie Morrison and Kathleen Finnegan, Stony Brook University, New York.

Figure 12.2 Spectrum of neutrophil maturation seen in CML.

seen. In the acute phase, the blast count increases and may be greater than 30%.

Examination of the bone marrow reveals a hypercellular marrow with marked myeloid **hyperplasia.** The myeloid-to-erythroid (M:E) ratio is 10:1 and can be as high as 25:1. A normal M:E ratio is 3:1. The bone marrow may become fibrotic as the disease progresses. Table 12.4 summarizes the peripheral blood and bone marrow findings in the three phases of CML.

Table 12.4 ● **Peripheral Blood and Bone Marrow Findings in the Three Phases of CML**			
	Chronic Phase	**Acceleratsed Phase**	**Blast Phase**
Peripheral blood	Leukocytosis with the presence of neutrophils in all stages of maturation Blasts >2% Increased basophils Increased eosinophils Thrombocytosis Mild anemia NRBs	Increase in promyelocytes Blasts increased Basophils >20% Increase in circulation NRBs Erythrocytes Persistent thrombocytopenia Anemia	Blasts >20% Increase in promyelocytes Increase in basophils and eosinophils Thrombocytopenia
Bone marrow	Hyperplasia myeloid Blasts <5% M:E ratio 10:1 Increased immature forms of basophils Reduced erythrocytes Increased megakaryocytes	Dysplasia Blasts >5% <20 Left shift of mature neutrophils Increased basophils Megakaryocytic proliferation in sheets and clusters Fibrosis	Blasts >20% Large clusters of blasts Increased fibrosis Marked dysplasia of all three cell lines

Diagnosis

CML must be distinguished from other myeloproliferative disorders. The presence of the Ph chromosome or *BCR-ABL* fusion gene and a low or absent leukocyte alkaline phosphate (LAP) score is diagnostic for this disorder. The LAP score is a cytochemical stain and is used to differentiate CML from a leukemoid reaction. Leukocyte alkaline phosphatase enzyme is located in the granules of the neutrophil and bands. LAP activity increases with the maturity of the neutrophil. One hundred mature neutrophils and bands are stained, counted, and scored for stain intensity and granulation. In a leukemoid reaction, the LAP score is high, and in CML, it is low. A leukemoid reaction is caused by a severe infection or inflammation. This reaction can resemble a leukemic process. Table 12.5 summarizes the differentiation of a neutrophilic leukemoid reaction and CML.

Treatment

The goal of treatment for CML is to achieve hematological remission, which consists of a normal CBC, no **organomegaly,** and a negative Ph chromosome or negative *BCR-ABL* fusion gene. The chronic phase can be controlled with hydroxyurea, interferon-alfa, or busulfan therapy.[10] This type of therapy is called myelosuppressive therapy, with the goal of controlling the hyperproliferation of the myeloid elements. The drug tries to decrease the WBC count by interfering with cell division. Neither cytotoxic drug can prevent the blast crisis. Another treatment is called leukapheresis. This therapy uses a cell separator to lower the WBC count rapidly (red cells are reinfused), and a cytotoxin drug is used to keep the patient in a longer remission.[5,7]

A new approach to treatment is to directly inhibit the abnormal molecular molecule, using a tyrosine kinase inhibitor. This inhibitor reacts to the BCL-ABL tyrosine kinase associated with the Ph chromosome. The drug is called imatinib mesylate (Gleevec), and it inhibits proliferation, slows down cell growth, and induces cell death.[11-13] An additional treatment for CML is an allogeneic bone marrow or stem cell transplantation. However, bone marrow transplant has a high mortality rate.[14] Allogeneic bone marrow transplant is currently the only curative therapy.[1] There are many clinical trials now being studied for better prognosis.

Prognosis

The chronic phase CML is highly responsive to treatment. The median survival is 4 to 6 years, with a range of 1 year to longer than 10 years. Survival after development of an accelerated phase is usually less than 1 year, and after blast crisis survival, is only a few months.[15] Poor prognosis in patients with CML is associated with several prognostic factors. These factors include

- Patient's age
- Phase of CML
- Amount of blasts in the peripheral blood and bone marrow
- Size of the spleen at diagnosis
- Marrow fibrosis
- Patient's general health

Table 12.5 ⊙ Differentiating a Neutrophilic Leukemoid Reaction and CML		
Criterion	**CML**	**Leukemoid Reaction**
Neutrophil	The whole spectrum of cells mature to the blast	A shift to the left, more bands, metas, blast very rare
Eosinophil	Increased	Normal
Basophil	Increased	Normal
Platelet	Increased with abnormal forms	Normal
Anemia	Usually present	Not typical
LAP score	Decreased	Increased
Philadelphia chromosome	Present	Absent
Toxic granulation	Absent	Increased
Döhle bodies	Absent	Increased

For patients lacking the Ph chromosome, median survival is about 1 year.[16]

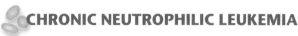CHRONIC NEUTROPHILIC LEUKEMIA

CNL is a rare chronic myeloproliferative disease characterized by an elevated neutrophil count. The bone marrow is hypercellular with an increase in the granulocytic proliferation. An enlarged spleen and liver are also presented. There is no significant dysplasia in any cell line, and bone marrow fibrosis is uncommon.[1] The Philadelphia chromosome or *BCR-ABL* fusion gene is absent.[17]

CHRONIC EOSINOPHILIC LEUKEMIA

CEL is a chronic myeloproliferative disease characterized by an elevation and proliferation of the eosinophil.[1] The eosinophil is increased in the peripheral blood, bone marrow, and peripheral tissue. There is tissue and organ damage from the overproduction of eosinophils. The diagnosis of CEL is made if the blood eosinophil count is greater than 1500/μL, there are no other causes of increased eosinophils, and there are clinical signs and symptoms of organ damage. There is no Ph chromosome or *BCL-ABL* fusion gene found.

Synonyms include hypereosinophilic syndrome (HES).

POLYCYTHEMIA VERA

Disease Overview

PV (polycythemia rubra vera) is a clonal disorder characterized by the overproduction of mature RBCs, WBCs, and platelets.[19,20] With the increased production of red cells, there is an increase in hemoglobin, hematocrit, and red cell mass (RCM). Erythrocytosis is the most prominent clinical manifestation of this disorder. The bone marrow is usually hypercellular with hyperplasia of all three bone marrow elements. This disorder usually occurs in the sixth or seventh decade of life. All causes of secondary erythrocytosis must be excluded before a diagnosis of PV can be made. Table 12.6 summarizes the key facts of polycythemia.

Pathophysiology

The etiology of polycythemia has become clearer. The primary defect involves the pluripotential stem cell that has the capability of differentiating into RBCs, WBCs, and platelet. Recently the JAK2 V617F mutation has been discovered in most patients with PV.[18] Erythroid precursors in PV are very sensitive to erythropoietin, which leads to an increased red cell production. The increased red cell production leads to an increase in RCM and increased blood viscosity. For this reason, patients are predisposed to arterial and venous thrombosis and/or increased bleeding. The elevated hematocrit and platelet counts are directly proportional to the number of thrombotic events.[18]

Clinical Features and Symptoms

Patients tend to be asymptomatic at the time of diagnosis. Symptoms are often insidious in onset. As the RBCs and platelet number increase, more symptoms are evident. The major symptoms are related to the hypertension, hyperviscosity, and the vascular abnormalities caused by the increased RCM. Symptoms of hyperviscosity and increased hematocrit include headache, lightheadedness, blurred vision or visual disturbances, fatigue, and plethora. **Plethora** is a condition of a red or ruddy complexion due to the expanded blood volume. Additionally, this manifests itself in the nail beds, hands, feet, face, and conjunctiva. Thrombosis in the small blood vessels leads to painful dilation of the vessels in the extremities. Sometimes ulceration or gangrene can occur in the fingers and toes. Thrombosis in the larger vessels can lead to myocardial infarction, **transient ischemic attacks,** stroke, and **deep vein thrombosis (DVT).**

Abnormalities in platelet function can lead to bleeding from the nose (epistaxis), easy bruising, and gingival bleeding. The increased blood cell turnover can cause hyperuricemia, **gout,** and stomach ulcers. As the disease progresses, the patients develop abdominal pain due to hepatomegaly and splenomegaly. Splenomegaly is present in 75% of the patients at the time of diagnosis, and hepatomegaly is present in about 30%.[20,21] **Pruritus,** which results from increased histamine levels released from the basophil, is a common extenuating symptom.

Peripheral Blood and Bone Marrow Findings

Polycythemia is characterized by an increased cell count in all three cell lines. The major characteristics of

---

Table 12.6 ● Key Facts of Polycythemia Vera

- Increase in all three cell lines
- Absolute increase in RCM
- Normal oxygen saturation
- Splenomegaly
- Recommended treatment is phlebotomy
- Thrombosis and hemorrhage

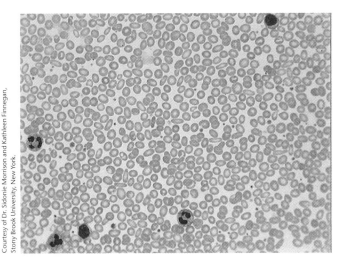

Figure 12.3 Increased RBCs in PV.

Table 12.7 ● Causes of Secondary Erythrocytosis
• Hypertension
• Arterial hypoxemia
• Impaired tissue oxygen delivery
• Smoking
• Renal lesions
• Renal disease
• Endocrine lesions
• Drugs
• Alcohol
• Hepatic lesions

PV are normoblastic erythroid proliferation in the bone marrow and an increased number of normocytic, normochromic RBCs in the peripheral blood. Figure 12.3 illustrates the increase in RBCs. The reticulocyte count tends to be normal or slightly increased. Neutrophilia with a "shift to the left" and basophilia are common in the blood smear.[1] At disease onset, the red cell count, hemoglobin, and hematocrit are increased. The red cell distribution width (RDW) tends to be higher than normal. The granulocyte and platelet counts are found to be increased. The leukocyte alkaline phosphatase (LAP) score is usually elevated. Platelet counts are increased and have abnormal morphology and function.

Characteristically, the bone marrow biopsy is hypercellular. Pancytopenia accounts for the increased cellularity. The increase in the number of erythroid and megakaryocytic precursors is more significant. The bone marrow biopsy shows increased reticulin or fibrosis. The amount of reticulin is directly proportional to the amount of cellularity. The iron stores of the bone marrow are usually depleted.

As the disease progresses, the erythroid activity in the marrow decreases. Immature WBC and RBC precursors are found in the peripheral blood with marked morphology. Microcytes, elliptocytes, and dacryocytes (teardrop cells) develop. Granulocytes and platelet morphology is abnormal with increases in younger and younger cells.

Diagnosis

The major diagnostic issue related to PV is distinguishing it from secondary and relative erythrocytosis. Secondary erythrocytosis is an increase in the RCM without evidence of changes in the other cell lines. Table 12.7 summarizes the causes of secondary erythrocytosis.

Relative erythrocytosis is due to dehydration and hemoconcentration. Elevated hematocrit and hemoglobin counts are a result of a high red cell count and a low plasma volume.

The National Polycythemia Vera Study Group (PVSG) diagnostic criteria are given in Table 12.8.[1,22] PV is present when a patient demonstrates all of the major or primary criteria (elevated hematocrit or RCM, normal arterial oxygen saturation, and splenomegaly) or together with the secondary or minor criteria (thrombocytosis, leukocytosis, elevated LAP, and increased serum B_{12}). In summary, the most significant finding in PV is increased RCM, splenomegaly, and the JAK2 mutation with the increase in leukocytes and platelets. Other tests that are helpful in the diagnosis of PV are a bone marrow aspirate and biopsy. However, these invasive procedures are not necessary to establish a diagnosis, but a hypercellular marrow with hyperplasia of erythroid, granulocytic, and megakaryocytic elements supports the diagnosis. Serum erythropoietin levels in patients with PV are often found to be low compared with patients with secondary and relative erythrocytosis.[20,23]

There is no consistent or unique cytogenetic abnormality associated with this disorder. Cytogenetic abnormalities are found in 8% to 20% of patients at the time of diagnosis.[24] The most frequent cytogenetic abnormality are **trisomy** of 1q, 8, 9 or 9p, del 3q, del 20q or interstitial deletions of 13 or 20.[24]

Treatment

Treatment begins with decreasing the hematocrit and hemoglobin, thereby reducing the plasma viscosity. Therapy recommendations are based on age, sex, clinical manifestations, and hematological findings. Treatment recommendations for patients are phlebotomy,

Table 12.8 ● Diagnostic Criteria for Polycythemia Vera

A1	Elevated RCM >25% above mean normal predicated Hgb >18.5 g/dL in men or 16.5 g/dL in women
A2	No cause or absence of secondary erythrocytosis
A3	Splenomegaly
A4	Prescence of JAK2 V617 F mutation or other cytogenetic abnormalities in hemopoietic cells
A5	Endogenous erythroid colony formation in vitro
B1	Thrombocytosis >400 × 10⁹/L
B2	WBC >12 × 10⁹/L
B3	Bone marrow biopsy presenting with panmyelosis with prominent and megakaryocytic proliferation
B4	Low serum erythropoietin levels

A1 + A2 + any other category A are present, diagnose PV.
   A1 + A2 + any two of category B are present, diagnose PV.
   Adapted from Jaffee ES, Harris NL, Stein H, Vardiman JW, eds. World Health Organization Classification of Tumors: Pathology and Genetics of Tumors of Haematopoietic Lymphoid Tissues. Lyon: IARC Press, 2001; and Pearson TC, Messinezy M, Westwoos N, Green AR, et al. A polycythemia vera update: Diagnosis, pathobiology and treatment. Hematology 1:51–68, 2000.

radioactive phosphorus (^{32}P), myelosuppressive agents, and interferon-alfa.[25] The target goal for therapy is to decrease the hematocrit. For men, the hematocrit target value is less than 45%, and for women, it is less than 40%.[26] **Therapeutic phlebotomy** is an immediately effective therapy and is usually the first choice of the recommended treatments.

Prognosis

PV is a chronic disease. The median survival is more than 10 years with treatment.[1] The major causes of death in untreated patients are hemorrhage and thrombosis. Other causes of death are complications of myeloid metaplasia or the development of leukemia.[1] The incidence of transformation into an acute leukemia is greater in patients treated with radioactive phosphate or alkylating agents.[26]

During the later stages of PV, a post–polycythemic myelofibrosis phase occurs, characterized by a leukoerythroblastic peripheral blood picture with an increase in immature WBCs and RBCs. The red cells will appear in a teardrop shape, with an increase in shape changes. The spleen will increase in size due to extramedullary hematopoiesis. The main characteristics of this stage are the increase in reticulin and fibrosis in the bone marrow.[27]

MYELOFIBROSIS WITH MYELOID METAPLASIA

Disease Overview

Myelofibrosis with myeloid metaplasia (MMM) is a CMPD characterized by bone marrow fibrosis, proliferation of megakaryocytic and granulocytic cells, and extramedullary hematopoiesis. MMM presents with an elevated WBC, teardrop RBCs, normocellular or hypercellular bone marrow, leukoerythroblastic anemia, splenomegaly, and the absence of the Philadelphia chromosome.[28,29] MMM is a clonal hematopoietic stem cell expansion in the bone marrow with the production of reticulin and bone marrow fibrosis.[30,31] Table 12.9 summarizes the key facts found in MMM.

There are many synonyms for this myeloproliferative disorder; they include agnogenic myeloid metaplasia, chronic idiopathic myelofibrosis, idiopathic myelofibrosis, primary myelofibrosis, leukoerythroblastic anemia, and myelosclerosis with myeloid metaplasia.

Pathophysiology

The etiology of this disorder is unknown, and the mechanism of myelofibrosis is poorly understood. The clonal proliferation of hematopoietic stem cell is thought to produce growth factors and an abnormal cytokine release that mediates a bone marrow reaction that leads to fibrosis of the bone marrow.[32,33] Platelets, megakaryocytes, and monocytes are thought to secrete cytokines, transforming growth factor beta (TGF beta), platelet-derived growth factor (PDGF), interleukin 1, and fibroblast growth factor, which may result in formation of the bone marrow matrix.[32,33]

Table 12.9 ● Key Facts of Myelofibrosis

- Leukoerythroblastosis
- Extramedullary hematopoiesis
- Fibrosis of the bone marrow/reticulin silver stain
- Teardrop RBCs
- Absence of the Philadelphia chromosome
- Hepatosplenomegaly

MMM has an evolution in the disease process. The initial phase is the prefibrotic stage, which is characterized by a hypercellular bone marrow with minimal reticulin. The second phase is the fibrotic stage, which is characterized by the bone marrow having marked reticulin or collagen fibrosis. Normal hematopoiesis is blocked as the bone marrow becomes more fibrotic. This stage is characterized by a leukoerythroblastic blood smear: immature white cells and nRBCs combined with teardrop RBCs. Patients become pancytopenic (decrease in all three cell lines). Extramedullary hematopoiesis contributes to the leukoerythroblastic blood picture, splenomegaly, and hepatomegaly. Myelofibrosis is a complicating reactive feature of the primary disease process.

Clinical Features and Symptoms

In the early stages of the disease, the patient may be asymptomatic. Patients with myelofibrosis exhibit splenomegaly, an anemia, and marrow fibrosis. Many of the signs and symptoms are attributed to the pancytopenia associated with the presence of a fibrotic bone marrow. Pancytopenia occurs as a result of decreased cell production because of the fibrosis marrow or ineffective hematopoiesis with increased spleen sequestration. Most patients exhibit symptoms of anemia. Patients who are thrombocytopenic and neutropenic tend to have bleeding tendencies and infection. Other symptoms include night sweats, low-grade fever, weight loss, and anorexia. Patients often complain of left upper quadrant discomfort due to the enlarged spleen and liver. Patients with myelofibrosis develop **osteosclerosis,** which can cause severe joint pain.

Peripheral Blood and Bone Marrow Findings

The peripheral blood and bone marrow biopsy provide information for diagnosis. The WBC and platelet counts may increase initially but will decrease as the disease progresses. The typical picture is a blood smear that shows leukoerythroblastosis and teardrop red cells (Fig. 12.4). Large platelets, megakaryocyte fragments, and immature blood cells may be found due to the crowding out of normal cell development by fibrosis in the bone marrow. A normocytic, normochromic anemia is present with hemoglobin of less than 10 g/dL.

The bone marrow is hypercellular with increased and abnormal megakaryocytes and megakaryocyte clusters. Bone marrow aspirates are sometimes dry taps in about 50% of the patients. This refers to the inability

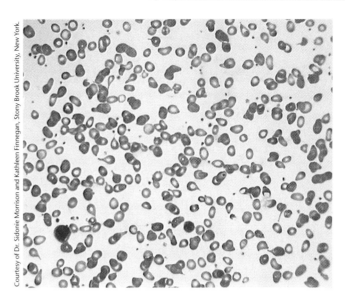

Figure 12.4   Teardrop RBCs in MMM.

of the physician to obtain a sample because the normal architecture of the bone marrow is disrupted by fibrotic tissue, reticulin.

Diagnosis

Diagnosis is made on the basis of detecting splenomegaly and of the result of the CBC. Splenomegaly is the most common finding, followed by hepatomegaly.[34] The PVSG has criteria for myelofibrosis as follows: splenomegaly, fibrosis of the bone marrow, a leukoerythroblastic blood picture, absence of increased RCM, absence of the Philadelphia chromosome, and exclusion of any other systemic disease. Table 12.10 summarizes the diagnostic criteria of MMM.[35]

There are no specific genetic defects. Cytogenetic abnormalities occur in about 60% of the patients.[36] Cytogenetics rule out CML, myelodysplastic syndrome, and other chronic myeloid disorders. Various chromosomal abnormalities may occur, with the most common being del(13q), del(20q), and partial trisomy 1q.[36]

Treatment

There are no available treatments to reverse the process of myelofibrosis. Asymptomatic patients are observed and require no treatment. Therapy for MMM is mainly supportive for the anemia and thrombocythemia. Hydroxyurea is used as a cytoreductive therapy to control leukocytosis, thrombocytosis, and organomegaly.[28] Interferon-alfa is used in patients younger than 45 years. Splenectomy may be considered for treating patients with symptomatic splenomegaly that is refractory to hydroxyurea.[37] Radiation may be used to treat

Table 12.10 ◉ Diagnostic Criteria for Myelofibrosis

Clinical Criteria

A1	No preceding or allied subtype of CMPDs
A2	Early clinical stages Normal hemoglobin Slight or moderate splenomegaly Thrombocythemia platelets $>400 \times 10^9$/L
A3	Intermediate clinical stage Anemia Definitive leukoerythroblastic blood picture/teardrop RBCs Splenomegaly No advance signs
A4	Advanced clinical stage Anemia One or more adverse signs

Pathological Criteria

B1	Megakaryocytic and granulocytic proliferation Reduction RBC precursors Abnormal giant-sized megakaryocytes

Adapted from Spivak JL, Barosi G, Tognoni G, et al. Chronic myeloproliferative disorders. Hematology 1:200–224, 2003.

symptomatic extramedullary hematopoiesis. A more aggressive approach is an allogeneic peripheral stem cell or bone marrow transplant.[38]

Prognosis

MMM has the worst prognosis of all the myeloproliferative disorders. The median survival is approximately 3 to 5 years from diagnosis.[29] The major causes of death are infection, cardiovascular disease, hemorrhage, thrombosis, progressive marrow failure, and transformation into an acute leukemia.[29,31] Prognostic factors that affect survival include age, anemia, leukopenia, leukocytosis, circulating blasts, and karyotype abnormalities. There is a shorter survival with poor prognostic values.[28,39]

ESSENTIAL THROMBOCYTHEMIA

Disease Overview

ET, or primary thrombocythemia, is a chronic MPD characterized by a clonal proliferation of megakaryocytes in the bone marrow. The peripheral blood platelet counts exceed 600,000/μL and can be greater than 1 million. This disease is characterized by an

Table 12.11 ◉ Key Facts for Essential Thrombocythemia

- Marked thrombocytosis (platelet count $>600 \times 10^9$/L)
- Usually no fibrosis
- Neurological manifestations
- Abnormal platelet function
- Megakaryocyte fragments in both peripheral blood and bone marrow
- Absent Philadelphia chromosome

increased platelet count, a megakaryocytic hyperplasia, and an absence of increased RCM. The clinical course is complicated by hemorrhage or thrombotic episodes. Etiology is unknown, and the disorder usually occurs between the ages of 50 and 70.[1] Table 12.11 summarizes the key factors for ET.

Pathophysiology

ET is considered to be a clonal disorder of the multipotential stem cell.[35] ET has many biological characteristics in common with PV and the other myeloproliferative disorders. This disorder can affect all three cell lines, but the main characteristic is the increase in the megakaryocyte. Bone marrow and peripheral blood are the principal sites of involvement in this disorder. Megakaryocytes are hypersensitive to several cytokines, including IL-3, IL-6, and thrombopoietin, which leads to increased platelet production.[40] Platelet survival and platelet aggregation studies are normal.

The increased platelet count can cause increased thrombotic and hemorrhagic episodes. Qualitative abnormalities in the platelet contribute to the increased risk of thrombotic and hemorrhagic complications. Age, previous thrombotic event, increased or greater than 600×10^9/L platelet counts, duration of diseases, and prior symptoms are considered high-risk factors. The increase in thrombotic risk with age has been attributed to vascular disease or hypercoagulable platelets.

Clinical Features and Symptoms

Most often, patients present asymptomatic at the time of diagnosis. The elevated platelet count is discovered on a routine CBC. The clinical signs and symptoms are similar to those of PV. The most frequent symptoms are weight loss, low-grade fever, weakness, pruritus, hemorrhage, headache, and dizziness. Bleeding is usually mild and may present as epistaxis and the tendency to bruise easily. The gastrointestinal tract is the primary site for bleeding complications. Patients who present with microvascular occlusion may have transient ischemic attacks with symptoms of unsteadiness, syncope, and seizures. Thrombosis of the large veins and main arteries is common. Occlusion of the leg arteries and renal arteries may be involved.

Approximately 50% of the patients at the time of diagnosis will present with an enlarged spleen and approximately 20% of patients will present with an enlarged liver.[1]

Peripheral Blood and Bone Marrow Findings

The hallmark for ET is an unexplained elevated platelet count. The blood platelet count is usually in excess of 1 million. The platelets will have anisocytosis ranging from small to large forms. Figure 12.5 illustrates the increased platelet count. The peripheral blood may reveal a leukocytosis with an occasional immature cell (myelocytes and metamyelocytes), erythrocytosis, and a mild normocytic, normochromic anemia. A mild basophilia and eosinophilia may be seen. Leukoerythroblastosis and teardrop cells are not features of ET.

The bone marrow shows an increase in cellularity. Megakaryocytic hyperplasia is the most striking feature. Giant megakaryocytes and clusters of megakaryocytes are frequently seen. The megakaryocytes have abundant, mature cytoplasm and hyperlobulated nuclei. Proliferation of erythroid precursors may be found in some cases. The network of reticulin fibers is normal or slightly increased.[1] Increased reticulin or collagen fibrosis points more toward MMM than ET. Stainable iron is present.

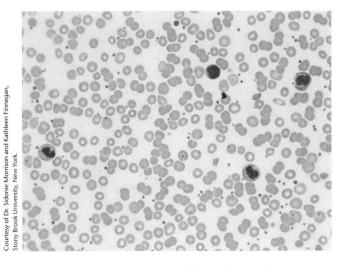

Courtesy of Dr. Sidonie Morrison and Kathleen Finnegan, Stony Brook University, New York.

Figure 12.5 Increased thrombocytes in ET.

Table 12.12 ◉ Causes of Relative Thrombocytosis

- Inflammatory states
- Infection
- Trauma
- Blood loss
- Postsplenectomy
- Acute hemorrhage
- Malignancy
- Postoperative
- Hemolytic anemia

Diagnosis

Discriminating ET from reactive thrombocytosis and the other myeloproliferative disorders is a diagnostic challenge. For the diagnosis of ET, reactive thrombocytosis needs to be excluded. Secondary or reactive thrombocytosis is associated with many acute and chronic infections. Table 12.12 summarizes the causes of relative thrombocytosis. In reactive thrombocytosis, the platelet count is less than 1 million and is transient. Leukocytes and erythrocytes are normal. Platelet function is normal, and the spleen and liver are not enlarged.

Diagnostic requirements for ET include a normal RBC mass (increased with PV), a hemoglobin of less than 13 g/dL (elevated in PV), absence of the Philadelphia chromosome (associated with CML), and the absence of teardrop RBCs or significant increase in bone marrow fibrosis (as seen in MMM). Diagnosis for ET follows the gold standard criteria of the PVSG.[3] Table 12.13 summarizes the diagnostic criteria for ET.[3,41]

There are no characteristic cytogenetic or molecular abnormalities associated with or that establish the diagnosis for patients with ET.[41,42]

Treatment

The goal of treatment of ET is to prevent or reduce the risk of complications from vaso-occlusion or hemorrhage. The treatment of ET can vary from no treatment, if patients are asymptomatic, to low-dose aspirin for low-risk patients, to treatment with hydroxyurea, anagrelide, or alfa-interferon to reduce the platelet count.[43,44] Patients with life-threatening hemorrhagic or thrombotic events should be treated with platelet phoresis in combination with myelosuppressive therapy to reduce the platelet count below 1 million.[40] The maintaining of a platelet count of less than 400,000/μL is needed to reduce the risk of a thrombotic event.

Table 12.13 ⊙ Diagnostic Criteria for Essential Thrombocythemia	
I.	Platelet count >600 × 10⁹/L
II.	Hematocrit <40 or normal RBC mass (males <36 mL/kg, females <32 mL/kg)
III.	Stainable iron in marrow or normal serum ferritin or normal RBC mean corpuscular volume
IV.	Absent Philadelphia chromosome or *BCR-ABL* gene rearrangement
V.	Collagen fibrosis of marrow A. Absent or B. <⅓ of biopsy involved and neither marked splenomegaly nor a leukoerythroblastic reaction
VI.	No cytogenetic or morphological evidence for a myelodysplastic syndrome
VII.	No cause for reactive thrombocytosis

Adapted from Murphy S, Peterson P, Iland H, Laszio J. Experience of the Polycythemia Vera Study Group with essential thrombocythemia: A final report on diagnostic criteria, survival and leukemic transition by treatment. Semin Hematol 34:29, 1997; and Nimer S. Essential thrombocythemia: Another "heterogeneous disease" better understood? Blood 93:415–416, 1999.

Prognosis

Prognosis is dependent on the age of the patient and the history of thrombotic events (Table 12.14). The survival rate is 10 years for 64% to 80% of the patients, particularly the younger patients.[4,46] Less than 10% of patients with ET will convert to AML and less than 5% will convert to MMM.[47] Most patients die from thrombotic complications.

Table 12.14 ⊙ Differentiation of Myeloproliferative Disorders				
Laboratory Findings	Chronic Myelogenous Leukemia	Myelofibrosis With Myeloid Metaplasia	Polycythemia Vera	Essential Thrombocythemia
Hematocrit	Normal/decreased	Decreased	Marked increased	Normal/decreased
WBC	Marked neutrophilia with a shift to the left Basophilia and eosinophilia	Increased Left shift with myeloblasts (occ) Basophilia and eosinophilia	Normal/increased Leukocytosis with neutrophilia and basophilia	Normal/increased Leukocytosis usually mild
RBC	Normal Few nRBCs	Teardrop reticulocytosis nRBCs	Normal morphology as disease progresses; iron deficient morphology	Normal morphology and maturation
Platelets	Normal/increased Enlarged and fragments	Normal/decreased/increased Giant and abnormal megakaryocytes present	Increased	Increased Platelet count >600,000/μL Giant size Bizarre shapes Micromegakaryocytes and megakaryocytic fragments
Immature granulocytes	Increased	Increased	Absent or shift	Rare
LAP	Decreased	Normal/increased	Increased	Normal

Laboratory Findings	Chronic Myelogenous Leukemia	Myelofibrosis With Myeloid Metaplasia	Polycythemia Vera	Essential Thrombocythemia
Ph chromosome	Present	Absent	Absent	Absent
Spleen	Normal/increased	Increased	Increased	Normal/increased
Bone marrow	Hypercellular predominantly granulocytic decreased iron stores	Increased fibrosis Megakaryocytic hyperplasia RBCs and WBCs usually normal Bone marrow aspirate DRY TAP	Hypercellular moderate to severe All three lines increased with normal maturation Deceased iron stores	Hypercellular mild to moderate Megakaryocytic hyperplasia Clusters and sheets of megakaryocytes Some marrow fibrosis
Diagnostic criteria	Complete rainbow of all stages of neutrophil maturation Less than 5% blasts in peripheral blood Ph chromosome present in 90% to 95% of cases Three clinical phases: Chronic Accelerated Blast	Leukoerythroblastic picture with teardrop RBCs Fibrotic marrow as disease progresses Enlarged spleen	Excessive RBC production Increased red cell volume, normal O_2 saturation, all three lines increased Enlarged spleen	Platelet count greater than 600,000/µL with no known cause for reactive thrombocytosis Complications of thrombosis and hemorrhage

Adapted from Finnegan K. Leukocyte disorders. In: Lehmann C, ed. Saunders Manual of Clinical Laboratory Science. Philadelphia: WB Saunders, 1998: 903–944.

CONDENSED CASE

A 44-year-old woman went to her physician as part of a physical examination for life insurance. Her medical history was unremarkable, but she did complain of loss of appetite with a full feeling in her upper abdomen. She appeared to be in good physical condition but her spleen was palpable. Her physician ordered a complete CBC. **What condition could cause an enlarged spleen?**

Answer

An enlarged spleen can occur primarily as a result of hemolysis and sequestered cells or as a result of extramedullary hematopoiesis. In this case, the CBC revealed a 50,000 white count and a differential that showed the entire family of white cells. An LAP was ordered, and it was negative. This patient was diagnosed with early-stage chronic myelocytic leukemia. She was in no acute distress, but she was cautioned that since her spleen was enlarged, her movements should be restricted so as not to cause a rupture.

Summary Points

- Chronic myeloproliferative disorders (CMPDs) are caused by abnormal stem cells that lead to unchecked autonomous proliferation of one or more cell lines.

- The most common CMPDs are chronic granulocytic leukemia, polycythemia vera (PV), myelofibrosis with myeloid metaplasia (MMM), and essential thrombocythemia (ET).

- The bone marrow in CMPDs may show hyperplasia or elements of fibrosis.

- Most of these disorders are seen in older adults and show a normochromic normocytic process.

- Individuals with chronic myelogenous leukemia (CML) show an extremely high white count, moderate anemia, and the entire spectrum of white cells in the peripheral smear.

- Ninety percent of CML individuals show the Philadelphia chromosome, which is a cytogenetic abnormality in which a small part of chromosome 9 is translocated to the broken arm of chromosome 22.

- A hybrid gene, *BCR-ABL,* is also manifested with Philadelphia chromosome, and this gene prevents natural cell death or apoptosis.

- In the accelerated phase of CML, a higher blast count may be present and eventually ends in blast crisis, all blasts in the bone marrow.

- PV is a clonal disorder of red cells in which the patient shows a pancytosis: high red count, high white count, and high platelet count.

- Patients with PV have symptoms related to hyperviscosity, including hypertension and vascular abnormalities.

- The leukocyte alkaline phosphatase score is usually elevated in PV and low in CML.

- Patients with PV must be distinguished from those with secondary or relative erythrocytosis.

- The major causes of death in patients with PV are hemorrhage and thrombosis.

- MMM is characterized by marrow fibrosis, extramedullary hematopoiesis, and the leukoerythroblastic blood smear.

- In patients with MMM, the accelerating fibrosis may contribute to leukopenia and thrombocytopenia.

- In 50% of patients with MMM, bone marrow aspirates are impossible because of increased fibrosis: the dry tap.

- MMM has the worst prognosis of all of the myeloproliferative disorders.

- ET is a clonal proliferation of megakaryocytes in the bone marrow.

- The peripheral count of patients with ET is extremely elevated, sometimes up to 1 million.

- The increased platelet count in ET can cause hemorrhagic and thrombotic episodes, including gastrointestinal bleeding, epistaxis, and transient ischemic attacks.

- Diagnosis for ET involves ruling out any other causes for reactive thrombocytosis other than the clonal proliferation of megakaryocytes.

CASE STUDY

A 45-year-old male police officer sustained a fall from his motorcycle while driving at low speed while on patrol. He started to experience light-headedness, headache, and left upper quadrant abdominal pain. He was brought to a local hospital emergency department. On the basis of a physical examination, he was scheduled for surgery for a ruptured spleen. A STAT CBC was performed prior to surgery, with the following results:

Laboratory Data		Differential	
WBC	199×10^9/L	Basophils	5%
Hgb	10.6 g/dL	Eosinophils	5%
Hct	32%	Metamyelocytes	15%
Platelets	850×10^9/L	Myelocytes	8%
Bands	17%	Promyelocytes	7%
Neutrophils	32%	Blasts	7%
Lymphocytes	3%		
Monocytes	1%		

Which conditions show a differential with these abnormalities?

Insights to the Case Study

Considering our case study, there are many pieces of abnormal laboratory data. Chief among these is the exorbitant white count and platelet count. When you combine this unexpected data with the police officer's enlarged spleen and the peripheral smear findings, a likely diagnosis is chronic granulocytic leukemia. The patient seems to be in the chronic phase of the disease, since his blast count is low. This phase can last months to years. Cytogenetic studies need to be run to determine if he is Philadelphia chromosome positive. Myelosuppressive therapy will probably be instituted to reduce his white count, and he will be followed closely to monitor his progress and the progress of the disease.

Review Questions

1. One of the hallmarks in the diagnosis of a patient with CML is:
   a. splenomegaly.
   b. presence of teardrop cells.
   c. thrombocytosis.
   d. an M:E ratio of 10:1 or higher.

2. The *BCR:ABL* fusion gene leads to:
   a. increased LAP activity.
   b. increased tyrosine kinase activity.
   c. increased organomegaly.
   d. increased platelet count.

3. Blast crisis in CML means that there are more than _____ blasts in the peripheral smear
   a. 10%
   b. 30%
   c. 5%
   d. 15%

4. The origin of the dry tap in MMM occurs as a result of:
   a. extramedullary hematopoiesis.
   b. the presence of teardrop cells in MMM.
   c. the infiltration of fibrotic tissue in MMM.
   d. the increase of megakaryocytes in MMM.

5. Thrombotic symptoms in PV are generally related to:
   a. hyperviscosity syndrome.
   b. increased M:E ratio.
   c. increased LAP.
   d. splenomegaly.

6. Pancytopenia in MMM may be caused by:
   a. an aplastic origin.
   b. increase in reticulin fiber in the bone marrow.
   c. extramedullary hematopoiesis.
   d. the Ph chromosome.

7. The diagnostic criteria for essential thrombocytes includes all EXCEPT which of the following criteria?
   a. Increased platelet count
   b. Absence of collagen fibers
   c. Increased hematocrit
   d. No cytogenic abnormalities

❍ TROUBLESHOOTING

How Do I Obtain a Valid White Count When My Patient's White Count Is Outside of the Linearity Range?

Consider the case study presented earlier in this chapter. The white count is 199×10^9/L, which is out of the linearity range. Special techniques must be used by the technologist to obtain a valid white count on this sample. The technologist will notice that the white count is seen as a vote out $++++$ on the automated screen, and this is the first alert that the count may be too high (out of the linearity range) to be recorded by the instrument. The first step is to dilute a small amount of the patient's sample, usually 1:2 dilution, and re-run it to see if a number can be obtained. If this dilution is still out of range then several more dilutions are tried until a reading can be obtained. Once a reading is obtained, then the technologist must remember to multiply by the dilution factor to obtain an accurate white count. The white count will be a critical value and must be called and reported to a responsible party. Additionally, each of the other parameters of the CBC must be examined to evaluate whether they are credible. The troubleshooting case in Chapter 11 outlines each of the steps necessary to resolve the total CBC on a troublesome patient such as this, examining each CBC parameter and the resolution steps. Although each of these procedures seems exhaustive, they are necessary to give the physician an accurate account of this patient's CBC.

WORD KEY

Clonal • Disease arising from a single cell

Deep vein thrombosis • Formation of a blood clot in the deep veins of the legs, arms, pelvis, etc.

Gout • Arthritic disorder marked by crystal formation (usually uric acid) in the joints or tissues

Hyperplasia • Increase in the number of cells in the bone marrow

Myelofibrosis • Increase in the reticulin or fibrotic tissue in the bone marrow.

Myeloproliferative • Disease that results in the uncontrolled overproduction of normal-appearing cells in the absence of an appropriate stimulus

Organomegaly • Enlargement of the organs

Osteosclerosis • Abnormal increase in the thickening or density of bone

Plethora • Excess blood volume

Pruritus • Itching

Therapeutic phlebotomy • Withdrawing blood for a medical purpose

Transient ischemic attack • Neurological defect, having a vascular cause, producing stroke symptoms that resolve in 24 hours

Trisomy • In genetics, having three homologous chromosomes instead of two

References

1. Jaffee ES, Harris NL, Stein H, Vardiman JW, eds. World Health Organization Classification of Tumors: Pathology and Genetics of Tumors of Haematopoietic Lymphoid Tissues. Lyon: IARC Press, 2001.
2. Vardiman JW, Harris NL, Brunning RD. The World Health Organization (WHO) classification of the myeloid neoplasms. Blood 100:2292–2302, 2002.
3. Murphy S, Peterson P, Iland H, Laszio J. Experience of the Polycythemia Vera Study Group with essential thrombocythemia: A final report on diagnostic criteria, survival and leukemic transition by treatment. Semin Hematol 34:29, 1997.
4. Berlin NI. Diagnosis and classification of the polycythemias. Semin Hematol 12:339–351, 1975.
5. Melo JV, Hughes TP, Apperley JF. Chronic myeloid leukemia. Hematology 1:132–152, 2003.
6. Drucker BJ, Sawyers CL, Kantarjian H, et al. Activity of a specific inhibitor of the BCR-ABL tyrosine kinase in the blast crisis of chronic myeloid leukemia and acute lymphoblastic leukemia with Philadelphia chromosome. N Engl J Med 344:1038–1042, 2001.
7. Goldman JM, Melo JV. Chronic myeloid leukemia-advances in biology and new approach in treatment. N Engl J Med 349:1451–1464, 2003.
8. Deininger MW, Goldman JM, Melo JV. The molecular biology of chronic myeloid leukemia. Blood 96: 3342–3356, 2000.
9. Calabretta B, Perrotti D. The biology of CML blast crisis. Blood 103:4020–4022, 2004.
10. Faderl S, Talpaz M, Estrov Z, Kantarjian HM. Chronic myelogenous leukemia: Biology and therapy. Ann Intern Med 131:207–219, 1999.
11. O'Brien SG, Guilhot F, Larson RA, et al. Imatinib compared with interferon and low-dose cytarabine for newly diagnosed chronic-phase chronic myeloid leukemia. N Engl J Med 348:994–1004, 2003.
12. Obrien SG, Tefferi A, Valent P. Chronic myelogenous leukemia and myeloproliferative disease. Hematology 1:146–162, 2004.
13. Sawyers CL, Hochhaus A, Feldman E, et al. Imatinib induces hematologic and cytogenetic responses in patients with chronic myelogenous leukemia in myeloid blast crisis: Results of a phase II study. Blood 99:3530–3539, 2002.
14. Reiffers J, Trouette R, Marit G, et al. Autologous blood stem cell transplantation for chronic granulocytic leukemia in transformation: A report of 47 cases. Br J Haematol 77:339–345, 1991.
15. Sawyers CL. Chronic myeloid leukemia. N Engl J Med 340:1330–1340, 1999.
16. Onida f, Ball G, Kantarjian HM, et al. Characteristics and outcome of patients with Philadelphia chromosome negative, BCR/ABL negative chronic myelogenous leukemia. Cancer 95:1673–1684, 2002.
17. Bohm J, Schaefer HE. Chronic neutrophilic leukemia: 14 new cases of an uncommon myeloproliferative disease. J Clin Pathol 55:862–864, 2002.
18. Campbell PJ, Green AR. Management of Polycythemia Vera and Essential Thrombo cythemia. Am Soc Hematol Educ Program 2005; 201–205.
19. Bilrami S, Greenburg BR. Polycythemia rubra vera. Semin Oncol 22:307–326, 1995.
20. Spivak JL. Polycythemia vera: myths, mechanisms, and management. Blood 100:4272–4290, 2002.
21. Streiff MB, Smith B, Spivak JL. The diagnosis and management of polycythemia vera since the Polycythemia Vera Study Group: A survey of American Society of Hematology practice patterns. Blood 99:114–119, 2002.
22. Pearson TC, Messinezy M, Westwoos N, Green AR, et al. A polycythemia vera update: Diagnosis, pathobiology and treatment. Hematology 1:51–68, 2000.
23. Cazzola M, Guarnone R, Cerani P. et al. Red blood cell precursor mass as an independent determinant of serum erythropoietin level. Blood 91:2139–2145, 1998.
24. Swolin B, Weinfeld A, Westin J. A prospective long term cytogenetic study in polycythemia vera in relation to treatment and clinical course. Blood 72:386–395, 1998.
25. Lengfelder E, Berger U, Hehlman R. Interferon alpha in the treatment of polycythemia. Hematology 79:103–109, 2000.
26. Berk PD, Goldberg JD, Donovan PB, et al. Therapeutic recommendations in polycythemia based on Polycythemia Vera Study Group protocols. Trans Assoc Am Physicians 99:132–143, 1986.
27. Georgii A, Buesche G, Kreft A. The histopathology of chronic myeloproliferative diseases. Baillieres Clin Haematol 11:721–749, 1998.
28. Barosi G. Myelofibrosis with myeloid metaplasia: Diagnostic definition and prognostic classification for clinical studies and treatment guidelines. J Oncol 17: 2954–2970, 1999.
29. Tefferi A. Myelofibrosis with myeloid metaplasia. N Engl J Med 341:1255–1265, 2000.
30. Tefferi A, Mesa RA, Schroeder G, Hanson CA, Li CY, Dewald GW. Cytogenetics findings and their clinical

relevance in myelofibrosis with myeloid metaplasia. Br J Haematol 113:763–761, 2001.

31. Manoharan A. Idiopathic myelofibrosis: A clinical review. Int J Hematol 68:355–362, 1998.

32. Mesa RA, Hanson CS, Rajkumar V, Schroeder G, Tefferi A. Evaluation and clinical correlations of bone marrow angiogenesis in myelofibrosis with metaplasia. Blood 96:3374–3380, 2000.

33. Reilly JT. Idiopathic myelofibrosis: Pathogenesis, natural history and management. Blood Rev 11:233–242, 1997.

34. Dickstein JI, Vardiman JW. Hematopathologic findings in the myeloproliferative disorders. Semin Oncol 22:355–373, 1995.

35. Spivak JL, Barosi G, Tognoni G, et al. Chronic myeloproliferative disorders. Hematology 1:200–224, 2003.

36. Dupriez B, Morel P, Demory JL, et al. Prognostic factors in agnogenic myeloid metaplasia: A report on 195 cases with a new scoring system. Blood 88:1013–1018, 1996.

37. Tefferi A, Mesa RA, Nagomey DM, Schroeder G, et al. Splenectomy in myelofibrosis with myeloid metaplasia: A single-institution experience with 223 patients. Blood 95:226–233, 2000.

38. Deeg HJ, Gooley TA, Flowers ME, et al. Allogenetic hematopoietic stem cell transplantation for myelofibrosis. Blood 102:3912–3918, 2003.

39. Cervantes F, Barosi G, Demoray JL, et al. Myelofibrosis with myeloid metaplasia in young individuals: Disease characteristics, prognostic factors and identification of risk groups. Br J Haematol 102:684–690, 1998.

40. Tefferi A, Solberg LA, Silverstein MN. A clinical update in polycythemia vera and essential thrombocythemia. Am J Med 109:141–149, 2000.

41. Nimer S. Essential thrombocythemia: Another "heterogeneous disease" better understood? Blood 93:415–416, 1999.

42. Harrison CN, Gale RE, Machin SJ, Linch DC. A large proportion of patients with a diagnosis of essential thrombocythemia do not have a clonal disorder and may be at lower risk of thrombotic complications. Blood 93:417–424, 1999.

43. Cortelazzo S. Finazzi G. Ruggeri M, Hydroxyurea for patients with essential thrombocythemia and a high risk of thrombosis. N Engl J Med 332:1132–1136, 1995.

44. Ruggeri M, Finazzi G, Tosetro A, et al. No treatment for low-risk thrombocythemia: Results from a prospective study. Br J Haematol 103:772–777, 1998.

45. Fenaux P, Simon M, Caulier MT. Clinical course of essential thrombocythemia in 147 cases. Cancer 66:549–556, 1990.

46. Hehlmann R, Jahn M, Baumann B. Essential thrombocythemia: Clinical characteristics: A study of 61 cases. Cancer 61:2487–2496, 1988.

47. Sterkers Y, Preudhomme C, Lai JL, et al. Acute myeloid leukemia and myelodysplastic syndromes following essential thrombocythemia treated with hydroxyurea. Blood 91:616, 1998.

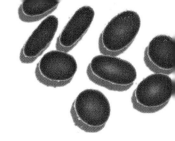

13

Lymphoproliferative Disorders and Related Plasma Cell Disorders

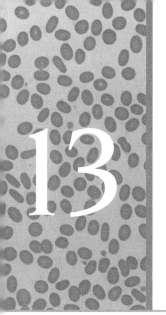

Betty Ciesla

Lymphoid Malignancies

Chronic Lymphocytic Leukemia

Hairy Cell Leukemia

Sezary Syndrome

Prolymphocytic Leukemia

Hodgkin's and Non-Hodgkin's Lymphoma (Briefly)

Plasma Cell Disorders

Normal Plasma Cell Structure and Function

Multiple Myeloma

Waldenstrom's Macroglobulinemia

Objectives

After completing this chapter, the student will be able to:

1. Define the common features of the chronic lymphoproliferative disorders.

2. Describe the symptoms, peripheral smear morphology, and treatment of individuals with chronic lymphocytic leukemia.

3. Evaluate the complications of chronic lymphocytic leukemias with respect to immunocompetency and bone marrow involvement.

4. Describe the pertinent features of hairy cell leukemia to include clinical presentation, peripheral smear, and pertinent cytochemical stains.

5. Define the clinical features of Sézary syndrome.

6. List the morphological features of the plasma cell.

7. Describe the basic immunoglobulin unit.

8. List the laboratory criteria used to diagnose the monoclonal gammopathies.

9. Differentiate the clinical and laboratory features that distinguish multiple myeloma and Waldenstrom's macroglobulinemia.

10. List the CD markers used to differentiate B-cell and T-cell disorders.

11. Compare and contrast the clinical and laboratory features of multiple myeloma and Waldenstrom's macroglobulinemia.

12. Briefly describe how molecular diagnostics aid in the diagnosis of lymphoid malignancies.

Lymphoproliferative disorders comprise those disorders of the B and T lymphocytes, in which there is a clonal, malignant proliferation of either cell subset. This chapter discusses the malignant lymphoproliferative disorders (with variants) and the plasma cell disorders. There are several common features of each of these groups. Primarily these diseases affect the elderly; they are chronic; most complications are related to a compromised immune ability; and these diseases progress slowly.

Hodgkin's and non-Hodgkin's lymphoma are covered briefly in this chapter. These diseases have complicated staging systems and are primarily diagnosed through lymph node biopsy, through bone marrow studies, and with molecular techniques. The laboratory involvement in these diseases is peripheral at best. Major plasma cell disorders such as multiple myeloma and Waldenstrom's macroglobulinemia will be presented. Molecular diagnostic techniques such as flow cytometry and chromosomal analysis with a molecular component provide essential data for diagnosis of the malignant disorders. These techniques will be mentioned throughout the text.

LYMPHOID MALIGNANCIES

Chronic Lymphocytic Leukemia

Chronic lymphocytic leukemia (CLL) is caused by a clonal proliferation of B lymphocytes. It is the most common chronic leukemia with a predilection for men over women. Most patients are older, over 50 years of age.[1] Small lymphocytes begin to accumulate in the spleen, lymph nodes, and bone marrow to a high degree and eventually spill into the peripheral blood. These malignant lymphocytes will show CD15, CD19, CD20, and CD22 antigen markers as well as exhibit a low level of surface immunoglobulin (SIg) and CD5, a marker usually reserved for T cells. Chromosomal abnormalities include chromosomes 11, 12, and 13 in over 82% of patients.[2] Trisomy 12 is reported in almost half of all CLL patients and is associated with a poor prognosis.[2] The presenting symptoms of this disease are fairly unremarkable (fatigue, pallor, weight loss), and for this reason, it is often discovered by accident, as a result of other complaints. However, lymphadenopathy is the most common initial symptom.[3] The white counts are exaggerated with many over $100,000 \times 10^9$/L. The M:E ratio is 10 or 20:1, and the bone marrow and peripheral blood present a monotonous tapestry of mature lymphocytes to the exclusion of other normal elements in the blood or bone marrow.

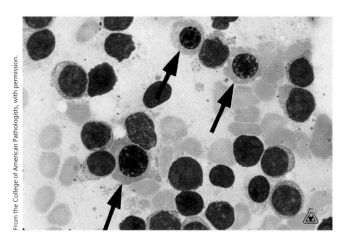

Figure 13.1 Bone marrow view of chronic lymphocytic leukemia. Compare the nRBCs at the *arrow* with mature lymphocytes.

Disease Progression in Chronic Lymphocytic Leukemia

The peripheral blood smear shows exclusively small lymphocytes intermixed with few lymphoblasts. The lymphocytes show certain homogeneity in morphology with a heavily clumped chromatin combined with round and at times slightly indented nucleus. Figure 13.1 provides a comparison of nucleated red blood cells (nRBCs) and lymphocytes in CLL. Smudge cells may be present in the peripheral smear and are visualized as pieces of lymphocyte chromatin splashed across the peripheral smear. Because lymphocytes are fragile, smudge cells may arise in the process of making a peripheral smear where the cytoplasm is disrupted and the nuclear chromatin strands are smudged across the smear in a basket shape or amorphous smudge (Fig. 13.2).

As the disease progresses, lymphocyte mass accumulates in the bone marrow and splenomegaly and

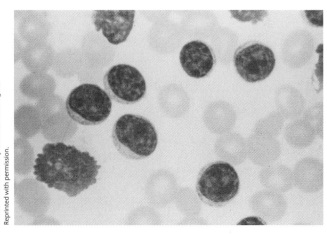

Figure 13.2 Chronic lymphocytic leukemia with smudge cells.

lymphadenopathy may develop. Anemia, thrombocytopenia, and neutropenia usually develop in the course of the disease, subsequent to lymphocytic involvement in the bone marrow. The altered immune function of the lymphocytes may lead to the complication of **autoimmune hemolytic anemia** in 10% to 30% of individuals with CLL. Spherocytes and nRBCs that appear in the peripheral smear of CLL individuals may be early indicators of the autoimmune hemolytic process. Erythroid hyperplasia is present in the bone marrow, and the **direct antiglobulin test** (which measures antibody coating of the red cells) is positive.

Immunological Function in Chronic Lymphocytic Leukemia and Treatment Options

The B lymphocytes present in CLL patients are long-lived and nonproliferating. Programmed cell death or apoptosis is a significant feature in most cell line progressions, but in 80% of CLL patients there is the presence of *Bcl2*, an antiapoptosis gene.[4] Therefore, the survival of the dysfunctional B-cell clone is guaranteed. Additionally, the immunological function of these lymphocytes is compromised, with over 50% of patients showing a hypogammaglobulinemia. Patients experience bacterial or skin infections, particularly herpes zoster (shingles) and herpes simplex (cold sores), that can be painful and debilitating.[5]

Treatment options for CLL patients include irradiation for enlarged spleen and lymph nodes as a means to reduce discomfort and related symptoms.[6] The most effective drug for reducing lymphocyte burden is fludarabine, a cytotoxic drug that induces apoptosis.[7] Other therapies include alkylating agents, monoclonal antibodies, and possibly allogeneic stem cell transplants. Table 13.1 depicts the Rai staging systems and survival projections. The Rai staging system was designed by Dr. Rai in 1970 and modified in 1987. These systems divide patients into risk categories and provide survival statistics. Staging systems are developed to analyze patient

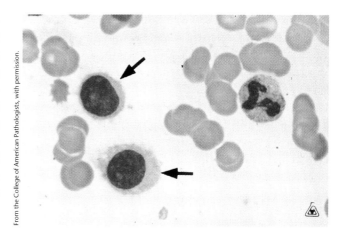

Figure 13.3   Hairy cell leukemia, showing hair-like projections in large mononuclear cells.

data in an attempt to project disease prognosis and risk factors.

Hairy Cell Leukemia

Hairy cell leukemia (HCL) is a rare B-cell malignancy in which the key morphological entity is a fragile appearing mononuclear cell with hair-like or ruffled projections of the cytoplasm (Fig. 13.3). The nuclear material in these cells is round or dumbbell shaped with a spongy appearance of the chromatin. Hairy cells represent approximately 50% of cells seen in the peripheral smear. These cells eventually infiltrate the bone marrow and spleen, leading to pancytopenia and thrombocytopenia. Most patients are older, in their fifth decade, with more males than females being affected. Abdominal discomfort is a frequent presenting symptom; more than 80% of patients show massive spleens that misplace the stomach. Bleeding, infections, and anemia develop as malignant cells predominate in the bone marrow and peripheral circulation. Neutrophils and monocytes are greatly reduced. Bone marrow aspirates are usually unsuccessful and lead to a dry tap. Dry taps occurs when the normal bone marrow architecture becomes filled

Staging	Lymphocytes	Lymph Nodes	Spleen	Platelet Count	Survival
0	Increased				12.5 years
I	Increased	Enlarged			8.5 years
II	Increased	Enlarged/some	Enlarged		6 years
III	Increased	Enlarged/some	Enlarged		1.5 years
IV	Increased			Decreased	1.5 years

Table 13.1 ◉ **Modified Rai Staging for Chronic Lymphocytic Leukemia**

with fibrotic material and liquid marrow is unable to be aspirated. A key item in the diagnosis of HCL is the cytochemical stain known as TRAP, or tartrate-resistant acid phosphatase stain. Most lymphocytes contain many isoenzymes, and isoenzyme 5 is especially abundant in hairy cells.[8] When blood smears from patients with HCL are stained with the acid phosphatase, most cells will take up the stain. Once tartrate is added, lymphocytes from HCL patients will remain stained while the staining in other cells will fade. This resistance to tartrate is directly related to the level of isoenzyme 5 activity in hairy cells. CD markers present in hairy cells are CD22, CD11c, CD25, and CD103 (Table 13.2).

Treatment for patients with HCL is individualized according to the progress and course of disease. Therapeutic splenectomy will provide an improvement in cytopenias and hypersplenism, as well as providing an improvement in physical symptoms such as abdominal fullness and satiety. Other treatments with interferon-alfa and 2-chlorodeoxyadenosine (2-CdA) have offered positive remissions.[9]

Sézary Syndrome

T-cell lymphomas may present with a cutaneous manifestation in some patients. The name for this is mycosis fungoides. Individuals with mycosis fungoides will show reddened itchy areas (generalized **erythroderma**) that become thickened, scaly, and pronounced. Skin biopsies of these areas will show an infiltration of lymphocytes. As this disease progresses, the spleen, bone marrow, and lymph nodes become involved, presenting the characteristic Sézary syndrome, which is the leukemic phase of T-cell lymphoma. Sézary cells can be identified in the peripheral blood as large cells, approximately 8 to 20 µm, with a convoluted, cerebriform, ovoid nucleus. Although they may be mistaken for monocytes, the concentration of chromatin is much thicker and more compact in Sézary cells. Sézary cells are **pathognomonic** for cutaneous T-cell lymphoma

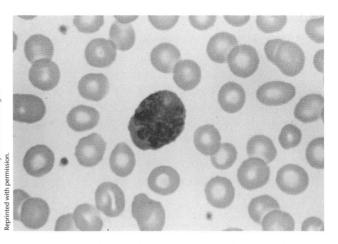

© 1967 American Society of Clinical Pathologists. Reprinted with permission.

Figure 13.4 Sézary cells. Note the folded or convoluted nuclear membrane that may appear cerebriform.

and individuals who progress to this phase have decreased survival rates. Sézary cells shown CD2, CD3, CD4, and CD5 markers[10] (Fig. 13.4).

Prolymphocytic Leukemia

Prolymphocytic leukemia (PLL) is a variant of chronic lymphocytic leukemia. A rare disorder, this peripheral smear of individuals with PLL shows a majority of circulating prolymphocytes. These cells of lymphoid origin have more abundant cytoplasm than mature lymphocytes, and their nuclear chromatin appears more mature and coarse. This leukemia has a poor prognosis and, in contrast to CLL patients, these patients have more severe symptoms such as splenic enlargement, liver involvement, and escalating white counts. Individuals with PLL will show strong CD20 markers and SIg activity and will also be positive for CD19 and CD20.

Hodgkin's and Non-Hodgkin's Lymphoma (Briefly)

Hodgkin's lymphoma represents a significant lymphoproliferative disorder with a bimodal incidence. It is one of the most common lymphomas in young males between the ages of 14 and 40, but it also may be seen in individuals older than 50 years. Most patients complain of a single lymph node in the cervical region that is firm to the touch and usually does not disappear. Symptoms of hypermetabolism such as low-grade fever and weight loss may be present. Individuals who have had previous exposure to Epstein-Barr virus or who have been exposed to environmental hazards may be more vulnerable to Hodgkin's lymphoma. Diagnosis is made based upon the cellular features seen in lymph node biopsy, which may feature a Reed-Sternberg cell, a large multinucleated cell resembling an "owl's eye." Other histo-

Table 13.2 ● CD Markers in Hairy Cell Leukemia
• CD19
• CD20
• CD22
• CD11c—membrane adhesion
• CD25
• CD103

logical classifications of lymphoma include lymphocyte predominant (5%), nodular sclerosing (60%), mixed cellularity (20%), and lymphocyte depleted (5%). The disease may spread across the lymphatic system and may involve the liver, spleen, and bone marrow. Prognosis is good, however, with a high cure rate.

Non-Hodgkin's lymphoma is three times more common than Hodgkin's lymphoma and may present as painless cervical lymph node involvement. The lymph nodes may be enlarged, and the disease may spread to the gastrointestinal and respiratory systems, skin, liver, and spleen. The range of spread may be more sporadic than that of Hodgkin's lymphoma, and lymphoma cells may be seen in the peripheral blood. Any history of congenital or acquired immunological disorder may be a predisposing factor in the development of non-Hodgkin's lymphoma. The diagnostic scheme is divided into low grade, intermediate grade, or high grade based on the different histological types of lymphocytic cells. Radiation and chemotherapy may be successful in obtaining remission, but relapses for non-Hodgkin's lymphoma are frequent.[11]

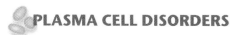 PLASMA CELL DISORDERS

Normal Plasma Cell Structure and Function

A normal plasma cell evolves as the last stage of a B lymphocyte. In structure and function, this is a unique cellular entity that comprises less than 5% of the cells in the bone marrow. Rarely do these cells make an appearance in the peripheral circulation, and when they do, they are in response to infectious, inflammatory conditions, or malignant proliferation (Table 13.3). A plasma cell is a medium-sized cell with an eccentric nucleus having a well-defined Golgi apparatus. Of particular

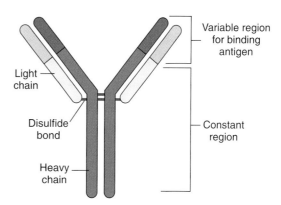

Figure 13.5   Basic immunoglobulin structure.

note is the color of the cytoplasm, which is a distinct sea blue or cornflower color. The chromatin, although clumped, is evenly arranged in a pinwheel structure. Plasma cells make immunoglobulins, the basic building blocks of antibody production (see Fig. 13.5). There are five types of immunoglobulin—IgG, IgM, Ig D, IgE, and IgA. Each immunoglobulin has:

- Four polypeptide chains
- Two H chains (heavy chains)
- Two L chains (light chains)

There are five different types of H chains
- Gamma (γ), alpha (α), mu (μ), epsilon (ε), and delta (δ)

There are two different types of L chains
- Kappa (κ) and lambda (λ)

Table 13.4 presents the specific function of each immunoglobulin type.

Table 13.3 ⊙ Increased Plasma Cells in Blood
• Streptococcal infections
• Syphilis
• Epstein-Barr virus
• HIV
• Tuberculosis
• Mumps
• Rubella
• Collagen vascular disease

Adapted from Glassy E. Color Atlas of Hematology: An Illustrated Guide Based on Proficiency Testing. Northfield, IL: College of American Pathologists, 1998.

Table 13.4 ⊙ Immunoglobulin and Range of Activity	
Immunoglobulin	**Range of Activity**
IgG	Secondary immune response, precipitating antibodies, hemolysins, virus neutralizing antibodies
IgA	Secretory antibody, protects airways and gastrointestinal tract
IgM	Primary immune response
IgD	Lymphocyte activator and suppressor
IgE	Antibody found in respiratory and gastrointestinal tract/parasitic infections

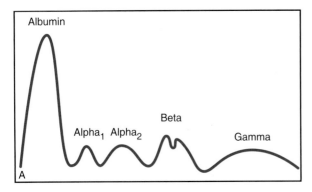

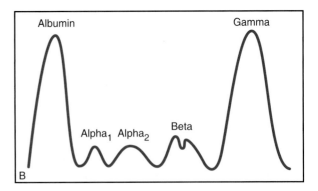

Figure 13.6   Serum protein electrophoresis showing patterns of (*A*) normal serum and (*B*) serum from patient with multiple myeloma; note the monoclonal spike in the gamma region.

Immunoglobulins are assessed either quantitatively or qualitatively. Serum protein electrophoresis gives a representation of all serum proteins: immunoglobulins, albumins, and some minor proteins (Fig. 13.6). Immunoelectrophoresis, on the other hand, separates the specific immunoglobulins by using antibodies directed against each fraction combined with an electrical field and a gel medium.

Multiple Myeloma

One of the premier disorders of plasma cells (Fig. 13.7) is multiple myeloma. This disorder has a well-defined pathophysiology that centers around the accumulation of plasma cells in the bone marrow and other locations. Multiple myeloma occurs in older age, among men more than among women, and with greater frequency in the African American population.

Several environmental and occupational factors are thought to contribute to the clonal proliferation of plasma cells. These include exposure to atomic radiation, work involving the use of organic solvents, work with toxins within the textile industries, and any occupation that may primarily or secondarily expose one to chemicals, pesticides, or herbicides.[12] Additionally, chromosome abnormalities have been defined in 18% to 35% of patients with multiple myeloma.[13] Aberrations in chromosome 13 have been particularly well studied and include **monosomy,** deletions, or translocations of the chromosome. Multiple myeloma patients with chromosomal damage have a worse prognosis, a higher rate of disease acceleration, and a decreased survival.[14] Screening for chromosomal abnormalities seems a prudent course of action in monitoring disease progress (Table 13.5).

Pathophysiology in Multiple Myeloma

Disease and clinical symptoms in multiple myeloma follow along three distinct pathways:

1. Acceleration of plasma cells in the bone marrow
2. Activation of bone resorption factors or osteoclasts
3. Production of an abnormal monoclonal protein

Figure 13.7   Plasma cells. Note basophilic cytoplasm and eccentric nucleus.

Table 13.5 ⊙ A Simplified list of Chromosomal Aberrations in Multiple Myeloma

- 13q14 deletions
- 14q32
- t(11:14)(q13:q32)
- t(4:14)

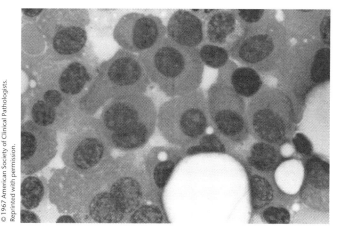

Figure 13.8   Sheets of plasma cells.

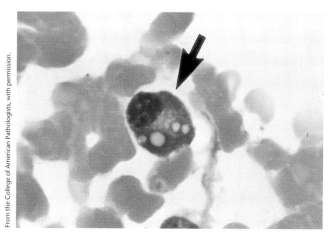

Figure 13.10   Plasma cell with inclusion.

To begin, plasma cells accelerate in multiple myeloma under the direction of the renegade cytokine interleukin (IL)-6. The plasma cells appear in clusters (Fig. 13.8) and may be morphologically normal, or they may appear binucleated and have a bizarre structure. Some may even develop colorless inclusions called Russell bodies or other crystalline inclusions (Figs. 13.9 and 13.10). Flame cells may also be visualized in IgA myelomas and appear as plasma cells with a striking deep pink cytoplasm (Fig. 13.11). Eventually, these clusters or sheets overtake the normal bone marrow structure, leading to the appearance of plasma cells in the peripheral smear as well as anemias, thrombocytopenia, and neutropenia. Plasma cell tumors may seed to other areas in the body, and plasmacytomas may occur in liver, spleen, gastrointestinal tract, or nasal cavities. Additionally, the increased plasma cell activity leads to commensurate increased osteoclast activity. Osteoclasts are

large multinucleated cells in the bone marrow that absorb bone tissue. With increased activity, bone loss is inevitable and this pathology usually brings forward the single most frequent complaint from MM patients— bone pain. Pain usually develops due to compressed vertebrae in the back, ribs, or sternum. This compression may lead to loss of sensation, fractures, and paralysis. Serum calcium is also greatly increased due to bone loss, and this event may lead to kidney failure or the formation of kidney stones.

Increased plasma cell production results in increased immunoglobulin production and usually the advent of a monoclonal gammopathy, a purposeless proliferation of one particular antibody, usually IgG. On serum immunoelectrophoresis (see Fig. 13.11), this is seen as an M spike. This excess globulin production may lead to complications from hyperviscosity in the plasma such as blurred vision or headache. Subsequent

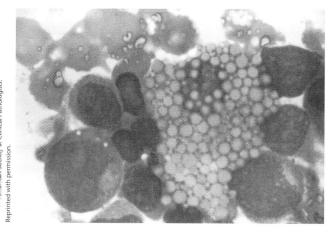

Figure 13.9   Russell bodies. These inclusions are derived from an accumulation of immunoglobulin.

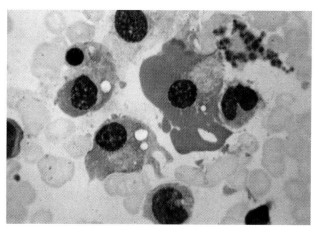

Figure 13.11   Flame cell; a plasma cell with a pink cytoplasm.

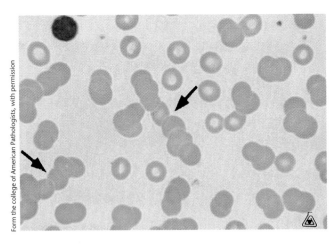

Form the college of American Pathologists, with permission

Figure 13.12   Rouleaux. Red cells form stacks of coins as a reaction to excess protein.

laboratory abnormalities such as **rouleaux** may also be seen. Red cells circulating in abnormal proteins like fibrinogen and globulin may cause rouleaux formation (Fig. 13.12), where red cells look like stacks of coins even in the thinner areas of the smear. Unlike red cell agglutination, where red cells are attracted to an specific antibody and appear in clumps, rouleaux is nonspecific binding of red cells where the net negative charge of red cells has been neutralized by excess protein (Fig. 13.13). Rouleaux may cause falsely decreased red counts and falsely increased MCV and MCHC. Red cell counts appear lower as the doublets and triplets caused by rouleaux pass through the red cell–counting aperture of automated equipment as one cell. MCV appears higher because the red cell volume is directly measured and red cells showing rouleaux appear larger. MCHC appears falsely increased because these parameters are calculated using red count. The peripheral smear may also show a blue coloration on macroscopic examination due to excess proteins. The ESR (refer to procedure section, Chapter 20) is usually elevated due to the increased settling of the red cells brought on the increased globulin content of the plasma (Table 13.6).

Bence Jones protein is a peculiar protein made by some individuals with MM as a result of an excess of kappa and lambda light chains. These light chains are small and can be filtered by the kidneys. They appear in the urine and have several unique properties. When urine is heated to 56°C, Bence-Jones protein precipitates out and will redissolve at higher temperature. As the urine is cooled, precipitates will once again appear, and will dissolve upon cooling. Bence-Jones protein is damaging to the kidneys.

Symptoms and Screening for Multiple Myeloma

Approximately 50,000 Americans are diagnosed with multiple myeloma each year.[15] Symptoms usually do not develop initially, but as the numbers of plasma cells accelerate, the individual may experience the following:

- Fatigue—due to anemia
- Excessive thirst and urination—due to excess calcium
- Nausea—due to excess calcium
- Bone pain in back and ribs—due to plasma cell acceleration
- Bone fractures—due to calcium leeching from bones into circulation
- Unexpected infections—due to compromised immunity
- Weakness and numbness in the legs—due to vertebrae compression

Screening and diagnosis of patients suspected of having MM include a CBC, possibly a bone marrow, urinalysis, and protein panel. Serum protein electrophoresis (SPE) and beta-microglobulin might also be ordered. Serum beta-microglobulin is a protein produced by the light chains. In the early stages of MM, this protein is at a low level. Elevated levels greater than 6 µg/mL are seen later in the disease and usually indicate higher tumor burden and poor prognosis.

Prognosis and Treatment in Multiple Myeloma

Patients with multiple myeloma face many difficulties especially with respect to their skeletal condition. Some individuals show punched-out lesions on initial radiographs. Chemotherapy and radiation may be used, with radiation providing some relief in painful bone areas. Agents used in chemotherapy include the glucocorticoids and interferon-alfa, yet survival times from

Table 13.6 ◉ Laboratory Findings of Multiple Myeloma
• Pancytopenia
• N/N anemia
• ↑ ESR
• ↑ Calcium
• ↑ Urine protein
• ↑ Uric acid
• Abnormal serum electrophoresis

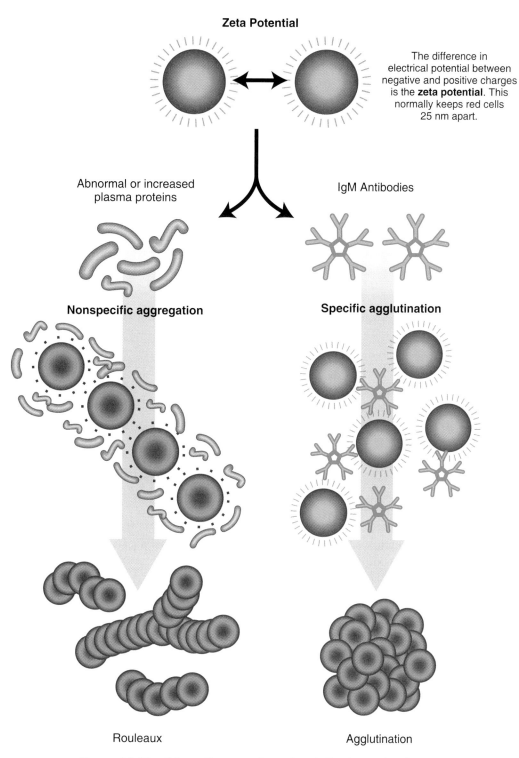

Zeta Potential

The difference in electrical potential between negative and positive charges is the **zeta potential**. This normally keeps red cells 25 nm apart.

Abnormal or increased plasma proteins

IgM Antibodies

Nonspecific aggregation

Specific agglutination

Rouleaux

Agglutination

Figure 13.13   Schematic comparison of agglutination and rouleaux.

diagnosis are usually 3 to 4 years. A newer therapy involves the use of thalidomide, an antinausea drug of the 1950s. This drug was banned from the market because its use in pregnant women to control nausea led to many birth defects, particularly with respect to the limbs. It is, however, effective in stalling the growth of myeloma cells, and it is used under close supervision.[12]

Plasma Cell Leukemia

Plasma cell leukemia is a complication of multiple myeloma in which there is an increased number of plasma cells in the circulating blood (Fig. 13.14). This condition is usually seen late in the progression of the disease as plasma cells overtake the normal bone marrow elements.

Waldenstrom's Macroglobulinemia

Waldenstrom's macroglobulinemia was discovered in 1944 by the Swedish physician Dr. Jan Waldenstrom. His original presentation described two patients who had abnormal mucosal bleeding, enlarged lymph nodes, anemia, and thrombocytopenia. No bone pain was evident and both patients showed an elevated ESR. He described an abnormal protein that we now know is an overproduction of IgM, which presents as a particular spike on SPE and produces the hyperviscosity syndrome. Patients tend to be older, but the condition affects both men and women equally, with more whites than blacks being affected. The overproduction of globulin is caused by abnormal B lymphocytes that manifest in the bone marrow and peripheral smear as having features of plasma cells—thus, the name plasmacytoid lymphocytes. Clinical issues related to hyperviscosity feature largely in the complications experienced by these patients. Because IgM is such a large molecule, an overproduction of this macromolecule has the ability to coat platelets, impeding their function, interfering with coagulation factors, and causing potential neurological or thrombotic complications. Although there is no unique profile of symptoms in these patients, most

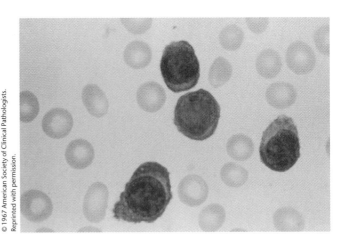

© 1967 American Society of Clinical Pathologists. Reprinted with permission.

Figure 13.14   Plasma cell leukemia.

experience headaches, dizziness, visual problems, and serious coagulation difficulties. The peripheral smear may show rouleaux and plasmacytoid lymphocytes. As a subset of the abnormal IgM protein, cryoglobulins may form in some patients, which leads to **Raynaud's phenomenon** and bleeding. Chemotherapy is available for these patients, and **plasmapheresis** may be used as a means to reduce the IgM concentration. In the plasmapheresis procedure, blood is removed from the patient, which separates the plasma from the cells. The cells are returned to the patient while the offending plasma, which contains the elevated IgM protein, is discarded. Treatment for many patients consists of plasmapheresis chemotherapy, immunotherapy with monoclonal antibodies, or possibly stem cell transplantation. Interferon may also be used to relieve symptoms. Table 13.7 provides a summary of the major lymphoproliferative disorders.

CONDENSED CASE

A 65-year-old grandmother, Ms. L. was recently bitten by mosquitoes while she was gardening. This time, her experience with mosquito bites was different than previously. She noticed that despite her normal routine of rubbing alcohol and Calamine lotion on her bites, her bites became suppurative, bumpy, and large. She decided to seek medical attention from her internist. After prescribing steroids and applying a topical antibiotic, the internist ordered a CBC just as a precaution. Two days later, Ms. L was called back into the office. Her results were WBC 65 × 10⁹/L, Hct 33, and platelets 150 × 10⁹/L. A differential was ordered as part of reflex testing and revealed 99% mature lymphocytes

Are the results of this differential in the normal reference range?

Answer

Clearly, this is an unexpected case of CLL. While it is unusual to have a severe cutaneous response to mosquito bites, the fact that the lymphocytic cells in CLL are compromised and unable to provide proper immune response certainly contributes to this unusual presentation. Ms. L will probably do well with little intervention. She will need to be followed as the disease progresses.

Table 13.7 ● Overview of Major Malignant Lymphoproliferative Disorders

	CLL	HCL	HL	NHL	MM	WM
Predominant cell type*	Mature lymphocyte	Hairy cell	Reed-Sternberg cell (in node)	Lymphocyte Lymphocyte variations	Plasma cells in marrow	Plasmacytoid lymphs
Main symptoms	Fatigue Weight loss	Infections Bleeding	Enlarged lymph node	Painless, enlarged lymph node	Bone pain, thirst, fatigue	Bleeding, lymphadenopathy Dizziness, blurred vision
Significant lab findings	↑↑WBC Peripheral smear shows 90% lymphs	TRAP + Pancytopenia	Variable presentations	Variable presentations	↑↑ Calcium, hyperviscosity (↑ESR), monoclonal gammopathy (IgG-M spike), rouleaux	Monoclonal gammopathy (Ig M), hyperviscosity (ESR ↑) Rouleaux
Organ involvement	Enlarged lymph nodes	↑↑↑Spleen	Possibly extra-nodal sites	Possible extranodal sites	Kidneys Bone marrow	Kidneys Bone marrow
Survival rate	Variable	Good	Good	Poor	Variable	Poor
Immunological markers	CD15, CD19, CD20, CD22	CD19, CD20, CD22, CD11c, D25, CD103	CD15	None	CD38	CD19, CD20, CD22

CLL, chronic lymphocytic leukemia; HCL, hairy cell leukemia; HL, Hodgkin's lymphoma; NHL, non-Hodgkin's lymphoma; MM, multiple myeloma; WM, Waldenstrom's macroglobulinemia; TRAP, Tartrate-resistant acid phosphatase stain; ESR, erythrocyte sedimentation rate.
*See text for appearance in bone marrow or peripheral smear.

Summary Points

- Lymphoproliferative disorders comprise the B and T lymphocytes in which there is a clonal malignant proliferation of either cell subset.

- Chronic lymphocytic leukemia (CLL) is a clonal proliferation of B lymphocytes that is seen in older patients and often discovered by accident.

- CLL shows an accumulation of mature lymphocytes in the bone marrow and eventually the lymph nodes, spleen, and peripheral blood.

- The white counts in CLL are extremely elevated and the M:E ratio is 10 to 20:1.

- Immune function is compromised in CLL, and 10% to 30% of individuals may experience autoimmune hemolytic anemia.

- Hairy cell leukemia (HCL) is a rare B-cell malignancy in which the cells have a lymphoid appearance but hair-like projections in the cytoplasm.

- Pancytopenia, splenomegaly, and dry tap are the key features of HCL.

- Sézary syndrome is the blood equivalent of cutaneous T-cell lymphoma that presents with a convoluted, cerebriform, ovoid nucleus.

- Multiple myeloma is a disorder of plasma cells that leads to a monoclonal gammopathy, bone involvement, and pancytopenia.

- Most of the abnormal proteins are an accumulation of IgG, which may lead to a hyperviscosity and rouleaux in the peripheral smear.

- Serum calcium is elevated in MM patients due to bone loss and increased distribution of calcium in the peripheral circulation.

- Bence-Jones protein may be seen in individuals with MM.

- Plasma cell leukemia is a complication of MM in which mature plasma cells are seen in increasing numbers in the peripheral circulation.

- Waldenstrom's macroglobulinemia is a rare disorder of plasma cells in which IgM is overproduced.

- Many of the symptoms of Waldenstrom's macroglobulinemia are related to hyperviscosity of the plasma, which accounts for coagulation abnormalities, rouleaux formation, and bleeding or thrombotic complications.

- Plasmapheresis, the therapeutic removal of plasma, may be used as a treatment to decrease the amount of abnormal IgM protein.

CASE STUDY

A 60-year-old woman complained of gastric pain and vomiting for 2 weeks. She had no fever, but a CAT scan was ordered and showed a slightly enlarged spleen. An enlarged lymph node was also discovered. The patient complained of severe itching, redness and scaling of the skin, and pitting edema. A bone marrow showed a hypocellular architecture with increased fat.

Laboratory findings are as follows:

		Differential:	
WBC	39.0×10^9/L		
RBC	4.25×10^{12}/L	Segs	29%
Hgb	11.7 g/dL	Lymphs	67%
Hct	38%	Eosinophils	4%
MCV	89 fL	Platelets	normal
MCH	27.5 pg	Technologist note: lympho-	
MCHC	30.6%	cytes appear abnormal with	
		rounded, clefted, folded or	
		bilobed nucleus; vacuoles in	
		some cells	

Considering the patient's symptoms, which are unusual, the increased white count and the differential reversal, what are the diagnostic possibilities?

Insights to the Case Study

Relative lymphocytosis is usually reported in conditions like infectious mononucleosis, hepatitis virus infection, or cytomegalovirus infection. These lymphocytes, however, showed a distinct morphology with a large cell and a small cell variant. Nuclear clefting or folding may be seen in lymphoma cells, but lymphoma cells rarely have vacuoles. An additional finding is that these cells were very large, some up to 20 μm, and the clefting manifestation is very pronounced. When clinical characteristics are included, the most likely diagnosis in this case is Sézary syndrome, a rare type of T-cell lymphoma. This disorder usually has serious skin manifestations, as shown in our patient, combined with an elevated white count and rising lymphocyte count. The abnormal lymphocyte morphology usually causes confusion when performing a differential due to the unusual nuclear manifestations of these cells. Sézary cells are usually confirmed by immunophenotyping and are usually CD4-positive T lymphocytes. The life expectancy for a patient with this condition is around 5 years.

(Adapted from Hematology Problem, November 1981, American Journal of Medical Technology.)

Review Questions

1. What is the most common presenting symptom in individuals with chronic lymphocytic leukemia?
   a. Massive spleens
   b. Thrombocytosis
   c. Increased calcium
   d. Enlarged lymph nodes

2. What are the peripheral cell indicators of an autoimmune hemolytic anemia in a patient with CLL?
   a. nRBCs and spherocytes
   b. Smudge cells and normal lymphs
   c. Howell-Jolly bodies and siderocytes
   d. Lymphoblasts and prolymphocytes

3. A dumbbell-shaped nucleus with fragile, spiny projections like cytoplasm best describes:
   a. Sézary cells.
   b. lymphoblasts.
   c. hairy cells.
   d. smudge cells.

4. In contrast to most of the other leukemias, which of these conditions presents with a pancytopenia?
   a. CLL

   b. HCL
   c. CGL
   d. PV

5. Hypercalcemia in patients with multiple myeloma is the direct result of:
   a. increased plasma cell mass.
   b. crystalline inclusions in the plasma cells.
   c. increased osteoclast activity.
   d. hyperviscosity.

6. Plasmapheresis is a possible treatment for:
   a. Waldenstrom's macroglobulinemia.
   b. HCL.
   c. PCL.
   d. CLL.

7. Patients with Waldenstrom's macroglobulinemia frequently encounter thrombotic complications due to:
   a. increased platelet count.
   b. increased megakaryocytes in the bone marrow.
   c. increased plasma cells.
   d. coating of platelets and clotting by increased IgM.

○ TROUBLESHOOTING

What Do I Do When the Hematology Analyzer Fails to Report a Differential Count?

An 82-year-old man came through the emergency department with altered mental status. His initial WBC through the hematology analyzer was 31.3 × 10⁹/L, but the instrument voted out the differential and gave a platelet clump warning message. The technologist proceeded with several corrective actions as she was beginning to doubt the reported white count. She took the following steps:

- She physically checked the specimen for clots; there were none.
- She vortexed the sample, because according to the SOP at this hospital this was the optimal method when the platelet clumping flag appeared and there were no visible clots.

The CBC was repeated, and the WBC increased to 39.1 × 10⁹/L and the platelet count was 178.0 × 10⁹/L. The technologist decided to hold the CBC for further study and proceeded to make a differential. When she observed the differential, the white cell count appeared

much lower, no platelet clumps were observed, but strange, foamy purple blobs were observed. While canvassing the laboratory for other specimens, the technologist noticed that the centrifuged coagulation samples on the same patient contained a 2-cm layer of what appeared to be lipemia but the rest of the plasma was clear. This is not the typical picture of lipemia. The technologist knew that something was wrong with the plasma, but she could not pinpoint the problem. At this point, the technologist cancelled the CBC and coagulation tests and called the emergency department to inform them of this action and inquire about the patient. Additional patient samples were also requested. The technologist was informed that the patient had Waldenstrom's macroglobulinemia. The samples were redrawn and run through the hematology analyzer again with a WBC of 12.1 × 10⁹/L. The instrument again gave messages such as platelet clumps and interfering substances. A slide examination was performed, and again the white cell estimate appeared lower than the instrument-reported WBC. As a last step, the technologist performed a *manual* white count and platelet

(continued on following page)

● TROUBLESHOOTING *(continued)*

count. The manual white count and platelet count were 5.6×10^9/L and 166.0×10^9/L, respectively. The technologist left a message for future shifts that a **manual** white count and platelet would be necessary for this patient. This case offers an insight into the level of interference possible with the increased IgM globulin in patients with Waldenstrom's macroglobulinemia. Because the level of IgM monoclonal antibody is so elevated (paraprotein), it is seen as an interfering substance with significant consequences to the white count and differential primarily. Many hours of investigation and trying alternatives were spent in obtaining results on this patient. An observant technologist combined with reliable information from the family eventually led to actions that would contribute to the credibility of the patient's hematology samples. The next day, the patient underwent plasmapheresis and the CBC was run through the instrument with no interferences.

WORD KEY

Autoimmune hemolytic anemia • Process by which cells fail to recognize self and consequently make antibodies that destroy selected red cells

Direct antiglobulin test • Laboratory test for the presence of complement or antibodies bound to a patient's red blood cells

Erythroderma • Abnormal widespread redness and scaling of the skin, sometimes involving the entire body

Monosomy • Condition of having only one of a pair of chromosomes, as in Turner's syndrome, where there is only one X chromosome instead of two

Pathognomonic • Indicative of the disease

Raynaud's phenomenon • Intermittent attacks of pallor or cyanosis of the small arteries and arterioles of the fingers as a result of inadequate arterial blood supply

Plasmapheresis • Plasma exchange therapy, involving the removal of plasma from the cellular material that is then returned to the patient

Rouleaux • Group of red cells stuck together that look like a stack of coins

Translocations • Alteration of a chromosome through the transfer of a portion of it either to another chromosome or to another portion of the same chromosome

References

1. Cutler S J, Axtell L, Hesiett H. Ten thousand cases of leukemia 1940-62. J Natl Cancer Inst 39:993, 1967.
2. Dohner H, Stilgenbauer S, Beuner A, et al. Genomic aberrations and survival in chronic lymphocytic leukemia. N Engl J Med 343:1910–1916, 2000.
3. Redaelli A, Laskin BL, Stephens JM, et al. The clinical and epidemiological burden of chronic lymphocytic leukemia. Eur J Cancer Care 13:279–287, 2004.
4. McConkey DJ, et al. Apoptosis sensitivity in chronic lymphocytic leukemia is determined by endogenous endonuclease content and related expression of BCL-2 and BAX. J Immunol 156:2624, 1996.
5. Holmer LD, Hamoudi W, Bueso-Ramos CD. Chronic leukemia and related lymphomproliferative disorders. In: Harmening D, ed. Clinical Hematology and Fundamentals of Hemostasis, 4th ed. Philadelphia: FA Davis, 2002: 303.
6. McFarland JT, Kuzma C, Millard FE, et al. Palliative irradiation of the spleen. Am J Clin Oncol 25:178–183, 2003.
7. Rosenwald A, Chuang EY, Dabis RE, et al. Fludarabine treatment of patients with CLL induces a p53-dependent gene expression response. Blood 104: 1428–1434, 2004.
8. Bradford C. Cytochemistry. In: Rodak B, ed. Hematology: Clinical Principles and Applications, 2nd ed. Philadelphia: WB Saunders, 2002: 391.
9. Jenn U, Bartl R, Dietzfelbinger H, et al. An update: 12 Year follow-up of patients with hairy cell leukemia following treatment with 2-chlorodeoxyadenosine. Leukemia 18:1476–1481, 2004.
10. Turgeon ML. Malignant lymphoid and monocytic disorders and plasma cell dyscrasias. In Turgeon ML, ed. Clinical Hematology: Theory and Principles, 4th ed. Baltimore: Lippincott Williams & Wilkins, 2005: 287.
11. Manner C. The lymphomas. In Steine-Martin EA, Lotspeich-Steininger CA, Keopke J, eds. Clinical Hematology: Principles, Procedures, Correlations, 2nd ed. Baltimore: Lippincott Williams & Wilkins, 1998: 490–497.
12. Bergsagel DE, Wong O, Bergsagel PL, et al. Benzene and multiple myeloma: Appraisal of the scientific evidence. Cancer Invest 18:467, 2000.
13. Dewald GW, Kayle RA, Hicks GA, et al. The clinical significance of cytogenetic studies in 100 patients with MM, plasma cell leukemia or amyloidosis. Blood 66:380–390, 1985.
14. Shaughnessy J, Jacobsin J, Sawyer J, et al. Continuous absence of metaphase-defined cytogenetic abnormalities, especially of chromosome 13 and hypodiploidy, ensures long-term survival in multiple myeloma treated with Total Therapy I: Interpretation in the context of global gene expression. Blood 101:3849–3854, 2003.
15. Multiple myeloma. Available at http://www.mayoclinic.com/health/multiple-myeloma/DS00415 from the Mayo Clinic. Accessed September 25, 2006.

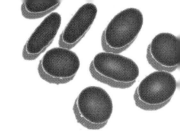

14

The Myelodysplastic Syndromes

Betty Ciesla

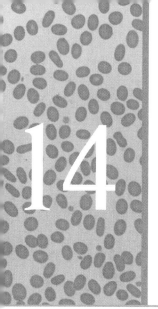

Pathophysiology

Chromosomal Abnormalities

Common Features and Clinical Symptoms
  How to Recognize Dysplasia

Classification of the Myelodysplastic Syndromes
  Specific Features of the World Health Organization
    Classification

Prognostic Factors and Clinical Management

Objectives

After completing this chapter, the student will be able to:

1. Define the *myelodysplastic syndromes* (MDSs).

2. Outline the possible causes of the MDSs.

3. Discuss the major cellular morphological abnormalities associated with MDSs.

4. Classify MDSs according to the World Health Organization.

5. List the disease indicators that contributed to prognosis of the MDSs.

6. Discuss the management of the MDSs.

The myelodysplastic syndromes (MDSs) are a group of hematology disorders that have eluded a firm designation for many decades. These disorders have been known by several other names, including preleukemia, dysmyelopoietic syndrome, oligoblastic leukemia, and the refractory anemias. In the past 20 years, considerable information has developed concerning the hematology of these disorders, the molecular biology, and the treatment protocols for patients with an MDS. What began as a group of cases with vague symptoms and morphology has become a recognized entity complete with classification and well-defined characteristics. Presently, 1 in 500 individuals over the age of 60 have an MDS, and it represents the most common hematological malignancy in this age group.[1]

PATHOPHYSIOLOGY

The MDSs are a clonal stem cell disorder, resulting from a lesion in the stem cell that leads to the formation of an abnormal clone of cells, a neoplasm. There are two types of MDS: de novo (new cases unrelated to any other treatment) and secondary cases related to prior therapy, usually **alkylating** therapy or radiation. Certain populations are at risk for MDS: those individuals exposed to benzene, radiation petrochemical employees, cigarette smokers, and patients with Fanconi's anemia.[2] Secondary cases are often seen following immunosuppressive therapy, and the transformation to MDS may occur within 2 to 5 years after the agent or agents have been administered.[3] From 30% to 40% of all MDS cases end in an acute leukemia.[4]

CHROMOSOMAL ABNORMALITIES

Chromosomal abnormalities play a large role in patients from both classifications of MDS. Typically, patients will exhibit partial or complete absence of chromosomes 5 and 7 and trisomy in chromosome 8. Other abnormalities may include a deletion of 17p or 20q and loss of the Y chromosome. Ninety percent of therapy-related MDS patients show some abnormality, whereas only 40% to 70% of patients with primary cases show chromosomal abnormalities.[5]

COMMON FEATURES AND CLINICAL SYMPTOMS

Key features that almost all MDS patients share are a macrocytic anemia that is **refractory**, cytopenias of one or more cell lines, and a hypercellular marrow. **Organomegaly** is not a frequent finding. The symptoms that patients experience—weakness, infection, and easy bruisability—are all explained from the perspective of the clonal abnormality, depending on which cell line is the most affected. The following is a likely sequence of events:

• Weakness develops from the anemia and shortened red cell survival.
• Infections develop due to white blood cells with poor microbicidal activity and decreased chemotaxis.
• Bruising develops due to lower numbers and abnormally functioning platelets.

In general, a diagnosis of MDS is made based on the percentage of blasts present, the type of dysplasia seen in the marrow and the peripheral smear, and the presence or absence of ringed sideroblasts (see Chapter 5). Classification into one of the six subtypes of MDS is made once all of the information from marrow, peripheral smear, cytogenetic studies, and immunological features is gathered.

How to Recognize Dysplasia

Dysplasia in the bone marrow and peripheral smear are hallmark features of the MDSs. Therefore, it is essential that the morphologist have an understanding of what is meant by this term with respect to variations in each cell line. Well-stained and well-distributed peripheral smears and bone marrow preparations are an essential ingredient to determining if dysplasia is present in the individual. Their importance cannot be underestimated. By definition, *dysplasia* means "abnormal development of tissue." In the bone marrow, this may manifest itself in the nuclear and cytoplasmic characteristics of precursor cells. Bone marrow nuclear changes may include multinuclearity, disintegration of the nucleus, asynchrony similar to megaloblastic changes, and nuclear bridging between cells. Bone marrow cytoplasmic changes include vacuolization or poor granulation. In the peripheral smear, similar changes may be seen like hypogranulated cells (Fig. 14.1), hypergranulated cells, hyposegmented cells, nuclear material that is too smooth, pseudo–Pelger-Huët cells, and red cell size changes (Fig. 14.2). Platelet abnormalities in the peripheral smear include abnormal size (Fig. 14.3), or megakaryocytic fragments. Degenerating neutrophils may also be seen (Fig 14.4). What usually comes to mind when these peripheral smear changes are first observed are technical factors like a poorly stained smear or a poorly made smear. The morphologist may not exercise the index of suspicion, feeling that what is

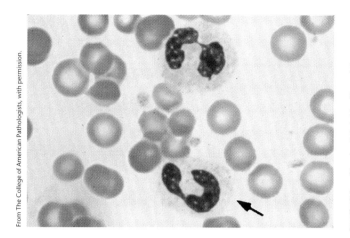

Figure 14.1   Hypogranular band.

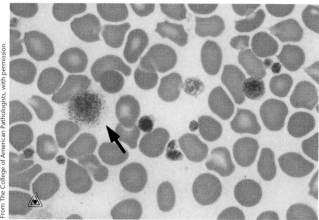

Figure 14.3   Giant platelet.

observed is **not** hematologically relevant. Yet when 10%[6] of a particular cell line starts manifesting any of the changes noted, the change is significant and due to a pathology (Table 14.1).

CLASSIFICATION OF THE MYELODYSPLASTIC SYNDROMES

The French-American-British (FAB) investigative group devised a working classification for the MDSs in 1981 based on a study of 50 cases.[7] This classification was groundbreaking work and presented the first formal body of knowledge on this group of disorders.In 1997, the World Health Organization (WHO) revised this work and presented their classification of the MDSs based on the additional knowledge gained from molecular, immunological, and cytogenetic studies. Although both classifications will be presented, only the WHO classification will be elaborated on[6] (Table 14.2).

Specific Features of the World Health Organization Classification

Refractory anemia (RA) is primarily a disorder of red cells, with an anemia resistant to treatment. Less than 1% myeloblasts in the peripheral blood and less than 5% myeloblasts are seen in the bone marrow. The marrow shows hyperplasia with megaloblastoid features, such as multinuclearity, etc.

Refractory anemia with ringed sideroblasts (RARS) is a refractory anemia in which 15% or more of red cell precursors are ringed sideroblasts (Fig. 14.5). The bone marrow shows erythroid hyperplasia and less than 5% myeloblasts, and the liver and spleen may show changes related to iron overload.

Refractory anemia with multilineage dysplasia shows bone marrow failure with two or more myeloid cell lines affected. Fifty percent of patients are

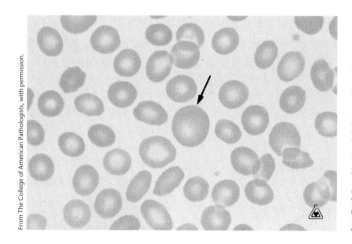

Figure 14.2   Macrocytic red cell.

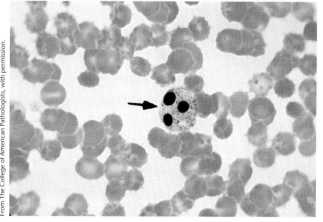

Figure 14.4   Degenerating neutrophil.

Table 14.1 ⊙ Dysplastic Changes in MDS

Dysplastic changes of the red cell—Dyserythropoiesis
- Nuclear budding
- Ringed sideroblasts
- Internuclear bridging
- Dimorphism
- Megaloblastoid asynchrony
- Multinuclearity

Dysplastic changes of the white cell—Dysgranu-lopoiesis
- Abnormal staining throughout the cytoplasm
- Hyposegmentation
- Hypersegmentation
- Nucleus with little segmentation
- Missing primary granules
- Granules that are poorly stained

Dysplastic changes of platelets—Dysthrombopoiesis
- Micromegakaryocytes
- Abnormal granules
- Giant platelets

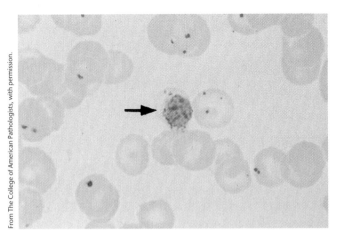

From The College of American Pathologists, with permission.

Figure 14.5 Ringed sideroblast.

affected with multiple chromosomal abnormalities, showing marked erythroid hyperplasia with nuclear and cytoplasmic dysplastic changes. There are less than 1% blasts in peripheral blood.

Refractory anemia with excess blasts (RAEB) shows anemia, thrombocytopenia, and neutropenia.

Table 14.2 ⊙ The FAB and WHO Classifications of Myelodysplastic Syndromes

The FAB Classification	The WHO Classification
Refractory anemia	Refractory anemia
Refractory anemia with ringed sideroblasts	Refractory anemia with ringed sideroblasts
Refractory anemia with excess blasts	Refractory cytopenia with multilineage dysplasia
Chronic myelomono-cytic leukemia	
Refractory anemia with excess blasts in transformation	Refractory anemia with excess blasts
	Myelodysplastic syndrome unclassifiable
	5(q) chromosome abnormality

There are abnormalities in all myeloid cell lines with 5% to 19% blasts in the bone marrow. Two subclasses are recognized: RAEB 1, which shows 5% to 10% blasts in bone marrow, less than 5% blasts in the peripheral blood, and RAEB 2, which shows 10% to 19% blasts in the bone marrow and less than 20% blasts in the peripheral blood, hypercellular marrow in most cases.

Myelodysplastic syndrome unclassifiable is a condition that shares features of the MDSs but not a clearcut classification. Neutropenia and thrombocytopenia are common.

Deleted 5q is seen in female patients primarily as a deletion of the long arm of chromosome 5. Normal or elevated platelet counts are seen. There is a marked anemia with macrocytes and less than 5% blasts in peripheral blood, associated with long survival times.

PROGNOSTIC FACTORS AND CLINICAL MANAGEMENT

Progression to an acute leukemia is always a concern for patients with an MDS. Low-grade disorders like RA or RARS have longer survival times and less tendency to develop into overt acute leukemias. These disorders are also unilineage. Disorders, however, like RAEB and the multilineage disorders are high grade with much shorter survival times and a greater incidence to progress to acute leukemia. Other factors such as multiple cytogenetic abnormalities, especially chromosome 7 abnormalities, have an unfavorable predictive influence (Table 14.3). Treatment of the MDS is difficult to manage. Issues such as quality of life, severe thrombocytopenia, and progression to more advanced disease are serious concerns. Patients with MDSs are classified into low- or high-risk categories based on their initial WHO

Table 14.3 ● Factors Indicating Progression to Leukemia in MDS

- Disease is stable if there is little increase in marrow blast count and the original karyotype is unchanged.
- Progressive rise in blast count usually indicates transition to acute leukemia.
- Sudden change in karyotype that may progress into acute leukemia.
- Abnormal karyotype develops without subsequent increase in blasts; acute leukemia may or may not develop.

Adapted from Bick RL, Laughlin WR. Myelodysplastic syndromes. Lab Med 11:712–716, 1993.

designation. Treatment protocols tailored to these designations range from transfusional support to erythropoietin (EPO) and G-CSF (granulocyte-colony stimulating factor), induction chemotherapy, and allogeneic stem cell transplant. Although stem cell transplants offer a potential cure, the morbidity and mortality associated with this procedure must be seriously considered.[8] Even in patients with allogeneic transplants there has only been a 30% to 50% long-term disease control.[9] Most patients are given supportive treatment such as red cells, antibiotics, or vitamins. The difficulty with this management is that the anemias are refractory, necessitating more transfusions, which may lead to iron overload. Iron chelating agents may be used but are more successful in younger patients. Recall that individuals with iron overload are usually attached to an iron chelating pump, which works to clear their blood of excess iron while they sleep. Generally, younger patients are more compliant than older individuals and are better able to cope with the constancy of this procedure. Oral iron chelators such as deferiprone and IL 670 will likely improve iron chelation therapy in this patient group.[10] Patients with cardiopulmonary complications due to progressive anemia must be handled carefully. EPO and G-CSF are important supplementary agents, and they are effective short-term measures during difficult episodes of cytopenias.[11] Several immunobiologic therapies are being considered in clinical trials such as anti-thymocyte globulin, anti-CD33 antibody, idarubicin, and fludarabine.[12] Additionally, a group of therapies known as anti**angiogenic** therapies are on the horizon. These agents direct their activities against microenvironmental factors such as vascular endothelial growth factor (VEGF) and tumor necrosis factor. It is thought that the increased production of these inflammatory factors amplify ineffective hematopoiesis, fuel the growth of certain premalignant or malignant cells, and suppress normal hematopoietic progenitor cells. Thalidomide (lenalidomide) and arsenic trioxide have both been studied.[13] Therapies for MDS will no doubt improve as the disease mechanisms become more clearly defined.

CONDENSED CASE

A 65-year-old recent retiree went to visit the nurse practitioner in her assisted living community. She complained of excessive fatigue, rapid heart rate, and bruising. A CBC and differential was performed and the results suggested a macrocytic anemia with a slightly decreased platelet count. No hypersegmented neutrophils were seen and no oval macrocytes were observed on the peripheral smear. **What other testing is worth considering in this case?**

Answer
Other causes for a nonmegaloblastic macrocytic anemia may be liver disease, reticulocytosis, or hypothyroid conditions. Each of these was ruled out on our patient, and she was referred for a hematology consult. A bone marrow and cytogenetic studies were ordered. The bone marrow showed a hypercellular marrow with slightly increased and dysplastic megakaryocytes. Cytogenetic studies show a deleted 5q. This patient progressed well with transfusion support and as of this date has not shown a progression to acute leukemia.

Summary Points

- The myelodysplastic disorders (MDSs) are a group of clonal disorders characterized by refractory anemias and cytopenias of one or more cell lines.

- The bone marrow and peripheral smear will show dysplastic changes in white cells, red cells, and platelets over time.
- Dyserythropoietic changes include multinuclear red cell precursors, bizarre nuclear

changes, nuclear bridging, macrocytes, and dimorphism.

- Dysgranulopoietic changes include abnormal granulation of mature cells, hypersegmentation, hyposegmentation, or complete lack of granulation.
- Dysthrombopoietic changes include micro-

megakaryocytes, abnormal granulation, no granulation, and giant platelets.

- The blast count in the MDS is less than 20%.
- Weakness, infections, and easy bruising are some of the symptoms that patients with MDS may manifest.
- According to the World Health Organization, there are six classifications of MDSs.

CASE STUDY

A 78-year-old man was referred to a hematology consult after complications from a total knee operation. After this surgery, the patient experienced bleeding from the operative site that was unexpected. His routine coagulation tests were normal at the time of preoperative review. No organomegaly was noted, and no petechiae were observed. Within 4 weeks, he was readmitted for wound oozing. His CBC and differential on the day of consult are as follows:

WBC	2.3×10^9/L	Segmented neutrophils 3%
RBC	3.14×10^{12}/L	Bands 4%
Hgb	10.8 g/dL	Metamyelocytes 2%
Hct	31%	Myelocytes 3%
MCV	81 fL	Lymphocytes 60%
MCH	26 pg	Monocytes 7%
MCHC	32 g/dL	Eosinophils 3%
Platelets	15.0×10^9/L	Blasts 18%

Based upon the patient's age, clinical presentation, CBC, and differential results, what are some of the diagnostic possibilities?

Insights to the Case Study

The CBC on this patient indicates a low platelet count combined with normocytic, normochromic anemia and differential indicating a left shift. The differential showed a fairly large number of blasts but not enough blasts to be called an overt acute leukemia (for acute leukemia, 20% or more blasts). A bone marrow was requested on this patient, but the hematologist was cautious given the low platelet count and decided to delay this procedure until the platelet count normalized. The patient was given platelets to boost his platelet count and was started on prophylactic antibiotics because his white count was depressed. A preliminary diagnosis of refractory anemia with excess blasts was made pending the bone marrow and cytogenetic studies.

Review Questions

1. Which one of the following is the predominant red cell morphology in patients with MDS?
   a. Schistocytes
   b. Macrocytes
   c. Target cells
   d. Bite cells

2. Which one of the MDS groups has the best prognosis?
   a. MDS with excess blasts
   b. Refractory anemia with ringed sideroblasts
   c. Refractory anemia
   d. 5q deletion

3. What is considered a significant number of ringed sideroblasts in the MDS classification?
   a. 15%
   b. 5%

   c. 10%
   d. 20%

4. Which mechanism accounts for the reticulocytopenia seen in most cases of MDS?
   a. Heavy blast tumor burden in the marrow
   b. Effects of toxins
   c. Marrow aplasia
   d. Ineffective erythropoiesis

5. What is the cutoff blast count used to distinguish a patient with MDS as opposed to a patient with acute leukemia?
   a. 50%
   b. 30%
   c. 20%
   d. 15%

○ TROUBLESHOOTING

What Influence Does the Patient's History Have on an Increased MCHC?

A patient had presented to the laboratory for 3 consecutive days with variability in his MCH and MCHC. At times his MCHC rose to 39%, prompting an investigation of this increased parameter. Cold agglutinins, lipemia, and spherocytes are each reasons why the MCHC might be elevated. Each of these was eliminated as a reason for the fluctuating MCHC. On day 4, the patient had another CBC, which again presented with an elevated MCHC.

WBC	16.9×10^9/L
RBC	2.71×10^{12}/L
Hgb	9.0 g/dL
Hct	22.9%
MCV	84.2 fL
MCH	33.2 pg
MCHC	39.3% H
Platelets	52×10^9/L
RDW	15.4

The technologist reviewed the previous results with the comments presented and decided that the patient's history might hold some clues to these variant results. It was noted that the Hgb and Hct had failed the correlation check (Hgb (3 = Hct ± 2). The technologist discovered that the patient had MDS. MDS has an unknown etiology but may *falsely increase the Hgb*,[14] thus elevating the indices (MCH and MCHC). With this in mind, the technologist decided to apply the laboratory procedure for correcting Hgb values that eliminates tedious manual procedures such as centrifugation, plasma blanks, and pipetting. The Hgb concentration is calculated with the following equation, which indicates that there is a ratio between the MCV and MCHC of 2.98[14]:

$$Hb \text{ (g/L)} = MCV \times RBC/2.98 \times 10 \text{ (29.8)}$$

Therefore, the corrected Hgb/L =

$$(84.2 \times 2.71)/29.8 = 7.7 \text{ g/L}$$

This calculation corrects the Hgb. As a result of this new value, the MCH and MCHC can be corrected with the new Hgb result.

The CBC now reports as

WBC	16.9×10^9/L
RBC	2.71×10^{12}/L
Hgb	7.7* corrected result
Hct	22.9%
MCV	84.2 fL
MCH	28.4 pg* recalculated result
MCHC	33.4%* recalculated result
Platelets	52×10^9/L
RDW	15.4

MDS is a classification of malignant clonal disorders that show cytopenias, dysplastic-looking cells in the peripheral smear, increasing numbers of blasts in the bone marrow, and a tendency to progress into a leukemic process. This case indicates a corrective action that is not often used but appropriate when all other causes of hemoglobin abnormality have been eliminated.

WORD KEY

Alkylating agent • Agent that introduced an alkyl radical into the compound in place of a hydrogen atom; these agents interfere with cell metabolism and growth

Angiogenesis • Development of blood vessels

Organomegaly • Enlargement of any organ

Refractory • Resistant to ordinary treatment

References

1. Hoffman WK, Ottmann OG, Ganser F, et al. Myelopdysplastic syndrome: Clinical features. Semin Hematol 33:177–178, 1996.
2. Willman CL. The biologic basis of myelodysplasia and related leukemias: Cellular and molecular mechanisms. Mod Pathol 12:101–106, 1999.
3. Kjeldsberg CR, ed. Practical Diagnosis of Hematologic Disorders, 3rd ed. Chicago: ASCP Press, 2000: 369–397.
4. Bick RL, Laughlin WR. Myelodysplastic syndromes. Lab Med 11:712–716, 1993.
5. West RR, Stafford DA, White AD, et al. Cytogenetic abnormalities in the myelodysplastic syndromes and occupational and environmental exposure. Blood 95:2093–2097, 2000.
6. Jaffe ES, Harris NL, Stein H, Vardiman JE, eds. World Health Organization Classification of Tumours. Pathology and Genetics of Tumours of Hematopoietic and Lymphoid Tissues. Lyon: IARC Press, 2001: 63–73.
7. Bennett HJM, Catovsky D, Daniel MT, et al. Proposals for the classification of the myelodysplastic syndromes. Br J Haematol 51:189–199, 1982.
8. Hellstrom-Lindberg E. Update on supportive care and new therapies: Immunomodulatory drugs, growth

factors and epigenetic acting agents. Hematology (Am Soc Hematol Educ Prog) 165, 2005.

9. Giralt S. Bone marrow transplant in myelodysplastic syndromes: New technologies, some questions. Curr Hematol Rep 3:165–172, 2004.

10. Hoffbrand VA. Deferiprone therapy for transfusional iron overload. Best Pract Res Clin Haematol 18: 299–317, 2005.

11. Negrin RS, et al. Maintenance treatment of patients with myelodysplastic syndromes using recombinant human granulocyte colony stimulating factor. Blood 78:36, 1992.

12. Appelbaum FR. Immunobiologic therapies for myelodysplastic syndromes. Best Pract Res Clinc Haematol 4:653–661, 2004.

13. Williams JL. The myelodysplastic syndromes and myeloproliferative disorders. Clin Lab Sci 17:227, 2004.

14. Kalache GR, Sartor MM, Hughes WG. The indirect estimation of hemoglobin concentration in whole blood. Pathologist 23:117, 1991.

Part IV

Hemostasis and Disorders of Coagulation

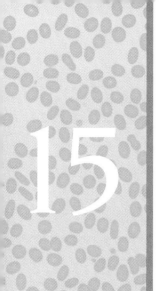
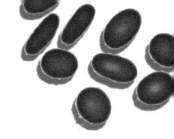

15 Overview of Hemostasis and Platelet Physiology

Donna Castellone

History of Blood Coagulation

Overview of Coagulation

Vascular System
Overview
Mechanism of Vasoconstriction
The Endothelium
Events Following Vascular Injury

Primary Hemostasis
Platelets: An Introduction
Platelet Development
Platelet Structure and Biochemistry
Platelet Function and Kinetics
Platelet Aggregation Principle

Secondary Hemostasis
Classification of Coagulation Factors
Physiological Coagulation (In Vivo)
Laboratory Model of Coagulation
Extrinsic Pathway
Intrinsic System
Activated Partial Thromboplastin Time
Common Pathway
Formation of Thrombin
Feedback Inhibition
Fibrinolysis
Coagulation Inhibitors
Kinin System
Complement System

Objectives

After completing this chapter, the student will be able to:

1. Describe the systems involved in hemostasis.

2. Describe the interaction of the vascular system and platelets with regard to activation, adhesion, and vasoconstriction.

3. Identify the process involved in the coagulation cascade from activation to stable clot formation.

4. Describe the role of platelets in hemostasis with respect to platelet glycoproteins, platelet biochemistry, and platelet function.

5. Define the difference between primary and secondary hemostasis.

6. Outline the intrinsic and extrinsic pathways, the factors involved in each, and their role in the coagulation system.

7. List the coagulation factors, their common names, and function.

8. Explain the interaction between the prothrombin time, activated partial thromboplastin time, and factor assays.

9. Identify the relationship of the kinin and complement systems to coagulation.

10. Identify the inhibitors and their role in hemostasis.

HISTORY OF BLOOD COAGULATION

The study of blood coagulation can be traced back to about 400 BC and the father of medicine, Hippocrates. He observed that the blood of a wounded soldier congealed as it cooled. Additionally, he noticed that bleeding from a small wound stopped as skin covered the blood. If the skin was removed, bleeding started again. Aristotle noted that blood cooled when removed from the body and that cooled blood initiated decay resulting in the congealing of the blood. If fibers were removed, there was no clotting. This was known as the cooling theory or blood coagulation. It was not until 1627 that Mercurialis observed clots in veins that were at body temperature. In 1770, William Hewson challenged the cooling theory and believed that air and lack of motion were important in the initiation of clotting. Hewson described the clotting process, demonstrating that the clot comes from the liquid portion of blood, the coagulable lymph, and not from the cells, disproving the cooling theory. It was Paul Morawitz in 1905 who assembled coagulation factors into the scheme of coagulation and demonstrated that in the presence of calcium and thromboplastin, prothrombin (II) was converted to thrombin, which in turn converted fibrinogen (I) into a fibrin clot. This theory persisted for 40 years until Paul Owren, in 1944, discovered a bleeding patient who defied the four-factor concept of clotting. Thus factor V was discovered. Owren also observed a cofactor that was involved in the conversion of prothrombin to thrombin. In 1952, Loeliger named this factor VII. Factor VIII was identified as classic hemophilia prior to the identification of VII in 1936/1937. In 1947, Pavlovsky reported that the blood from some hemophiliac patients corrected the abnormal clotting time in others. In 1952, this was called Christmas disease, after the family in which it was discovered, or factor IX. Factor X deficiency was described in 1957 in a woman named Prower and a man named Stuart. Factor XI was described in 1953 as a milder bleeding tendency. In 1955, Ratnoff and Colopy identified a patient, John Hageman, with a factor XII deficiency who died from a stroke—a thrombotic episode, not a bleeding disease. In 1960, Duckert described patients who had a bleeding disorder and characteristic delayed wound healing. This fibrin stabilizing factor was called factor XIII. Prekallikrein (1965) discovered from four siblings in the Fletcher family demonstrated no bleeding tendencies, as well as high-molecular-weight kininogen (1975). These were both identified as contact activation cofactors that participated in the activation of factor XI by factor XII.[1]

Testing of blood plasma factors and platelets depended on seeing the clotting process directly or microscopically. The first whole blood clotting time was done in 1780 by William Hewson, who noted that blood taken from healthy people clotted in 7 minutes while in some disease states, blood took from 15 to 20 minutes up to $1\frac{1}{2}$ hours to form a clot.

In 1897, Brodie and Russel begin observing the process on a glass slide. A drop of blood was placed on a glass cone, in a temperature-controlled glass chamber agitated by an air jet. Blood no longer moved microscopically but clotted in 3 minutes and was completed at 8 minutes. In 1905, Golhorm used a wire loop attached to a glass tube. In 1910, Kottman observed an increased **viscosity** in clotting blood in a Koaguloviskosimeter. Blood was rotated at 20 degrees 12 to 15 times per minute. In 1936, Baldes and Nygaard added photoelectric tracings called a coagelogram, depicting shape change by light transmittance.

In the 1960s, BBL introduced the Fibrometer. This instrument provided mechanical registration of clots that allowed more reproducible timing and an expression of the clotting process.[2]

OVERVIEW OF COAGULATION

Coagulation is a complex network of interactions involving vessels, platelets, and factors. The ability to form and to remove a clot is truly a system dependent on many synergistic forces. Hemostasis depends on a system of checks and balances between thrombosis and hemorrhage that includes both procoagulants and **anticoagulants.** This scale needs to be kept in balance. Thrombosis is an activation of the hemostatic system at an inappropriate time in a vessel. Thrombi formed in this fashion are pathologic and beyond the normal hemostatic mechanism. If physiological anticoagulants are decreased in the circulation there will be a clot. If procoagulants or clotting factors are decreased, the scale will tip toward bleeding. Hemorrhage or excessive bleeding may be due to blood vessel disease, rupture, platelet abnormalities, and acquired or congenital abnormalities. Hemostasis is comprised of the vascular system, platelets, and a series of enzymatic reactions of the coagulation factors. The role of hemostasis is to arrest bleeding from a vessel wall defect, while at the same time maintaining fluidity within circulation. Under physiological conditions, fluidity is maintained by the anticoagulant, profibrinolytic, and antiplatelet properties of the normal endothelium.[3]

Coagulation is divided into two major systems: the primary and secondary systems of hemostasis. The primary system comprises platelet function and **vasoconstriction.** The secondary system involves coagulation proteins and a series of enzymatic reactions. Once the coagulation proteins become involved, fibrin is formed and this reinforces platelet plug formation until healing is complete. The product of the coagulation cascade is the conversion of soluble fibrinogen into an insoluble fibrin clot. This is accomplished by the action of a powerful coagulant, thrombin. Thrombin is formed by a precursor circulating protein, prothrombin. Dissolution of the platelet plug is achieved by the fibrinolytic process.

VASCULAR SYSTEM

Overview

The vascular system prevents bleeding through vessel contraction, diversion of blood flow from damaged vessels, initiation of contact activation of platelets with aggregation, and contact activation of the coagulation system.[4] The vessel wall contains varying amounts of fibrous tissue such as collagen and elastin, as well as smooth muscle cells and fibroblasts. Arteries are the vessels that take blood away from the heart and have the thickest walls of the vascular system. Veins return blood to the heart, and are larger with a more irregular **lumen** than the arteries. Veins, however, are thin walled, with elastic fibers found only in larger veins. Arterioles are a smaller subdivision of arteries, and venules are smaller subdivisions of veins. Capillaries are the thinnest walled and most numerous of the blood vessels. They are composed of only one cell layer of endothelium that permits a rapid rate of transport materials between blood and tissue.[5]

Mechanism of Vasoconstriction

The process in which coagulation occurs begins with injury to a vessel. The first response of a cut vessel is vasoconstriction or narrowing of the lumen of the arterioles to minimize the flow of blood from the wound site. The blood is ordinarily exposed to only the endothelial cell lining of the vasculature. When this is invaded, the exposed deeper layers of the blood vessel become targets for cellular and plasma components. Vasoconstriction occurs immediately and lasts a short period of time. It allows for increased contact between the damaged vessel wall, blood platelets, and coagulation factors. Vasoconstriction is caused by several regulatory molecules including serotonin and thromboxane A_2, which interacts with receptors on the surface of cells of the blood vessel wall. These are products of platelet activation and endothelium. Endothelial cells lining the

lumen of the blood vessel are the principal elements regulating vascular functions. Physiologically, the surface of endothelial cells is negatively charged and repels circulating proteins and platelets, which are negatively charged.[6] Vasoconstriction occurs very quickly and is effective in stopping bleeding in small blood vessels but cannot prevent bleeding in larger vessels. Other systems are required for this task.

The Endothelium

The endothelium contains connective tissue such as collagen and elastin. This matrix regulates the permeability of the inner vessel wall and provides the principal stimuli to thrombosis following injury to a blood vessel. Circulating platelets recognize and bind to insoluble subendothelial connective tissue molecules. This process is dependent on molecules that are in plasma and on platelets. Two factors, von Willebrand (vWF) and fibrinogen, participate in the formation of the platelet plug and the insoluble protein clot, resulting in the activation of the coagulation proteins. Receptor molecules not only adhere to platelets and damaged vessel components but also allow platelets to use vWF and fibrinogen to bind platelets and form a plug. Blood flows out through the wall and comes in contact with collagen. Collagen is an insoluble fibrous protein that accounts for much of the body's connective tissue. Vessel injury leads to the stimulation of platelets. Platelets contain more of the contractile protein actomyosin than any cells, other than muscle cells, giving them the ability to contract. Basically platelets adhere to collagen and other platelets adhere to them. A plug is built and the platelets' ability to further contract compacts the mass.[7]

In forming the initial plug, platelets have now built a template on a lipoprotein surface, which in turn activates tissue factor. The balance between coagulation proteins and anticoagulants now leans toward coagulation. This process will accelerate vasoconstriction, platelet plug development, and the formation of cross-linked fibrin clot (Fig. 15.1).

Events Following Vascular Injury

1. Thromboresistant properties of a blood vessel maintain blood in a fluid state.
2. After vascular injury, subendothelial components of collagen induce platelet aggregation, which is mediated by vWF and platelet receptor glycoprotein Ib.
3. Further platelet recruitment occurs as a result from fibrinogen binding to its platelet receptor, glycoprotein IIb/IIIa.

INJURY TO VESSEL

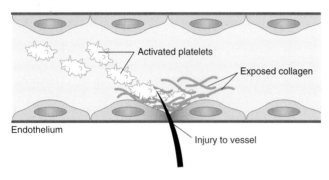

PLATELET RESPONSE

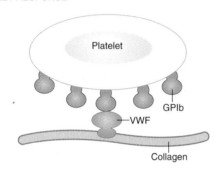

Figure 15.1   Platelet response to vascular injury.

4. Tissue factor generates thrombin, which results in cross-linked fibrin strands that reinforce the platelet plug.
5. Platelet actomyosin mediates clot retraction to compact the platelet mass.[8]

PRIMARY HEMOSTASIS

Platelets: An Introduction

Platelets were recognized in 1882 by Bizzozero as a cell structure different from red and white cells. However, it was not until 1970 that platelets' relationship to hemostasis and thrombosis became so important.[9] Every cubic millimeter of blood contains one-fourth of 1 billion platelets, resulting in approximately a trillion platelets in the blood of an average woman. Each platelet makes 14,000 trips through the bloodstream in its life span of 7 to 10 days.[7]

Platelet Development

Platelets, or thrombocytes, are small discoid cells (0.5 to 3.0 μm) that are synthesized in the bone marrow and stimulated by the hormone thrombopoietin. They are developed through a pluripotent stem cell that has been influenced by colony-stimulating factors (CSF) produced by macrophages, fibroblasts, T-lymphocytes, and stimulated endothelial cells. The parent cells of platelets

are called megakaryocytes (Fig. 15.2). These large cells (80 to 150 μm) are found in the bone marrow. Megakaryocytes do not undergo complete cellular division but undergo a process called endomitosis or endoreduplication creating a cell with a multilobed nucleus. Each megakaryocyte produces about 2000 platelets. Thrombopoietin is responsible for stimulating maturation and platelet release. This hormone is generated primarily by the kidney and partly by the spleen and liver.[10] There is no reserve of platelets in the bone marrow: 80% are in circulation and 20% are in the red pulp of the spleen. Platelets have no nucleus but do have granules: alpha granules, and dense granules. These granules are secreted during the platelet release reaction and contain many biochemically active components such as serotonin, ADP, and ATP. They are destroyed by the reticuloendothelial system (RE).

Platelet development occurs in the following sequence:

1. *Megakaryoblasts* are the most immature cell (10 to 15 μm) with a high nuclear to cytoplasmic ratio and two to six nucleoli.
2. *Promegakaryocyte* is a large cell of 80 μm with dense alpha and lysosomal granules.
3. *Basophilic megakaryocyte* shows evidence of cytoplasmic fragments containing membranes, cytotubules, and several glycoprotein receptors.
4. The *megakaryocyte* is composed of cytoplasmic fragments that are released by a process called the budding of platelets.

Platelet Structure and Biochemistry

Platelets have a complex structure comprised of four zones: the peripheral zone, the sol gel zone, the

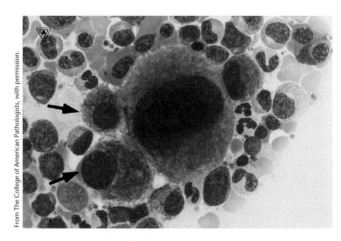

Figure 15.2   Megakaryocyte, the platelet parent cell.

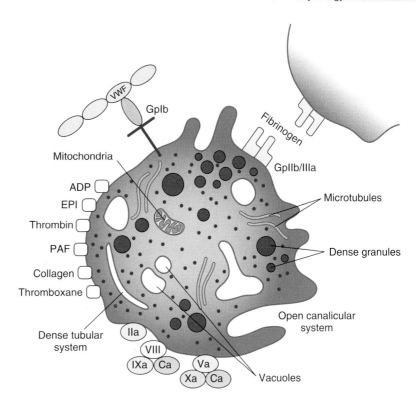

Figure 15.3   Schematic diagram of platelet morphology.

organelle zone, and the membrane system (Table 15.1). Figure 15.3 is a diagram of platelet morphology.

Platelet Function and Kinetics

Platelets play an important role in both the formation of a primary plug as well as the coagulation cascade. The formation of a plug at the site of a cut vessel serves as the initial mechanical barrier. The lumen of the vessel is lined with endothelial cells; a break in this will initiate a series of reactions.

There are four phases to platelet function:

- REACTION 1 (ADHESION): Platelets adhere to collagen and undergo shape change from disc to spiny spheres. Glycoprotein (GP) Ib and vWF aid in adhesion. This is primary aggregation and is reversible. This reaction is mediated by the release of platelet granules.
- REACTION 2 (AGGREGATION): In response to chemical changes, these events lead to platelet aggregation in which platelets adhere to other platelets. Platelet shape change occurs.
- REACTION 3 (RELEASE): Platelets release the contents of their dense granules. The release of these granules constitutes a secondary aggregation that is irreversible. Thromboxane A_2 is released by platelets, which promotes vasoconstriction. ADP amplifies the process.
- REACTION 4 (STABILIZATION OF THE CLOT): This reaction is responsible for thrombus formation. The adherent and aggregated platelets release factor V and expose platelet factor 3 to accelerate the coagulation cascade and promote activation of clotting factors and ultimately stabilize the platelet plug with a fibrin clot.

The platelet membrane contains important receptors called GPs on the platelet surface. Further interactions are mediated by both plasma protein receptors of vWF and fibrinogen. Other activators of platelets are thrombin, ADP, thromboxane A_2, serotonin, epinephrine, and arachidonic acid.

Table 15.1 ● The Four Functional Platelet Zones
1. The peripheral zone is associated with platelet adhesion and aggregation.
2. The sol gel zone provides a cytoskeletal system for platelets and contact when the platelets are stimulated.
3. The organelle zone contains three types of granules: alpha, dense bodies, and lysosomes.
4. The membrane system contains a dense tubular system in which the enzymatic system for the production of prostaglandin synthesis is found.

The receptor for vWF is GPIb-IX. GPIIb/IIIa are receptors for **fibronectin,** vWF, fibrinogen, and factors V and VIII. This interaction recruits more platelets to interact with each other.[11] Adhesion of platelets to collagen and each other can occur without contraction or shape change. Contraction causes shape change into a spiny sphere. Exposure of a negatively charged membrane leads to secretion of granular contents. These activated platelets release ADP and synthesized thromboxane A_2, which mediate activation of additional platelets, resulting in the formation of a platelet plug.[12]

Platelet Aggregation Principle

Aggregation defines the ability of platelets to stick to one another. The formation of aggregates is observed with a platelet aggregometer. This is a photo-optical instrument connected to a chart recorder. Light transmittance through the sample is increased and converted into electronic signals, which are amplified and recorded. A characteristic curve is formed with each aggregating agent. Primary aggregation is the first wave of aggregation and is preceded by a shape change except when platelets are stimulated with epinephrine (Fig. 15.4). Primary aggregation is a reversible process. The second phase of platelet aggregation occurs when platelet granule contents are secreted. Secondary aggregation is irreversible. Epinephrine, collagen, ADP, and arachidonic acid are the aggregating agents most frequently used in clinical platelet aggregation.

1. *Epinephrine* (EPI): When added to platelet rich plasma (PRP), it will stimulate platelets to aggregate. Normal platelets will respond by releasing endogenous ADP from their granules. Both primary and secondary aggregation is seen. An abnormal response is due to an absent or decreased release of nucleotides from dense granules.

2. *Adenosine diphosphate* (ADP): When added to PRP, it will stimulate platelets to change their shape and aggregate. Aggregation is induced by exogenous ADP at a high dose of 20 μmol/L. The primary and secondary wave aggregations are indistinguishable. Reversible aggregation may occur due to an inadequate

Platelet Aggregation Tracings

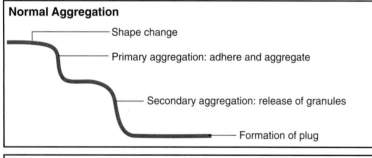

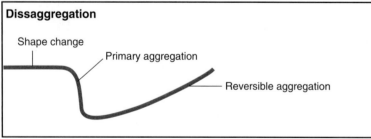

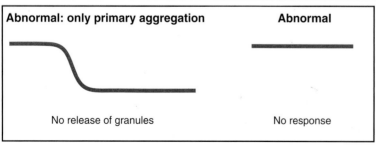

Figure 15.4 Platelet aggregation. Note the stages of aggregation, which include primary and secondary aggregation as well as shape change and plug formation.

release of nucleotides. Lack of a secondary wave is indicative of defective thromboxane production and/or a defective granule pool.

3. *Collagen:* When added to PRP, the platelets adhere to the collagen, followed by shape change, release of endogenous ADP, and then aggregation. An abnormal response to collagen may be seen if thromboxane production is deficient. Aggregation is slower and less complex, resulting in a decreased response.

4. *Arachidonic acid* (AA): This is a fatty acid present in membranes of human platelets and liberated from phospholipids. In the presence of the enzyme cyclooxygenase, oxygen is incorporated to form the endoperoxide prostaglandin G_2 (PGG_2). PGG_2 is then converted to thromboxane A_2, a potent inducer of platelet aggregation.

SECONDARY HEMOSTASIS

Secondary hemostasis involves a series of blood protein reactions through a cascade-like process that concludes with the formation of an insoluble fibrin clot. This system involves multiple enzymes and several cofactors as well as inhibitors to keep the system in balance. Coagulation factors are produced in the liver, except for factor VIII, which is believed to be produced in the endothelial cells. When the factors are in a precursor form, the enzyme or zymogen is converted to an active enzyme or a protease.

The initiation of clotting begins with the activation of two enzymatic pathways that will ultimately lead to fibrin formation: the intrinsic and extrinsic pathways. Both pathways are necessary for fibrin formation, but their activating factors are different. Intrinsic activation occurs by trauma within the vascular system, such as exposed endothelium. This system is slower and yet more important versus the extrinsic pathway, which is initiated by an external trauma, such as a clot and occurs quickly.

Classification of Coagulation Factors

Coagulation factors may be categorized into substrates, cofactors, and enzymes. Substrates are the substance upon which enzymes act. Fibrinogen is the main substrate. Cofactors accelerate the activities of the enzymes that are involved in the cascade. Cofactors include tissue factor, factor V, factor VIII, and Fitzgerald factor. All of the enzymes are serine proteases except factor XIII, which is a **transaminase**.[13]

There are three groups in which coagulation factors can be classified:

1. The *fibrinogen* group consists of factors I, V, VIII, and XIII. They are consumed during coagulation. Factors V and VIII are labile and will increase during pregnancy and inflammation.

2. The *prothrombin* group: Factors II, VII, IX, and X all are dependent on vitamin K during their synthesis. This group is stable and remains preserved in stored plasma.

3. The *contact* group: Factor XI, factor XII, prekallikrein, and high-molecular-weight kininogen (HMWK) are involved in the intrinsic pathway, moderately stable, and not consumed during coagulation.[5]

The coagulation factors and their actions are listed in (Table 15.2).

Factor I, Fibrinogen

Substrate for thrombin and precursor of fibrin, it is a large globulin protein. Its function is to be converted into an insoluble protein and then back to soluble components. When exposed to thrombin, two peptides split from the fibrinogen molecule, leaving a fibrin monomer to form a **polymerized** clot.

Factor II, Prothrombin

Precursor to thrombin, in the presence of Ca^{2+}, it is converted to thrombin (IIa), which in turn stimulates platelet aggregation and activates cofactors protein C and factor XIII. This is a vitamin K–dependent factor.

Factor III, Thromboplastin

Tissue factor activates factor VII when blood is exposed to tissue fluids.

Factor IV, Ionized Calcium

This active form of calcium is needed for the activation of thromboplastin and for conversion of prothrombin to thrombin.

Factor V, Proaccelerin or Labile Factor

This is consumed during clotting and accelerates the transformation of prothrombin to thrombin. A vitamin K–dependent factor, 20% of factor V is found on platelets.

Table 15.2 ◉ Factor Facts

Factor	Inheritance	Half-life (hr)	Clinical Picture If Deficient	Factor for Hemostasis	Screening Tests
I	Autosomal dominant	64 to 96	Bleed with trauma, stress, mucosal, umbilical stump, intracranial, gastrointestinal	40 to 50 mg/dL	↑ PT and aPTT
II	Autosomal recessive	48	Severe bleed, mucous membrane, spontaneous	20% to 30%	↑ PT and aPTT
V	Autosomal recessive	12	Moderate-severe bleed, mucosal, large ecchymoses	10% to 15%	↑ PT and aPTT
VII	Autosomal recessive	4 to 6	Intra-articular bleed, severe mucosal, epistaxis, hemarthrosis, genitourinary, gastrointestinal, and intrapulmonary	10% to 15%	↑ PT
VIII	Sex-linked recessive	15 to 20	Severity based on levels, hematuria, hemarthrosis, intra-articular, intracranial	>10%	↑ aPTT
IX	Sex-linked recessive	24	Severe mucous membrane, deep tissue, intra-muscular	>10%	↑ aPTT
X	Autosomal recessive	32	Mucous membrane, skin hemorrhages	10% to 15%	↑ PT and aPTT
XI	Autosomal recessive	60 to 80	Severity of bleeds vary, not proportional to factor level	30%	↑ aPTT
XII	Autosomal recessive and dominant	50 to 70	Hemorrhage is rare, risk for thrombosis	?	↑ aPTT
XIII	Autosomal recessive	40 to 50	Only homozygotes bleed, deep tissue muscle, intracranial bleed	10%	Normal PT and aPTT

Factor VI, Nonexistent

Factor VII, Proconvertin or Stable Factor

This is activated by tissue thromboplastin, which in turn activates factor X. It is a vitamin K–dependent factor.

Factor VIII, Antihemophilic

This cofactor is used for the cleavage of factor X-Xa by IXa. Factor VIII is described as VIII/vWF:VIII:C active portion, measured by clotting, VIII:Ag is the antigenic portion, vWF:Ag measures antigen that binds to endothelium for platelet function; it is deficient in hemophilia A.

Factor IX, Plasma Thromboplastin Component

A component of the thromboplastin generating system, it influences amount as opposed to rate. It is deficient in hemophilia B, also known as Christmas disease. It is sex linked and vitamin K–dependent.

Factor X, Stuart-Prower

Final common pathway merges to form conversion of prothrombin to thrombin, activity also related to factors VII and IX. It is vitamin K–dependent and can be independently activated by Russell's viper venom.

Factor XI, Plasma Thromboplastin Antecedent

Essential to intrinsic thromboplastin generating of the cascade, it has increased frequency in the Jewish population. Bleeding tendencies vary, but there is the risk of postoperative hemorrhage.

Factor XII, Hageman factor

This surface contact factor is activated by collagen. Patients do not bleed but have a tendency to thrombosis.

Factor XIII, Fibrin Stabilizing Factor

In the presence of calcium, this transaminase stabilizes polymerized fibrin monomers in the initial clot. This is the only factor that is not found in circulating plasma.

High-Molecular-Weight Kininogen

This surface contact factor is activated by kallikrein.

Prekallikrein, Fletcher Factor

This is a surface contact activator, in which 75% is bound to HMWK.

Physiological Coagulation (In Vivo)

The original theory of coagulation used a cascade or waterfall theory. This description depicted the generation of thrombin by the soluble coagulation factors and the initiation of coagulation. This theory identified two starting points for the generation of thrombin: the initiation of the Intrinsic pathway with factor XII and surface contact, and the extrinsic pathway with factor VIIa and tissue factor. These two pathways meet at the common pathway, where they both generate factor Xa from X, leading to a common pathway of thrombin from prothrombin and the conversion of fibrinogen to fibrin. This process holds true under laboratory conditions (Fig. 15.5). The discovery of a naturally occurring inhibitor of hemostasis, tissue factor pathway inhibitor (TFPI), is able to block the activity of the tissue factor VIIa complex, soon after it becomes active.[14]

Laboratory Model of Coagulation

Laboratory testing looks at the in vitro effect of the coagulation process which is measured by the prothrombin time (PT), activated partial thromboplastin time (aPTT), thrombin time (TT), fibrin degradation products (FDPs), and D-dimer. This section will focus on PT and a PTT, while Chapter 20 will concentrate on the other routine tests mentioned. While the coagulation cascade does not reflect what goes on in vivo, it provides a model in which the laboratory relates to for testing. However, the coagulation cascade reflects the mechanisms that the laboratory uses for results. The screening tests provide a tremendous amount of information to the physician. They can be performed both quickly and accurately (Fig. 15.6).

Extrinsic Pathway

The extrinsic pathway is initiated by the release of tissue thromboplastin that has been expressed after damage to

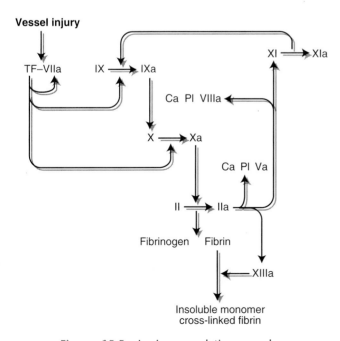

Revised Coagulation Cascade: **In Vivo**

Figure 15.5   In vivo coagulation cascade.

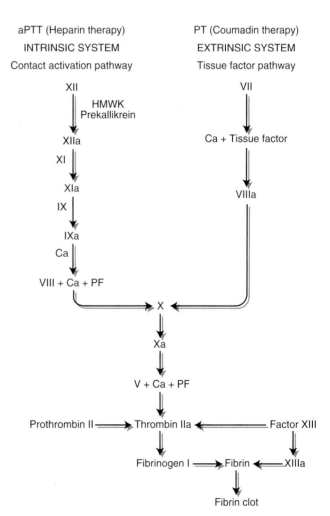

Figure 15.6   In vitro coagulation cascade.

a vessel. Factor VII forms a complex with tissue thromboplastin and calcium. This complex converts factors X and Xa, which in turn converts prothrombin to thrombin. Thrombin then converts fibrinogen to fibrin. This process takes between 10 and 15 seconds.

Prothrombin time (PT) developed by Armond Quick in 1935 measures the extrinsic system of coagulation. It is dependent upon the addition of calcium chloride and tissue factor. It uses a lipoprotein extract from rabbit brain and lung.[1]

PT uses citrate anticoagulated plasma. After the addition of an optimum concentration of calcium and an excess of thromboplastin, clot detection is measured by an automated device for fibrin clot detection. The result is reported in seconds. PT is exclusive for factor VII, but this test is also sensitive to decreases in the common pathway factors. Therefore, if a patient presents with a prolonged PT and there is no other clinical abnormality or medication, the patient is most likely factor VII deficient. The PT is also used to monitor oral anticoagulation or warfarin therapy used to treat and prevent blood clots. In many instances, patients are placed on life-long therapy and the dosage is monitored by the PT test. The attempt in anticoagulant therapy is to impede thrombus formation without the threat of **morbidity** or **mortality** from hemorrhage.

Warfarin is an oral anticoagulant, which means it must be ingested. It was discovered in 1939 at the University of Wisconsin quite by accident. It seems that a farmer found that his cattle were hemorrhaging to death, for what appeared to be no reason. The cattle were grazing in a field eating sweet clover. This contains dicumarol, actually bis-hydroxy coumadin, which caused the cattle to bleed.[6]

There are several compounds of coumadin: dicumarol, indanedione, and warfarin. Dicumarol works too slowly, and indanedione has too many side effects. Warfarin or 4-oxycoumarin is the most commonly used oral anticoagulant. Coumadin works by inhibiting the y-carboxylation step of clotting and the vitamin K–dependent factors.[15] Laboratory monitoring of oral anticoagulation therapy will be discussed in Chapter 19.

Intrinsic System

Contact activation is initiated by changes induced by vascular trauma. Prekallikrein is required as a cofactor for the autoactivation of factor XII by factor XIIa. XI is activated and requires a cofactor of HMWK. XIa activates IX to IXa, which in the presence of VIIIa converts X to Xa. Also present are platelet phospholipids PF3.

Calcium is required for the activation of X to proceed rapidly. The reaction then enters the common pathway where both systems involve factors I, II, V, and X. This results in a fibrin monomer polymerizing into a fibrin clot. Factor XIII, or fibrin stabilizing factor, follows activation by thrombin. This will convert initial weak hydrogen bonds, cross-linking fibrin polymers to a more stable covalent bond.

Activated Partial Thromboplastin Time

aPTT measures the intrinsic pathway. The test consists of recalcifying plasma in the presence of a standardized amount of platelet-like phosphatides and an activator of the contact factors. It will detect abnormalities to factors VIII, IX, XI, and XII. The aPTT is also used to monitor heparin therapy. Heparin is an anticoagulant used to treat and or prevent acute thrombotic events such as deep vein thrombosis (DVT), pulmonary embolism (PE), or acute coronary syndromes. The action of heparin is to inactivate factors XII, XI, and IX in the presence of antithrombin. Laboratory monitoring of heparin therapy will be discussed in Chapter 19.

Common Pathway

The common pathway is the point at which the intrinsic and extrinsic pathways come together and factors I, II, V, and X are measured. It is important to note that the PT and the aPTT will not detect qualitative or quantitative platelet disorders, or a factor XIII deficiency. Factor XIII is fibrin stabilizing factor and is responsible for stabilizing a soluble fibrin monomer into an insoluble fibrin clot. If a patient is factor XIII deficient, the patient will form a clot but will not be able to stabilize the clot and bleeding will occur later. Factor XIII is measured by a 5 mol/L urea test that looks at not only the formation of the clot but also if the clot lyzes after 24 hours.

Formation of Thrombin

When plasma fibrinogen is activated by thrombin, this conversion results in a stable fibrin clot. This clot is a visible result that the action of the protease enzyme thrombin has achieved fibrin formation. Thrombin is also involved in the XIII-XIIIa activation due to the reaction of thrombin cleaving a peptide bond from each of two alpha chains. Inactive XIII along with Ca^{2+} ions enables XIII to dissociate to XIIIa. If thrombin were allowed to circulate in its active form (Ia), uncontrollable clotting would occur. As a result thrombin circulates in its inactive form prothrombin (II). Thrombin, a protease enzyme, cleaves fibrinogen (factor I) which results in a fibrin monomer and fibrinogen peptides A and B. These initial monomers polymerize end to end due to hydrogen bonding.

Formation of fibrin occurs in three phases:

1. *Proteolysis:* Protease enzyme thrombin cleaves fibrinogen resulting in a fibrin monomer, A and B fibrinopeptide.
2. *Polymerization:* This occurs spontaneously due to fibrin monomer that line up end-to-end due to hydrogen bonding.
3. *Stabilization:* This occurs when the fibrin monomers are linked covalently by XIIIa into fibrin polymers forming an insoluble fibrin clot.

Feedback Inhibition

Some activated factors have the ability to destroy other factors in the cascade. Thrombin has the ability to temporarily activate V and VIII, but as thrombin increases it destroys V and VIII by proteolysis. Likewise, factor Xa enhances factor VII, but through a reaction with tissue factor pathway inhibitor (TFPI), it will prevent further activation of X by VIIa and tissue factor. Therefore, these enzymes limit their own ability to activate the coagulation cascade at different intervals.

Thrombin feedback activation of factor IX can possibly explain how intrinsic coagulation might occur in the absence of contact factors. Tissue factor is expressed following an injury forming a complex with VIIa, then activating X and IX. TFPI prevents further activation of X. Thrombin formation is further amplified by factors V, VIII, and XI, which leads to activation of the intrinsic pathway. This feedback theory helps to enforce why patients with contact factor abnormalities (factors XI and XII) do not bleed.[8] See Figure 15.7 for a diagram of feedback inhibition.

Fibrinolysis

The fibrinolytic system is responsible for the dissolution of a clot. Fibrin clots are not intended to be permanent. The purpose of the clot is to stop the flow of blood until the damaged vessel can be repaired. The presence or absence of hemorrhage or thrombosis depends on a balance between the procoagulant and the fibrinolytic system. The key components of the system are plasminogen, plasminogen activators, plasmin, fibrin, fibrin/FDP, and inhibitors of plasminogen activators and plasmin.[6] Fibrinolysis is the process by which the hydrolytic enzyme plasmin digests fibrin and fibrinogen, resulting in progressively reduced clots. This system is activated in response to the initiation of the activation of the contact factors. Plasmin is capable of digesting either fibrin or fibrinogen as well as other factors in the cascade (V, VIII, IX, and XI). Normal plasma contains the inactive form of plasmin in a precursor called plasminogen. This precursor remains dormant until it is activated by proteolytic enzymes, the kinases, or plasminogen activators. Fibrinolysis is controlled by the plasminogen activator system. The components of this system are found in tissues, urine, plasma, lysosomal granules, and vascular endothelium.

An activator, tissue-plasminogen activator (tPA) results in the activation of plasminogen to plasmin resulting in the degradation of fibrin. The fibrinolytic system includes several inhibitors. Alpha-2-antiplasmin is a rapid inhibitor of plasmin activity and alpha-2-macroglobulin is an effective slow inhibitor of plas-

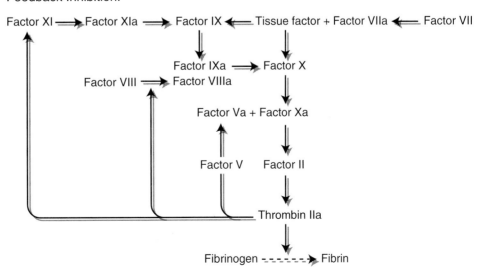

Feedback Inhibition:

Figure 15.7 Feedback inhibition. Note the role of thrombin in the activation and deactivation of coagulation factors.

min activity. This system is in turn controlled by inhibitors to tPA and plasmin-plasminogen activator inhibitor 1 (PAI-1) and alpha-2-antiplasmin. Reduced fibrinolytic activity may result in increased risk for cardiovascular events and thrombosis.

Pharmacologic activators are currently used for therapeutic **thrombolysis**, including streptokinase, urokinase, and tPA.

Urokinase directly activates plasminogen into plasmin, and streptokinase forms a streptokinase plasminogen complex, which then converts plasminogen into plasmin.[16]

Coagulation Inhibitors

Inhibitors are soluble plasma proteins that are natural anticoagulants. They prevent the initiation of the clotting cascade. There are two major inhibitors in plasma that keep the activation of coagulation under control. These inhibitors are:

1. Protease inhibitors: inhibitors of coagulation factors, which include
   • Antithrombin
   • Heparin cofactor II
   • Tissue factor pathway inhibitor
   • Alpha-2-antiplasmin
   • C1
2. The protein C pathway: inactivation of activated cofactors, which includes
   • Protein C and protein S

Each will be discussed in detail in Chapter 19. Table 15.3 has a listing on inhibitor and target reaction sites.

Table 15.3 ⬤ Serine Protease Inhibitors	
Inhibitor	**Specificity**
Antithrombin (AT)	IIa, Xa, IXa
Alpha-2-macroglobulin	Nonspecific
Tissue factor pathway inhibitor	Xa, VIIa/TF complex
Heparin cofactor II	IIa
Alpha-2 protease inhibitor	XIa, elastase
CI inhibitor	XIIa, kallikrein, XIa, CI (complement system)

Kinin System

Another plasma protein system in coagulation is the kinin system. This system is capable of vascular dilatation leading to hypotension, shock, and end-organ damage by its capability to increase vascular permability.[16] The kinins are peptides of 9 to 11 amino acids. The kinin system is activated by factor XII. Hageman factor XIIa converts prekallikrein (Fletcher factor) into kallikrein, and kallikrein converts kininogens into kinins. The most important is bradykinin (BK). This is an important factor in vascular permeability as well as a chemical mediator of pain. BK is capable of reproducing many characteristics of an inflammatory state such as changes in blood pressure, edema, and pain, resulting in vasodilation and increased microvessel permeability.[13]

Complement System

This system has a role in inflammation and the immune system as well as important thrombohemorrhagic disorders such as disseminated intravascular coagulation (DIC). Activated complement fragments have the capacity to bind and damage self tissues. Regulators of complement activation are expressed on cell surfaces. These protect the cell from the effects of cell-bound complement fragments. If this regulation process is abnormal, it may participate in the pathogenesis of autoimmune disease as well as inflammatory disorders. This system includes 22 serum proteins that play a role in mediating immune and allergic reactions and the lysis of cells due to a production of membrane attack complex (MAC). The lysis and disruption of red blood cells and platelets lead to the release of procoagulant material. This system is a sequential activation pathway. Complement is activated by plasmin through the cleavage of C3 into C3a and C3b. C3 causes increased vascular permeability, and because of the degranulation or lysis of mast cells, which in turn results in the release of histamine, C3b causes immune adherence.[13]

The interrelationship between the complement, kinin, and the coagulation system is complex and revealing. Coagulation and the elements that contribute to the success of the hemostatic system are multifactorial, and with each decade, more knowledge about this versatile system is learned. Figure 15.8 illustrates the important interrelationships between the coagulation, fibrinolytic, complement, and kinin systems.

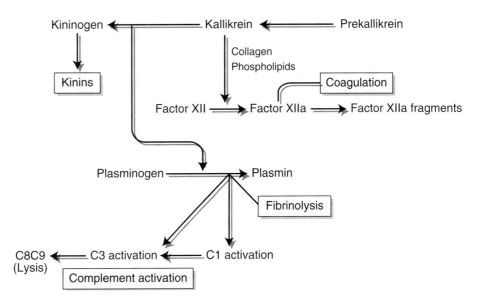

Figure 15.8 Interrelationships between the coagulation, fibrinolytic, complement, and kinin systems.

CONDENSED CASE

A 35-year-old woman needs to have an ovarian cyst removed. She had one delivery that was uneventful. Her mother has a history of bleeding after tooth extraction. The physician needs to determine if there is a bleeding disorder. The coagulation test results are as follows:

PT	12.5 seconds (Reference range, 10.5 to 13.3)
aPTT	32.1 seconds (Reference range, 28.7 to 35.5)
Platelets	320,000/mm^3 (Reference range, 150,000 to 400,000/mm^3)
Bleeding time	11 minutes (Reference, 8 minutes)

What is the most significant abnormal result in the coagulation panel?

Answer

The bleeding time is the only abnormal test, since it is greater than 8 minutes. This suggests a disorder within primary hemostasis. This can be caused by any disorder of platelets, such as von Willebrand disease, or a problem due to platelet secretion. Or it can be caused by several medications. Tests to rule out von Willebrand disease include factor VIII assay, a vWF antigen and activity, as well as platelet aggregation testing. Upon performing a platelet aggregation, there was only a primary wave for epinephrine, and no response for arachidonic acid. The patient was taking 81 μg of aspirin a day as a preventive measure. This resulted in a prolonged bleeding time. The patient was removed from aspirin and the bleeding returned to normal.

Summary Points

- Hemostasis depends on a system of checks and balances between thrombosis and hemorrhage that involve procoagulants and anticoagulants.
- The systems involved in hemostasis are the vascular system, platelets, coagulation system, and fibrinolytic system.
- Primary hemostasis is composed of platelet function and vasoconstriction.

- Secondary hemostasis is composed of fibrin clot formation and fibrin clot lysis.
- Platelet aggregation is mediated by von Willebrand's factor (vWF) and platelet glycoprotein Ib (GP1b).
- Platelets are small discoid cell fragments that are synthesized in the bone marrow and stimulated by the hormone thrombopoietin.
- There are four phases to platelet function at the site of injury: platelet adherence to collagen, platelet

aggregation, platelet granule release, and stabilization of the clot.

- Coagulation factors are produced in the liver with the exception of a portion of factor VIII, produced in the endothelial cells.

- The traditional coagulation pathway is divided into the intrinsic, extrinsic, and common pathways.

- The extrinsic pathway is monitored by the prothrombin time, while the intrinsic pathway is monitored by the partial thromboplastin time.

- The intrinsic pathway is initiated by factor XII and surface contact with the endothelial cells.

- Tissue factor pathway inhibitor is able to block the activity of the tissue factor: factor VII complex soon after it becomes active.

- Plasma fibrinogen activated by thrombin results in a stable fibrin clot.

- The key components of the fibrinolytic system are plasminogen, plasminogen activators, plasmin, fibrin, fibrin degradation products, and inhibitors of plasminogen and plasmin.

- Streptokinase, urokinase, and tissue plasminogen activator are activators of the plasmin-plasminogen system.

- Tissue plasminogen activator is available as a pharmacological product to break up pathologically formed clots.

- Serine protease inhibitors and the protein C pathway are the major physiologic inhibitors of coagulation.

- The kinin system is activated by factor XII and contributes to vascular permeability.

- The complement system once activated may contribute to the release of procoagulant material.

CASE STUDY

A 15-year-old boy with chronic strep throat has presented with excessive bruising. His coagulation results were as follows:

PT	15.5 seconds (Reference range, 10.8 to 13.5)
aPTT	42.1 seconds (Reference range, 28.5 to 35.5)
Platelets	325,000 (Reference range, 150,000 to 400,000)
Bleeding	5 minutes (Reference, 8 minutes)

Which coagulation tests are abnormal, and how should this physician proceed in his treatment of this patient?

Insights to the Case Study

In this case, two parameters, the PT and aPTT, are elevated. The patient is not bleeding, but he shows a history of recent bruising. Since both the PT and the aPTT are affected, one can assume the problem is in the common pathway, specifically factors I, II, V, and X. Factor assays could be performed to assess the level of activity of each of these clotting factors; however, a closer examination into the patient's history might reveal an additional feature. Since this patient has had chronic strep throat, it is logical to assume that he has been on long-term antibiotics. Antibiotics may deplete the normal flora, a source of vitamin K synthesis. Factors II, VII, IX, and X are vitamin K–dependent factors. Vitamin K is the essential cofactor for the gamma carboxyglutamic acid residues necessary to activate these factors. When vitamin K is in short supply or depleted, these factors fail to function properly. In our patient, vitamin K can be given by mouth to resume normal coagulation and correct bruising.

Review Questions

1. The factor with the longest half-life is:
   a. II.
   b. V.
   c. VII.
   d. X.

2. If a patient has a prolonged PT, the patient is most likely deficient in factor:

   a. VIII.
   b. II.
   c. VII.
   d. X.

3. Receptors that are found on the platelets are called:
   a. glycoproteins.
   b. vWF.

c. fibrinogen.

b. beta-thromboglobulin.

4. Vasoconstriction is caused by several regulatory molecules, which include:
   a. fibrinogen and vWF.
   b. ADP and EPI.
   c. Thromboxane A_2 and serotonin.
   d. Collagen and actomyosin.

5. The vitamin K–dependent factors are:
   a. I, II, V, and X.
   b. II, VII, IX, and X.
   c. I, VII, V, and VIII.
   d. II, IX, XI, and X.

6. The life span of a platelet is:
   a. 5 to 8 days.
   b. 7 to 10 days.
   c. 6 to 9 days.
   d. 9 to 12 days.

7. Alpha granules are found in:
   a. the peripheral zone.
   b. the sol gel zone.
   c. organelles.
   d. membranes.

8. If a patient has just a prolonged aPTT, the patient may be deficient in the following factors:
   a. VIII, X, II, and I
   b. VIII, IX, XI, and XII
   c. VIII, X, XI, and XII
   d. VIII, XI, II, and XII

9. The factor that is responsible for stabilizing a soluble fibrin monomer into an insoluble clot is:
   a. II.
   b. X.
   c. XII.
   d. XIII.

10. An inhibitor of plasmin activity is:
    a. tPA.
    b. PAI-1.
    c. alpha-2-antiplasmin.
    d. plasminogen.

11. Protein C and its cofactor protein S proteolytically inactivate factors:
    a. VIIa and Xa.
    b. Va and VIIIa.
    c. IXa and VIIa.
    d. VIIIa and XIIa.

○ TROUBLESHOOTING

What Do I Do When the Coagulation Sample Is Drawn Incorrectly?

Preanalytic variables represent important sources of error in patient testing and accuracy of results. In hemostasis testing, sample integrity is paramount. Areas in which sample integrity are most affected are in phlebotomy practices, transport and handling of specimens, choice of coagulation tubes, and patient variables.

Phlebotomy Practices

The sample must be provided from an atraumatic draw, on a properly identified patient, and the tube must be inverted three to four times for proper mixing of anticoagulant. The order of draw in coagulation testing is important to avoid contamination of the sample with tissue thromboplastin. Therefore, if multiple tubes are drawn, the coagulation tube should be last. If only a coagulation sample is requested and the sample is drawn through a butterfly, then a discard tube should be drawn first. If a syringe is needed for phlebotomy, a needle gauge of 12 to 19 is optimal. Additionally, the tubes must be filled to 90% capacity to preserve a 1:9 anticoagulant-to-blood ratio.

Transport and Handling of Specimens

There are several coagulation proteins that are labile, namely factors V and VIII. The activity of these factors will be lost if the sample is not tested in an appropriate time span. For maximum activity, testing should be performed within 4 hours for aPTT and up to 24 hours for PT. Plasma can be removed from the sample and stored at −20°C for up to 2 weeks. Additionally, samples must be centrifuged for a period of time that enables them to become platelet poor plasma. Platelet poor plasma is defined as having a platelet count of less than 10,000, which depends upon proper centrifugation. If samples are not platelet poor, falsely shortened results may occur as a result of activation of platelet factor 4. Activation of platelet factor 4 may also occur in heparinized samples that are allowed to sit on red cells for longer than 4 hours. In this case the platelet factor 4 may inactivate the heparin giving a falsely shortened PTT result.

(continued on following page)

⊙ TROUBLESHOOTING *(continued)*

Which Tubes to Use?

Most facilities are using blue top tubes, which contain 3.2% sodium citrate. The reasons for this are many and include the fact that this concentration provides a closer osmolality to plasma, has less binding of calcium, and provides a more favorable environment for heparinized samples.

Patient Variables

Many variables affect coagulation results such as medication, physical and emotional stress, and patient age and personal habits. These factors cannot be controlled by the laboratory. A patient's hematocrit, however, is something that can be adjusted for when drawing a coagulation sample. For patients who have hematocrits that are >60% (neonated, polycythemia), falsely prolonged results will occur if the anticoagulant is not adjusted, since there is too much anticoagulant for plasma. For patients who have hematocrits of less than 22%, results will be falsely decreased as a result of too little anticoagulant because of increasing plasma volume. The standard formula for adjusting the volume of anticoagulant is:

$$\text{New volume of sodium citrate} = (1.85 \times 10)^{-3} \times (100 - \text{Hct}) \times \text{volume of sample}$$

WORD KEY

Anticoagulant • Delaying or preventing blood coagulation

Fibronectin • Protein involved in wound healing and cell adhesion

Lumen • Space within an artery, vein, or intestine or tube

Morbidity • State of being diseased

Mortality • Death

Polymerize • Process by which a simple chemical substance or substances are changed into a substance of a much higher molecular weight but with the same proportions

Thrombolysis • Breaking up of a clot

Transaminase • Aminotransferase (an enzyme)

Vasoconstriction • Decrease in the diameter of the blood vessels that decreases the blood flow

Viscosity • State of being sticky or gummy

References

1. Owen CA. A History of Blood Coagulation. Rochester, MN; Mayo Foundation for Medical Education and Research, 2001.
2. Hougie C. Fundamentals of Blood Coagulation in Clinical Medicine. New York: McGraw-Hill Book Company, 1963.
3. Schetz M. Coagulation disorder in acute renal failure. Kidney Int S53(suppl 66):96–101, 1998.
4. Harmening D. Clinical Hematology and Fundamentals of Hemostasis, 3rd ed. Philadelphia: FA Davis, 1997.
5. Turgeon ML. Clinical Hematology, Theory and Procedures, 2nd ed. Boston: Little, Brown and Co, 1993.
6. McKenzie SB. Textbook of Hematology. Baltimore: Williams and Wilkins, 1996.
7. Zucker M. The functioning of blood platelets. Sci Am 242:86–89, 1980.
8. Kjeldsberg C. Practical Diagnosis of Hematologic Disorders, 2nd ed. Chicago: ASCP Press, 1995.
9. Plaut D. Platelet Function Tests. ADVANCE for the Administrators of the Laboratory, July 2003.
10. Southern D, Leclair S. Platelet Maturation and Function. In: Rodak B, ed. Diagnostic Hematology. Philadelphia, WB Saunders, 1995.
11. Kolde H.-J. Haemostasis pentapharm. Basel: 2001.
12. Rodgers G. Hemostasis Case Studies. Chicago: ASCP Press, 2000.
13. Ogedegbe HO. An overview of hemostasis. Lab Med 33: December 2002.
14. Fass D. Overview of Hemostasis, Mayo Clinic Coagulation Conference, Mayo Clinic, August 2004.
15. Kandrotis RJ. Pharmacology and pharmacokinetics of antithrombotic agents. Clin Appl Thromb/Hemost 3:157–163, 1997.
16. Bick R. Disorders of Thrombosis and Hemostasis. Chicago: ASCP Press, 1991.

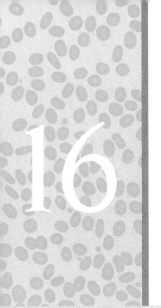

16

Quantitative and Qualitative Platelet Disorders

Betty Ciesla

Quantitative Disorders of Platelets

Thrombocytopenia Related to Sample Integrity/ Preanalytic Variables

Thrombocytopenia Related to Decreased Production

Thrombocytopenia Related to Altered Distribution of Platelets

Thrombocytopenia Related to the Immune Effect of Specific Drugs or Antibody Formation

Thrombocytopenia Related to Consumption of Platelets

Thrombocytosis

Inherited Qualitative Disorders of Platelets

Disorders of Adhesion

Platelet Release Defects

Acquired Defects of Platelet Function

Vascular Disorders Leading to Platelet Dysfunction

Objectives

After completing this chapter, the student will be able to:

1. Define the *quantitative platelet disorders*.

2. Identify the types of bleeding that are seen in platelet disorders.

3. List four laboratory tests that are helpful in evaluating platelet disorders.

4. State how preanalytic variables may affect the platelet count.

5. Describe three characteristics of the qualitative platelet disorders von Willebrand disease, Bernard Soulier, and Glanzmann's thrombasthenia.

6. Identify drugs that are implicated in immune thrombocytopenia.

7. Evaluate conditions that may cause thrombocytosis.

8. Compare and contrast acute versus chronic idiopathic thrombocytopenic purpura.

9. Describe the effect of ristocetin on platelet aggregation.

10. Define *hemolytic uremic syndrome* in terms of incidence, key clinical features, and patient management.

11. Define *thrombotic thrombocytopenic purpura* in terms of incidence, key clinical features, and severity.

12. Describe platelet abnormalities due to acquired defects: drug induced, nonimmune, or vascular.

QUANTITATIVE DISORDERS OF PLATELETS

A normal platelet count is 150 to 450 $\times$ 10^9/L. In this range, an individual will have properly functioning platelets that assist in the coagulation process by creating a platelet plug and stimulating the formation of a solid fibrin clot. A decrease in platelet count will cause bleeding from the mucous membranes such as gum bleeding (gingival bleeding), nose bleeding (epistaxis), extensive bruising (ecchymoses), or petechiae (pinpoint hemorrhages). A patient with a platelet count of 60,000 will bleed in surgery and a patient with a platelet count of 30,000 may have petechial bleeding At less than 5000 platelets, there is a risk of bleeding into the central nervous system. Laboratory tests that are helpful in the evaluation of platelet function are the evaluation of the peripheral smear for platelet number and morphology, the bleeding time test (or similar platelet function tests), platelet aggregation by one of several methods, or other methods that assess platelet function and aggregation. Thrombocytopenia or a decreased platelet count is caused by a number of factors. Decreased production of platelets or increased destruction of platelets usually accounts for the pathophysiology of most *quantitative* defects in platelets. Additionally, sample related conditions or preanalytic variables may lead to falsely decreased platelet counts.

Thrombocytopenia Related to Sample Integrity/Preanalytic Variables

Coagulation samples are drawn into blue top tubes containing sodium citrate. Sodium citrate anticoagulates a specimen by binding calcium in a 1:9 anticoagulant-to-blood ratio. Sample tubes must be at least 90% full and the phlebotomy must be nontraumatic. The blue top tube must be inverted at least three or four times for proper mixing of the anticoagulant. If this does not happen, there is a possibility of small clots being formed on the top of the tube. Platelet satellitism is another condition related to samples that may give a falsely decreased platelet count. First reported in 1963,[1] this condition is an in vitro phenomenon in which the patient's platelets rosette around segmented neutrophils, monocytes, and bands. This phenomenon occurs only in EDTA (ethylenediaminetetraacetic acid) samples and produces a pseudo-thrombocytopenia unrelated to medication or any other disease state (see Fig. 10.21). If platelet satellitism is observed on the peripheral smear, the sample should be redrawn in sodium citrate and cycled through the automated hematology counter for a more accurate platelet count.

Thrombocytopenia Related to Decreased Production

Any condition that leads to bone marrow aplasia or a lack of megakaryocytes, the platelet forming cell, will lead to a thrombocytopenia. Most patients with leukemia will exhibit a thrombocytopenia as a result of infiltration of the bone marrow with blast cells. Blasts of any cellular origin crowd out normal bone marrow elements leading to thrombocytopenia. Defects in platelet synthesis can occur in the megaloblastic anemias that show a pancytopenia, a decrease in all cell lines. **Cytotoxic** agents or chemotherapy usually interferes with the cell cycle, thereby reducing the number of active platelets. Patients undergoing chemotherapy are carefully monitored for platelet count and may need to be given platelet support if the count drops too far below 20.0 $\times$ 10^9/L.

Megakaryocytic function is impaired during the infectious process. Infections with several viral agents such as cytomegalovirus, Epstein-Barr virus, varicella, and rubella and certain bacterial infections may cause a thrombocytopenia. The mechanism at work in viral infections is thought to be megakaryocytic suppression; in bacteria, the mechanism is direct toxicity of circulating platelets.[2]

Thrombocytopenia Related to Altered Distribution of Platelets

The normal spleen holds one third of the platelet volume. Several hematological conditions may lead to an enlarged spleen as part of their pathological process: the myeloproliferative disorders, extramedullary hematopoiesis, and hemolytic anemias. As the spleen enlarges, blood pools in this organ withholding platelets from the peripheral circulation. If the organ is removed, then large numbers of platelets may spill into the circulation, causing possible thrombotic complications.[3] An additional scenario in which platelet distribution is altered is in massive transfusion. Once the total blood volume (10 units) has been replaced with two or three volume exchanges, the platelet and the coagulation factors become diluted leading to a transient thrombocytopenia.[4]

Thrombocytopenia Related to the Immune Effect of Specific Drugs or Antibody Formation

Drug-induced immune thrombocytopenia produces a reduced platelet count that can be severe and dangerous. Several drug classifications are particularly relevant and include quinines, NSAIDs (nonsteroidal anti-inflammatory drugs), sulfonamides, and diuretics.[5] The mechanism for thrombocytopenia is 2-fold. On the one hand, ingestion of the drug will cause an antidrug antibody formation that will bind to a glycoprotein on the platelet surface and be removed by the reticuloendothelial system (RES). The second mechanism involves the drug combining with a larger carrier protein to form an antigen that triggers an antibody response and subsequent platelet destruction, potentially in the spleen. The incidence of drug-induced thrombocytopenia is 10 cases per 1 million.[5]

Additionally, there are two rare conditions in which thrombocytopenia may be quite dramatic. Fortunately, these are rare. The first, posttransfusion purpura (PTP), occurs after transfusion of platelet-containing products in which the recipient has developed an antibody. The antibody is directed against an antigen on the platelet Pl[1A], a primary platelet antigen, and therefore when donor platelets are transfused containing this antigen, the platelets are coated and removed by the spleen. The resultant thrombocytopenia is quite long lasting, and treatment is directed toward delaying antibody production. The second condition, neonatal isoimmune thrombocytopenia, occurs as a result of maternal antibody made against a previous exposure to platelet antigens from an earlier pregnancy. The antibody is usually directed against the Pl[1A]. Since this antibody can cross the placenta, it can coat the baby's platelets in utero. Infants born to mothers carrying these antibodies will often show a normal platelet count initially but within days they will develop petechiae and skin hemorrhages with decreasingly low platelet counts. Infants are carefully observed and treatment is only begun when there is a risk of central nervous system hemorrhage.[2]

Thrombocytopenia Related to Consumption of Platelets

Hematological conditions studied under this category usually include idiopathic thrombocytopenia purpura, thrombotic thrombocytopenic purpura, and hemolytic uremic syndrome. In these conditions, excessive clots are formed throughout the body, which consume platelets. Each of these conditions is serious and can produce significant life-altering complications.

Idiopathic (Immune) Thrombocytopenic Purpura

Patients with idiopathic (immune) thrombocytopenic purpura (ITP) show a decreased platelet count that is thought to be a result of immune destruction of platelets. In 66% of cases, the antibody is an autoantibody directed against specific sites on glycoprotein (GP) IIb-IIIa or GP Ib-IX. Additionally, megakaryocytes

may be increased in the marrow; however, they are poorly functioning.[2] There are two types of ITP: chronic and acute. Patients with acute ITP are usually children between the ages of 2 and 6 who have just recovered from a viral illness.[2] The platelet counts may drop precipitously, some as low as 20×10^9/L. In this range, the child will usually show bruising, nose bleeding, or petechiae but will not usually show life-threatening hemorrhage. Fortunately, this low platelet count usually resolves in less than 6 weeks as the child fully recovers from the viral illness. Treatment, if necessary, may consist of intravenous immunoglobulin (IvIg or WinRho, anti–D immune globulin), splenectomy, or platelet transfusion.[2] Chronic ITP, on the other hand, shows a platelet count between 30 and 60×10^9/L in a much older age range of between 20 and 50 years of age. For these patients, an IgG antibody is produced that coats the platelets, causing them to be sequestered and subsequently destroyed in the spleen. Splenomegaly is a frequent physical symptom. Most patients are treated with prednisone, which suppresses the antibody response, increases the platelet count, and decreases the hemorrhagic episodes. For those who are nonresponsive, anti-CD20, Rituximab, has been shown to provide a sustained platelet response.[6] Splenectomy is a therapeutic option, but it must be carefully considered. Recently, immune thrombocytopenia related to infections has been investigated. Patients infected with HIV, hepatitis C, and *Helicobacter pylori* show thrombocytopenia at some point during their disease. The precise mechanism, thought to be immune derived, is under study.[7] Table 16.1 compares acute and chronic ITP.

Table 16.1 ◉ Chronic and Acute Idiopathic Thrombocytopenic Purpura		
	Acute Idiopathic Thrombocytopenic Purpura	**Chronic Idiopathic Thrombocytopenic Purpura**
Age	Young children	Adults
Prior infection	History of rubella, rubeola, or chickenpox	No prior history
Platelet count	<20,000	30,000 to 80,000
Duration	2 to 6 weeks	Months to years
Therapy	None	Steroids, splenectomy

Thrombotic Thrombocytopenic Purpura

This devastating platelet disorder described by Moschowitz in 1925 is acute and nonpredictable. More prevalent in women than in men, thrombotic thrombocytopenic purpura (TTP) can occur in women postpartum or near delivery[8] in those who have suffered from other immune disorders like SLE (systemic lupus erythematosus), and in those with previous viral infections or gastric carcinomas. Platelet counts are less than 20 × 10^9/L but other coagulation testing such as PT and PTT are within reference range. Platelet thrombi are dispersed throughout the arterioles and capillaries subsequent to the accumulation of large von Willebrand multimers made by the endothelial cells and platelets. The etiology for this pathological accumulation of multimers and subsequent thrombocytopenia is thought to be related to a deficiency of ADAMTS-13, a large metalloprotease.[9,10] This protein is responsible for cleaving large von Willebrand factor (vWF) multimers into smaller proteins. Large vWF multimers have increased binding sites for platelets as compared to smaller vWF portions. If large vWF are not cleaved and allowed to circulate, then excessive platelet clots may be formed. Schistocytes are seen in the peripheral smear and are directly related to shear stress as fragments of red cells are removed once the cells try to sweep past the thrombi. Patients experience a severe anemia with a high level of hemolysis, with increased lactate dehydrogenase (LDH). Some of the hemolysis may be intravascular with hemoglobinuria. Decreased haptoglobin may be seen. **Microangiopathic** hemolytic anemia (MHA) is the term used to describe this process of severe anemia combined with schistocytes (Fig. 16.1). Oftentimes patients will present with neurological complications. These complications may include mild presentations of visual impairment and intense headache ranging to more severe presentations such as coma and **paresthesias.** Renal dysfunction may occur, and patients with renal impairment experience an increased protein and possibly some blood in the urine. Treatment for TTP patients presents a dilemma for most physicians, as they watch their patients spiral rapidly downhill. Diagnosis is often difficult and often represents a diagnosis of exclusion. Once made, the patient's condition has usually dramatically worsened. Corticosteroids are often used in conjunction with plasma exchange, a dramatic procedure performed over a 3- to 5-day period in which the patient's plasma is removed and replaced by ABO matched fresh frozen plasma that is **cryoprecipitate** poor (lacking fibrinogen and vWF). The use of plasma exchange has dramatically improved the survival rate from a low of 3% before 1960

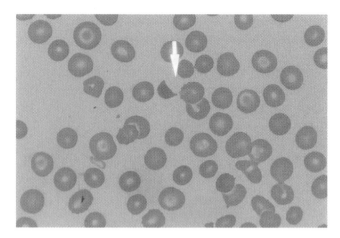

Figure 16.1   Schistocyte.

to 82% presently.[11] Few hospital facilities provide plasma exchange capabilities. Specialty teams of medical professionals using equipment designed for plasmapheresis are usually called upon. Timing is essential to the patient's welfare and long-term recovery. Recovery for TTP patients has improved in the past decade, with more than 80% surviving.[11]

Hemolytic Uremic Syndrome

Hemolytic uremic syndrome (HUS) frequently occurs in children between the ages of 6 months and 4 years. This clinical condition mimics TTP, with the exception that the renal damage is more severe. The kidney is the primary site of damage by the toxin *Escherichia coli* O157:H7 or the *Shigella* toxin.[11] The endotoxin produced by this particular strain of *E. coli* inevitably leads to cell death, particularly in the renal environment, where platelet thrombi predominate.[12] A child may initially present with bloody diarrhea and vomiting; however, hemolytic anemia, thrombocytopenia, and renal failure soon follow. Patients may also experience fever and abdominal pain, and the hemolytic anemia is microangiopathic with schistocytes present. The illness in children is usually self-limiting once the toxin is eliminated from the body; however, there have been reports of patients relapsing. Renal dialysis may be needed for those children suffering from acute renal failure. Most children make a complete recovery, but some have residual kidney problems into adulthood. HUS may occur in adults, but it is more similar to TTP in course of disease (Table 16.2).

Disorders such as heparin-induced thrombocytopenia and disseminated intravascular coagulation also lead to thrombocytopenia. These will be covered in subsequent chapters.

Table 16.2 ◉ Hemolytic Uremic Syndrome Versus Thrombotic Thrombocytopenic Purpura		
	Hemolytic Uremic Syndrome	Thrombotic Thrombocytopenic Purpura
Platelet count	<20,000	<20,000
Organ(s) affected	Kidney	Neurological manifestations Kidney
Age group	Children	Adults (more females than males)
Symptoms	Fever, bloody diarrhea MHA with schistocytes	Fever, headaches Visual impairment, coma MHA with schistocytes
Treatment	Renal dialysis, blood transfusions	Plasmapheresis

MHA, microangiopathic hemolytic anemia.

Thrombocytosis

Thrombocytosis is defined as a platelet count greater than 450×10^9/L. The cause for an increased platelet count may be primary or secondary. A primary thrombocytosis is seen in the myeloproliferative disorders (see Chapter 12), in which case platelets are high in number but have an impaired function. Of all of the myeloproliferative disorders, essential thrombocythemia has the highest platelet value, at times exceeding 1 million platelets. Secondary causes of thrombocytosis include acute and chronic blood loss, chronic inflammatory diseases, postsplenectomy, and iron deficiency anemia. In these cases, the platelet function is normal, although the increase in platelet numbers may last days to weeks. In severe iron deficiency anemia, the platelet count may increase to 2 million, as a result of marrow stimulation.[13] Once iron therapy is initiated, the platelet count usually returns to normal.

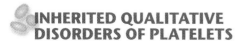

INHERITED QUALITATIVE DISORDERS OF PLATELETS

Inherited qualitative platelet disorders are those in which platelet function is impaired usually due to an intrinsic defect of platelets. Many of these disorders (with the exception of vWD) are rare, and in most cases the bleeding time is prolonged. Often, the qualitative defects are separated into disorders of adhesion and platelet release or storage pool defects.

Disorders of Adhesion

von Willebrand's Disease

The most important disease of platelet adhesion is von Willebrand disease (vWD). Discovered in 1926 by Dr. Eric von Willebrand, vWD is the most prevalent inherited bleeding disorder worldwide, affecting 1% to 3% of the world population by conservative estimates. In random studies of children investigated for epistaxis and women investigated for **menorrhagia,** vWD was the most frequent cause of bleeding.[14,15] von Willebrand initially described a family of 12 children of which 10 had excessive nosebleeds, gum bleeds, and menorrhagia. One of the youngest girls died at age 13 during her fourth menstrual cycle of uncontrollable bleeding. vWD is an autosomal dominant disorder marked by easy bruising, nosebleeds, heavy menses, and excessive bleeding after tooth extraction or dental procedures. Type O individuals have a lower plasma concentration of vWF than other blood types. For many patients, the variabilities in clinical symptoms and laboratory presentations have contributed to the underdiagnosis of this disorder. Women may represent a significant yet underserved subset of individuals affected by vWD, since menorrhagia is a frequent presenting feature of this disease. According to Luscher, vWD may be the underlying cause in 9% to 11% of cases of menorrhagia,[16] yet it is often not considered as a possible diagnosis by obstetricians and gynecologists.

As a disease entity, vWD is fairly complex with few clear-cut and consistent diagnostic clues. The basic pathophysiology in vWD is a qualitative or quantitative defect in vWF. vWF is a large multimeric glycoprotein derived from two sources: endothelial cells and megakaryocytes (Table 16.3). This protein is coded for by chromosome 12 and is carried into plasma circulation by factor 8, one of the clotting factors. vWF serves as an intermediary for platelet adhesion, providing a receptor molecule for GP Ib of the platelets and the subendothelium. With this platform in place, platelets, once activated by injury, adhere to the subendothelium forming a platelet plug, recruiting more platelets to the site of injury and eventually leading to platelet aggregation and the formation of an insoluble fibrin clot. Without a fully functioning vWF, platelet adhesion is impaired. Additionally, vWF binds GP IIb/IIIa. There are three *primary* levels of vWD: type 1, type 2, and type 3. Seventy percent of all individuals with vWD have the type 1 disorders characterized by an abnormal bleeding time and an increased PTT in most patients. Type 2 vWD is the result of a qualitative defect of wVF, and type 3, the rarest type, is characterized by a total absence of vWF multimers and is autosomal recessive in its presentation. Type 2 vWD has many subtypes: type 2A, type 2B, type 2M, and type 2N. See Table 16-4 for a description of vWD and its variants. The vWF protein can be measured by several methods; those that assess its role in adhesion, its secondary role in aggregation, and its role in clotting factor activity. Ristocetin co-factor activity is the single best predictive assay[17] and relies on the use of reagent platelets rather than patient's platelets during ristocetin-induced aggregation studies. Table 16.3 gives a description of a typical testing profile for vWD.

Treatment is usually tailored to the particular type or subtype of vWD. Some of the products that may be considered are desmopressin acetate (DDAVP), which causes the release of endothelial vWF. DDAVP may be given as an injectable agent or as a nasal spray, which makes it portable and convenient. For patients who are nonresponsive, vWF can be raised by giving high purity factor 8 products that contain a sufficient amount of vWF.

Bernard Soulier Syndrome

Bernard Soulier syndrome (BSS) is a rare adhesion defect of platelets that involves the GP Ib/IX complex. Once an injury has occurred, vWF acts as a medium through which the platelet membrane GP Ib has a receptor that allows its binding to collagen. As indicated

Table 16.4 ○ **Primary von Willebrand's Disease Derivatives***			
	Type 1	**Type 2**	**Type 3**
Frequency	70% to 80%	15% to 20%	Rare
Genetics	Autosomal dominant	Autosomal dominant	Autosomal recessive
Bleeding time	↑ or N	↑	↑
PTT	↑ or N	↑ or N	↑
RIPA	↑ or N	↑	↑
vWF agn.	↓	↓	Absent

*Secondary vWD variants include types 2A, 2B, 2M, and 2N: these are not discussed.

in Chapter 15, platelet glycoproteins play a significant role in hemostasis. The receptor for vWf is GP Ib-IX. This complex, Ib-IX, serves as a site for thrombin binding as well as regulating platelet shape and reactivity.[18] GP IIb and IIIa are receptors for fibronectin (an adhesive protein for platelets), vWF, fibrinogen, and factors V and VIII. BSS is inherited as an autosomal recessive disorder, with near normal amounts of GPIb in heterozygotes. If the disorder is inherited homozygously, however, moderate or severe bleeding may occur. Epistaxis, gingival bleeding, menorrhagia, and purpura are the usual bleeding manifestation. Additionally, there is a thrombocytopenia with giant platelets observed on the peripheral smear. Ristocetin-induced platelet aggregation is absent in BSS patients since there are no receptors to bind to vWF, a key ingredient in ristocetin induced platelet aggregation. Platelet aggregation with other agents such as epinephrine, thrombin, and collagen appears normal. The bleeding time test is prolonged.

Platelet transfusions are the treatment of choice for active bleeding but they should be used prudently to prevent the stimulation of platelet antibodies. To date, over 30 mutations of the glycoproteins involved in the GP Ib-IX complex have been described.[19]

Glanzmann's Thrombasthenia

Glanzmann's thrombasthenia (GT) is an autosomal recessive disorder, first described in 1918, most often associated with **consanguinity.** Homozygous individuals may experience variable bleeding patterns. When bleeding does occur, it is usually from birth as umbilical cord or circumcisional bleeding and may proceed to gingival bleeding, purpura, or prolonged bleeding from

Table 16.3 ○ **Basic Test Profile for vWD**

- Platelet count—measured by automated methods
- PTT—measures anticoagulant portion of the factor VIII molecule
- Bleeding time—measures adhesion of platelets to site of injury
- vWF activity—measured by ristocetin-induced platelet aggregation (RIPA)
- vWF antigen—measured by immunoassay

Most patients will have variable test results. It is recommended that this test profile be performed multiple times within a time period to aid in diagnosis.

minor cuts or childhood events. The defect in GT is a deficiency or abnormality of GP IIb and IIIa. These glycoproteins serve as the intermediary for fibrinogen binding to platelets, a necessary step in platelet aggregation. Aggregation cannot occur if GP IIb/IIIa is absent or if there is an absence of fibrinogen or calcium.[20] Patients with GT will have a prolonged bleeding time, normal platelet count and morphology, and abnormal aggregation with all aggregating agents except ristocetin. Ristocetin-induced aggregation depends upon the interaction of vWF and platelet GP Ib. The GP IIb/IIIa complex does not play a role in this type of aggregation. Treatment in GT depends upon the severity of the bleeding episode. Platelet transfusions may be considered but **HLA**-matched or ABO-matched transfusion may reduce the possibilities of platelet **alloimmunization.** Oral contraceptives may be used to control menorrhagia, and agents such as ethyleneaminocaproic acid (EACA) are effective topical thrombin-inducing agents for procedures such as tooth extractions.[21]

Platelet Release Defects

Once platelets adhere to an injured surface, the contents of the platelets are released. Platelets contain alpha and dense granules, which are highly metabolic substances containing procoagulant materials, vasoconstrictors ATP and ADP. The disorders that are described are inherited, usually have abnormal secondary phases of platelet aggregation, and show postoperative bleeding combined with menorrhagia and easy bruisability. In most of these disorders, the bleeding time is abnormal, but the platelet count may be normal.

Hermansky-Pudlak syndrome: An autosomal recessive disorder characterized by a severe deficiency of dense granules. Patients show albinism and may have hemorrhagic events.

Chediak-Higashi syndrome: An autosomal recessive disorder, in which patients show albinism and giant lysosomal granules in neutrophils. Not only are the white cells in these patients qualitatively flawed, but platelet release is impaired. Patients show frequent infections because of impaired phagocytic ability and death usually occurs in childhood. Patients manifest thrombocytopenia and increased liver and spleen.

Wiskott-Aldrich syndrome: This is an X-linked recessive disorder in which patients show severe eczema, recurrent infections, immune defects, and thrombocytopenia.

Thrombocytopenia with absent radii (TAR): A rare disorder of the skeletal system in which patients have no radial bones and other skeletal and cardiac abnormalities. Thrombocytopenia is seen in most patients.

Gray platelet syndrome: Platelets show a lack of alpha granules and are noted in the peripheral smear as appearing larger, having a gray or blue-gray color. Patients may show thrombocytopenia, bleeding tendencies, and bruisability.

ACQUIRED DEFECTS OF PLATELET FUNCTION

Included in this category of platelet defects are those factors that are external to the platelet and that are nonimmune, such as drug-related platelet abnormalities, extrinsic platelet abnormalities, or as a sequel to an underlying disorder. Of all the drugs that affect platelet function, aspirin is the most popular. Ingestion of aspirin irreversibly inhibits cyclooxygenase (COX-1 inhibitors) by inhibiting the formation of prostaglandin synthesis. Both of these chemicals are necessary for the production of thromboxane A_2, a potent platelet aggregator. Without the production of proper amount of thromboxane A_2, platelet aggregation is impaired. This effect lasts for the entire life span of the platelet, 7 to 10 days, and patients on aspirin will show a prolonged bleeding time. Patients should be queried about their aspirin use or use of aspirin-containing products prior to any surgical event, elective or nonelective, to avoid any unexpected bleeding complications. The effect of aspirin on platelets is fairly rapid, occurring 45 minutes after ingestion.[22] Additionally, aspirin as an antiplatelet agent is used as a preventive for patients susceptible to strokes, heart attacks, or other cardiovascular events. Other drugs such as NSAIDs and the class of COX-2 inhibitors such as naproxen and ibuprofen may affect platelet function. Certain antiplatelet agents such as ticlopidine and clopidogrel inhibit fibrinogen binding to GP IIb and IIIa. The plasma expander dextran also alters platelet function. The coating of platelets with dextran gives an antiplatelet effect by inhibiting the action of the platelet membrane and its surface receptors.

Platelet function may also be impaired by plasma conditions that are less than favorable to the platelet. In most cases, disorders in platelets are secondary to the main disorder but may not be present in the initial presentation. Conditions that may lead to disturbed platelet function include uremia due to renal disease and the paraproteinemias such as multiple myeloma and Waldenström's macroglobulinemia. The pathophysiology involved in the platelet defect in these acquired disorders is not clear-cut. Patients with renal disease are

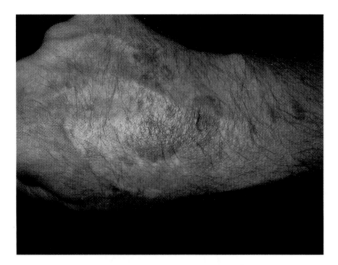

Figure 16.2   Purpura.

known to exhibit purpura (Fig. 16.2), epistaxis, and hemorrhage at times. A few of the factors involved in platelet dysfunction in uremia include decreased thromboxane synthesis, decreased adhesion, decreased platelet release, and decreased aggregation. Most of these patients will undergo peritoneal or hemodialysis, which usually improves platelet function.

Multiple myeloma and Waldenström's macroglobulinemia represent a group of plasma cell disorders in which a normal immunoglobulin is produced in excess leading to **hyperviscosity** syndrome and a paraproteinemia. Platelets circulating in abnormal amounts of protein are unable to fully participate in the activation of coagulation factors and in the fibrin formation. Patients will show a prolonged bleeding time and may show postoperative bleeding and ecchymoses. Table 16.5 displays a list of drugs that affect platelet function.

VASCULAR DISORDERS LEADING TO PLATELET DYSFUNCTION

Skin, collagen, and blood vessels are essential elements in the hemostatic system. Any abnormality, inherited or acquired, in any one of these components of the vascular system will lead to mucosal bleeding such as: purpura, petechia, ecchymoses, or **telangiectasia** (Fig. 16.3). Tests of platelet function and numbers in these individuals will be normal. Senile purpura is a condition of aging in which skin loses its elasticity. Oftentimes, older individuals will bruise more easily and more prominently. Allergic purpura is seen in rare childhood disorders such as Henoch-Schönlein purpura, an immune complex disease that involves the skin, gastrointestinal tract, heart, and central nervous system. The purpura is often seen in the lower extremities. Purpura may occur due to infectious agents such as meningococcemia, Rocky Mountain spotted fever, staphylococci, or streptococcal infections.[23] Conditions such as amyloidosis, vitamin C deficiency (scurvy), or Cushing syndrome may result in purpura.

Inherited collagen disorders provoking the formation of purpuric lesions or telangiectasia are hereditary hemorrhagic telangiectasia (Osler-Weber-Rendu disease), an autosomal dominant disorder of the blood vessels. In this condition, small pinpoint hemorrhagic lesions are seen on the tongue, roof of the mouth, palate, face, and hands.[23] In addition to these lesions, nosebleeds are prominent and the lesions in general become more fragile with age. Kasabach-Merritt syndrome is a rare congenital disorder featuring giant **hemangiomas,**[23] bleeding, and thrombocytopenia. Hemangiomas may be found on the liver, skin, or spleen, and they are deep and bleed easily and profusely. DIC may develop if thromboplastic substances are released when the blood vessels burst.

Table 16.5 ●	Modified List of Drugs that Affect Platelet Function

- Penicillin
- Ampicillin
- Carbenicillin
- Cephalosporin
- Ticlopidine
- Clopidogrel
- Ibuprofen
- Aspirin
- Nitroglycerin
- Propranolol
- Nitroprusside

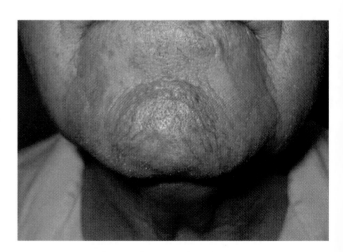

Figure 16.3   Telangiectasia.

CONDENSED CASE

A 14-year-old girl had a tooth extracted and was noted to have unexpected bleeding following extraction. She bled for 24 hours before the bleeding could be stopped. The dentist recommended that she have a hematology evaluation for the unexpected bleeding. **What questions concerning family history should be asked, and what baseline coagulation tests should be considered?**

Answer

This patient is exhibiting signs of mucosal bleeding, the type of bleeding seen in platelet adhesion defects such as vWD and BSS. The family of the patient should be asked about the bleeding history of family members, such as umbilical cord bleeding, circumcision bleeding, bleeding from minor cuts and abrasions, or gum or nose bleeding. The patient's mother revealed that her sibling had serious bleeding after a tonsillectomy procedure. This fact points to an autosomal defect. Routine studies that should be ordered are bleeding time (platelet function assay), PT, and aPTT. Factor assay should be considered if the PT or PTT are prolonged.

Summary Points

- A normal platelet count is 150 to 450 $\times 10^9$/L.

- Decreased platelet counts will lead to mucosal membrane bleeding such as gingival bleeding, epistaxis, purpura, and petechiae.

- Preanalytic variables that may lead to thrombocytopenia include improper mixing of tubes, improper anticoagulant used, and improper amount of sample collected.

- Acute idiopathic thrombocytopenia purpura is often a condition of children recovering from viral illness who show a dramatic drop in platelet count.

- Chronic idiopathic thrombocytopenia purpura occurs in adults as a result of an IgG antibody produced against platelets.

- Thrombotic thrombocytopenic purpura (TTP) and hemolytic uremic syndrome (HUS) are consumptive disorders of platelets.

- Individuals with TTP present with fever, a microangiopathic hemolytic anemia, neurological complications, thrombocytopenia, and renal failure.

- Individuals with HUS are predominantly children, with fever, bloody diarrhea, microangiopathic hemolytic anemia, thrombocytopenia, and renal failure.

- von Willebrand's disease (vWD) is a disorder of platelet adhesion in which von Willebrand factor is decreased or absent.

- vWD is the most common inherited qualitative platelet disorder, affecting 1% to 3% of the world's population.

- There are three primary types of vWD: type 1, type 2A, and type 3.

- Bernard Soulier syndrome is a platelet adhesion defect in which glycoprotein Ib is decreased or absent.

- Glanzmann's thrombasthenia is a defect of platelet aggregation that shows an absence of glycoprotein IIb/IIIa.

- Platelets from patients with vWD disease and Bernard Soulier syndrome will NOT aggregate with ristocetin.

- Aspirin impairs platelet function by interfering with the synthesis of thromboxane A_2, a potent platelet-aggregating agent.

- The platelet release function is impaired in the inherited disorders: Chediak-Higashi, Hermansky-Pudlak, Wiskott-Aldrich, gray platelet syndrome, and thrombocytopenia with absent radii syndrome.

- External conditions that alter platelet function include drugs, paraproteinemias, uremia, and the use of plasma expanders, like dextran.

- Skin, collagen, and blood vessels are essential elements in the hemostatic system.

- Any abnormality, inherited or acquired, in any one of these components of the vascular system will lead to mucosal bleeding such as purpura, petechiae, ecchymosis, or telangiectasia.

CASE STUDY

A 24-year-old woman was being evaluated by her gynecologist for menorrhagia. She gave a history of excessive menses since the age of 12. A CBC revealed a microcytic anemia and she began a course of ferrous sulfate therapy. Three months later, she had a follow-up visit with her gynecologist, and although her anemia was being corrected, she still complained of excessive menses. Her physician recommended her for a hematology consult. When asked about her family history, she revealed that her brother and mother had recurrent epistaxis and that her first cousin had a postpartum hemorrhage. The consulting physician ordered a CBC, PT, PTT, platelet aggregation studies, and bleeding time. ***Based upon this patient's history, what is the most likely outcome of this testing and what additional tests are to be considered?***

Insights to the Case Study

This patient gives a strong family history of mucosal bleeding. Although no member of her family has received a diagnosis of a bleeding disorder, it seems likely that she and some of them may have von Willebrand's disease, an autosomal dominant disorder. The patient's CBC and platelet count is normal; however, the PTT is slightly prolonged at 42 seconds. Factor assays for factor VIII and factor IX should be considered. Aggregation studies with collagen, ADP, and epinephrine were normal. Ristocetin aggregation was absent and the bleeding time test was abnormal with a result of 12 minutes (reference range, 3 to 9 minutes). A preliminary diagnosis of type 1 von Willebrand's disease was made pending the result of the vWF: AG by immunoassay. The hematologist recommended contraceptives as a way to control the patient's menstrual bleeding, and the patient was counseled on therapy alternatives such as DDAVP should she need dental extractions or minor surgery.

Review Questions

1. Which of the following are defects of platelet adhesion?
   a. Hermansky-Pudlak syndrome
   b. Glanzmann's thrombasthenia
   c. Bernard Soulier syndrome
   d. Wiskott-Aldrich

2. Which one of the conditions will produce a thrombocytopenia due to an altered distribution of platelets?
   a. Platelet satellitism
   b. Iron deficiency anemia
   c. Splenomegaly
   d. Chemotherapy

3. One of the main differences between TTP and HUS is:
   a. neurological involvement.
   b. kidney failure.
   c. thrombocytopenia.
   d. microangiopathic hemolytic anemia.

4. Nose bleeding, deep bruising, and gum bleeding are usually manifestations of which type of coagulation disorder?
   a. Clotting factor disorder
   b. Platelet defect
   c. Thrombosis
   d. Vascular disorder

5. The presence of thrombocytopenia and giant platelets best describes:
   a. classic von Willebrand's disease.
   b. Wiskott-Aldrich
   c. Glanzmann's thrombasthenia.
   d. Bernard Soulier syndrome.

6. Chronic idiopathic thrombocytopenia purpura (ITP):
   a. is found in children.
   b. usually spontaneously remits within several weeks.
   c. affects males more commonly than females.
   d. involves the immune destruction of platelets.

7. Aspirin prevents platelet aggregation by inhibiting the action of:
   a. PF 3.
   b. GP II.
   c. TXA_2.
   d. GP Ib.

⊙ TROUBLESHOOTING

What Do I Do When Preoperative Coagulation Studies Are Abnormal?

Preoperative testing was ordered on a 43-year-old woman scheduled for an elective hysterectomy. She has suffered with dysfunctional uterine bleeding for 6 months. Rather than go to the hospital setting, she went to a physician office laboratory that accepted her insurance. Her surgeon ordered a CBC with platelet count and a PT and PTT. Her CBC was within reference range but the results of her PT and aPTT were:

PT   10.6 seconds (Reference range, 10 to 14)

aPTT 53 seconds (Reference range, 28 to 38)

The elevated PTT was an unexpected result. Possibilities for an elevated PTT include a factor deficiency, the presence of a circulating anticoagulant, or a patient on heparin. Heparin was eliminated as a possible contributor to the prolonged PTT since there was no patient history of anticoagulation therapy. Mixing studies are familiar screening tests in the clinical laboratory to determine whether there is a factor deficiency or a circulating anticoagulant. The technologist decided to perform mixing studies on this patient and proceeded with the laboratory protocol. In mixing studies, the patient's plasma is mixed with pooled normal plasma, in a 1:1 ratio and the elevated test is repeated. Pooled normal plasma contains all clotting factors and technologists use normal quality control material as the source of pooled plasma. Once the test is repeated, if the result returns to the normal range, then it is assumed that the source of aPTT elevation was a clotting factor deficiency and factor assay tests on the plasma should be ordered. If the repeated test does not return to the reference range, then it is assumed that the patient plasma contains a circulating anticoagulant. As an additional screening procedure, the aPTT test was incubated for 1 to 2 hours. The rationale behind this additional step is to determine if there is a weak or time-dependent circulating inhibitor. Certain inhibitors such as factor VIII inhibitor have a stronger inhibitory effect with prolonged incubation. These pathological circulating inhibitors will be thoroughly discussed in Chapter 19.

WORD KEY

Alloimmunization • Antibodies that occur as a result of antigens introduced to the body through blood and tissue

Consanguinity • Relationships among close blood relatives

Cryoprecipitate • Product derived from fresh frozen plasma that is rich in factor VIII, von Willebrand factor, and fibrinogen

Cytotoxic • Antibody or toxin that attacks the cells of particular organs

Hemangiomas • Benign tumor of dilated blood vessels

HLA • Human leukocyte antigens, which are found in white blood cells and are part of the major histocompatibility complex

Hyperviscosity • Excessive resistance to the flow of liquids

Menorrhagia • Excessive menstrual bleeding

Microangiopathic • Related to pathology of small blood vessels

Paresthesias • Abnormal sensation that results from an injury to one or more nerves, described as numbness or prickly or tingling feeling

Telangiectasia • Vascular lesion formed by dilation of a group of small blood vessels, most frequently seen on face and thighs

References

1. Glassy E, ed. Color Atlas of Hematology: An Illustrated Field Guide based on Proficiency Testing. Illinois: Chicogo College of American Pathologists, 1998: 206.
2. Bruce L. Quantitative disorders of platelets. In: Rodak B, ed. Hematology: Clinical Principles and Applications, 2nd ed. Philadelphia: WB Saunders, 2002: 686.
3. Wolf BC, Neiman RS. Disorders of the Spleen. Philadelphia: WB Saunders, 1989: 22.
4. Blaney KD, Howard PR. Basic and Applied Concepts of Immunohematology. Boston: Mosby, 2000: 304.
5. vanden Bent PM, Meyboom PH, Egberts AC. Drug induced thrombocytopenia. Drug Saf 27:1243–1252, 2004.
6. Bengston K, Skinner M, Ware R. Successful use of anti-CD20 (Rituximab) in severe life threatening childhood ITP. J Pediatr 143:670–673, 2003.
7. Michel M, et al. Does *Helicobacter pylori* initiate or perpetuate immune thrombocytopenia purpura? Blood 103:890, 2004.
8. Ezra Y, Rose M, Eldor H. Therapy and prevention of thrombotic thrombocytopenia purpura during pregnancy: A clinical study of 16 pregnancies. Am J Hematol 51:1–6, 1996.
9. Zheng X, Chung D, Tekayama TK, et al. Structure of von Willebrand factor cleaving protease (ADAMS-13), a metalloprotease involved in thrombotic thrombocytopenic purpura. J Biol Chem 270:41059–41063, 2001.
10. Levy GC, Nicolas WC, Lian EC, et al. Mutations in a member of the ADAMTS gene family causing thrombotic thrombocytopenic purpura. Nature 413:488–494, 2001.

11. Kwaan HC, Soff GA. Management of thrombotic thrombocytopenic purpura and hemolytic uremic syndrome. Semin Hematol 34:159–166, 1997.

12. Bell A. Extracorpuscular defects leading to increased erythrocyte destruction: Nonimmune causes. In: Rodak B, ed. Hematology: Clinical Principles and Applications, 2nd ed Philadelphia: WB Saunders, 2002: 67.

13. Bruce L. Quantitative disorders of platelets. In Rodak B, ed. Hematology: Clinical Principles and Applications, 2nd ed. Philadelphia: WB Saunders, 2002: 697.

14. Sondoval C, Dong S, Visintainer P. Clinical and laboratory features of 178 children with recurrent epistaxis. J Pediatr Hematol 24:47–49, 2002.

15. Saxena R, Gupta M, Gupta PC. Inherited bleeding disorders in Indian women with menorrhagia. Hemophilia 9:193–196, 2003.

16. Lusher J. An underlying cause of menorrhagia. Mod Med 63:30–31, 1995.

17. Philips MD, Santhouse A. von Willebrand disease: Recent advances in pathophysiology and treatment. Am J Med Sci August:77–86, 1998.

18. Liles DK, Knupp CL. Quantitative and qualitative platelet disorders and vascular disorders. In: Harmening D, ed. Clinical Hematology and Fundamentals of Hemostasis. Philadelphia: FA Davis, 2002: 481.

19. Kunishima S, Kamiya T, Saito H. Genetic abnormalities of Bernard-Soulier syndrome. Int J Hematol 76: 319–327, 2002.

20. Rogers RL, Lazarchick J. Identifying Glanzmann's thrombasthenia. Lab Med 27:579–581, 1996.

21. Paper R, Kelley LA. A Guide to Living With von Willebrand Disease. Pennsylvania: Aventis Bering, 2002: 53.

22. Castellone D. Down and Dirty Coagulation: Practical Solutions and Answers. ASCP Workshop, May 7, 2004, Abstract 5799, Baltimore, MD.

23. Bick RL, Scates SM. Qualitative platelet defects. Lab Med 23:95–103, 1992.

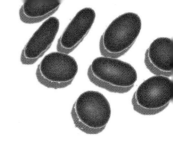

17

Defects of Plasma Clotting Factors

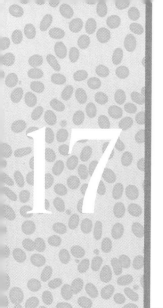

Betty Ciesla

Evaluation of a Bleeding Disorder and Types of Bleeding

The Classic Hemophilias

The Factor VIII Molecule

Symptoms in the Hemophilia A patient

Laboratory Diagnosis of Hemophilia Patients

Treatment for Hemophilia A Patients

Quality of Life Issues for Hemophilia A Patients

Hemophilia B or Christmas Disease

Congenital Factor Deficiencies With Bleeding Manifestations

Congenital Factor Deficiencies Where Bleeding Is Mild or Absent

Factor XIII Deficiency

Bleeding Secondary to a Chronic Disease Process

The Role of Vitamin K in Hemostasis

Vitamin K Deficiency and Subsequent Treatment

Objectives

After completing this chapter, the student will be able to:

1. Describe the variable types of bleeding found in patients with clotting factor deficiencies versus platelet disorders.

2. Define the factor VIII molecule.

3. Outline the genetics of the hemophilia disorders.

4. Describe the symptoms of an individual with hemophilia A and B.

5. Define the laboratory results in an individual with hemophilia A and B.

6. Describe the management and treatment of an individual with hemophilia A and B.

7. Distinguish the clotting factor disorders with little or no bleeding.

8. Distinguish the acquired factor disorders with regard to symptomatology and treatment.

EVALUATION OF A BLEEDING DISORDER AND TYPES OF BLEEDING

Patients who experience recurrent bleeding episodes are a select group of individuals that need to be evaluated for the source of their bleeding disorder. Bleeding may occur due to an inherited clotting factor defect or an acquired deficiency secondary to some other cause. Factors that should be considered in evaluating a bleeding disorder are the patient history, physical examination, laboratory testing, and family bleeding history. Often, the abnormal bleeding that they experience is not perceived as abnormal because that is all that they have ever known. Therefore, the questions that are asked relative to the types of and frequency of their bleeding need to be extremely specific and nonthreatening. Bleeding comes under two main categories: open bleeds and closed bleeds.

Open bleeds are those types of bleeding such as tongue bleeding, tonsil bleeding, gum bleeding, epistaxis, menorrhagia, umbilical cord bleeding, and circumcisional bleeding. Closed bleeds are soft tissue bleeds, genitourinary bleeding, gastrointestinal bleeding, and bleeding into the muscle, joints, skin, bone, or skull. Not every patient experiences all types of bleeding; some patients with clotting factor deficiencies never experience a bleeding episode. Yet, it is prudent to gather as much information as can be obtained to assess an individual with a history of bleeding.

Plasma clotting factors are inactive enzymes that circulate in plasma awaiting activation when injury occurs. They represent a significant ingredient to the proper clotting mechanism. Clotting factors that are poorly synthesized, inactivated by inhibitors, consumed by a rogue clotting process or functionally impaired will lead to faulty hemostasis.

THE CLASSIC HEMOPHILIAS

For most individuals the word *hemophilia* is at least a recognizable term. Many negative perceptions arise with this bleeding disorder including deep dark family secrets, profuse bleeding from small wounds, excruciating pain, and early death. By definition, *hemophilias* represent *any* of a group of disorders in which a particular clotting factor is decreased. With 13 clotting factors necessary for clot formation, there should be a wide range of hemophilias. Classically, however, only two disorders are referred to by the name *hemophilias*: hemophilia A, factor VIII deficiency and hemophilia B, factor IX deficiency. Both of these disorders are sex-linked recessive disorders, meaning that the mother carries the abnor-

mal gene and passes the gene to her sons. Not every male child will be affected, only those who inherit the abnormal gene. Likewise, if daughters inherit the abnormal gene, they are obligatory carriers. History is rich with accounts of hemophilia from the Talmud to British monarchy. Queen Victoria carried the abnormal gene and passed it through her offspring (nine births, five living children) into the Russian royal family, the Spanish dynasty, and the German royal family (Fig. 17.1). Victoria herself had no family history of hemophilia so her abnormal gene was acquired as a result of spontaneous mutation, which occurs in 30% of cases.

The Factor VIII Molecule

Factor VIII is the only one of the clotting factors that is not synthesized exclusively by the liver. It is unique among clotting factors for two reasons. Factor VIII is genetically controlled by the X chromosome (it is sex-linked), and it forms a complex with von Willebrand factor (vWF), which transports the factor into the circulation and is synthesized by an autosomal chromosome (Fig. 17.2). This clotting factor is also labile and unstable in stored plasma. In individuals with hemophilia A, the vWF level will be normal so that bleeding time will be normal; however, the aPTT will be abnormal because of the reduced level of factor VIII.

Symptoms in the Hemophilia A Patient

Clotting factors are measured in terms of their percent activity as well as their function in coagulation tests. Most clotting factors need to be available in the body at a minimum of 30% to achieve hemostasis. Bleeding manifestation in hemophilia A individuals are related to the level of factor VIII. There are three levels of clotting factor activity in hemophilia:

- Severe, <1%
- Moderate, 1% to 5%
- Mild, 6% to 24%

Patients with severe hemophilia A will manifest early bleeding manifestations such as circumcisional bleeds or umbilical cord bleeding. As they become more mobile, ordinary activities such as crawling, walking, or running may present challenges. It is not uncommon to see the severe hemophiliac child in protective gear (knee pads, ankle pads, helmet) for outside play. Bleeding may occur in other areas such as the gastrointestinal tract, the kidneys (hematuria), or gums or in **hematomas.** It is not accurate to say that individuals with hemophilia bleed more profusely. Rather, bleeding continues for a longer period of time due to the

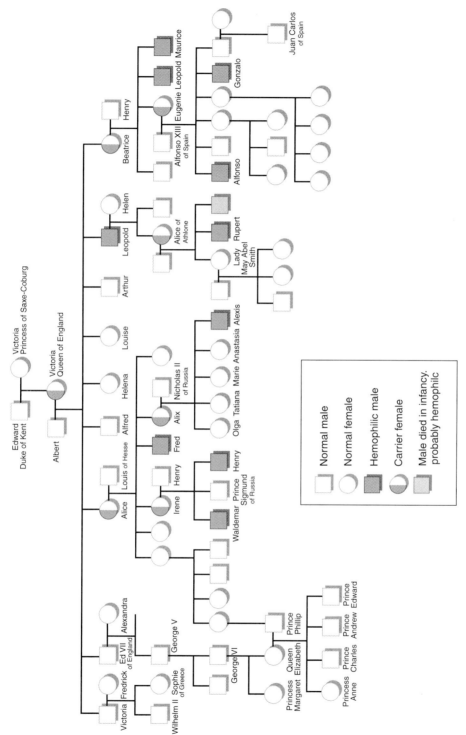

Figure 17.1 Queen Victoria carried the abnormal gene for thalassemia and passed it through her offspring into the Russian royal family, the Spanish dynasty, and the German royal family.

259

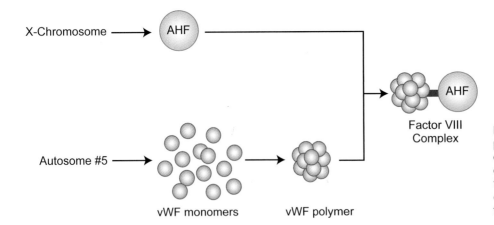

Figure 17.2 Factor VIII complex is controlled by the X chromosome and an autosomal chromosome. This complex transports factor VIII into the circulation. vWF, von Willebrand factor; AHF, antihemophilic factor.

decreased level of clotting factor. Platelet counts are normal and blood vessel function is adequate. Perhaps the most debilitating bleeds are muscle bleeds or joint bleeds, which have the potential for causing long-term disability, reduced range of motion, and intense pain. Joints become painful, swollen, and engorged with blood. **Hemarthrosis** occurs in the joints as pooled blood damages the surrounding tissue while a clot eventually forms. The joint become less and less mobile, limiting physical activity (Fig. 17.3). Internal hemorrhages into the muscles and deep soft tissues may compress and damage nerves. Intracranial bleeding is a leading cause of death in hemophilia A individuals, and other complications like paralysis, coma, memory loss, or stroke may precede an eventual fatality. Female carriers for the hemophilia gene rarely have symptoms, yet there are occasions when carrier females may become symptomatic. The union of a hemophilia patient and a female carrier would likely produce a symptomatic female.

Laboratory Diagnosis of Hemophilia Patients

Laboratory diagnosis of hemophilia patients is fairly uncomplicated. Laboratory tests which are ordered include bleeding time, PT, aPTT, and factor assays. In hemophilia, the bleeding time test is normal, the PT is normal, and aPTT is elevated, due to the reduced factor VIII. Single factor assays provide a means of assessing the percent activity of a clotting factor. These assays are performed using the aPTT test. A standard curve is created using serial dilutions of normal plasma of known factor levels and assigning a 1:10 dilution of normal plasma as 100% activity. Commercially prepared factor deficient plasma is then mixed with a 1:10 dilution of patient plasma and aPTT is performed. An aPTT that is

abnormal when mixed with a specific factor-deficient plasma suggests that the patient is missing the same clotting factor as that specific factor-deficient plasma. If the patient and deficient plasma give a normal result, then obviously the patient supplied the factor missing in the factor-deficient plasma. The aPTT result is plotted on the factor-activity curve, and the level of factor activity is derived from the standard curve.

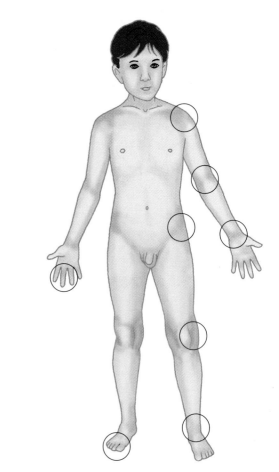

Figure 17.3 Hemarthrosis occurs in the joints as pooled blood damages the surrounding tissues.

Treatment for Hemophilia A Patients

Treatment options for hemophilia patients span decades and present one of the saddest treatment histories of any patient group with an inherited disorder. Factor VIII was discovered in 1937 and was termed antihemophilic globulin.[1] In the early days, treatment of hemophilia A patients consisted of giving whole blood units to relieve symptoms. Not until 1957 was it realized that the deficient coagulation protein was a component of the plasma portion of blood. Cryoprecipitate, a plasma derivative, was discovered in 1964. This product is produced as an insoluble precipitate that results when a unit of fresh frozen plasma is thawed in a standard blood bank refrigerator. Cryoprecipitate contains fibrinogen, factor VIII, and vWF. This product is extracted from plasma and usually pooled before it is given to the patient according to weight and level of factor VIII. This product presented a major breakthrough for the hemophilia population because it was an easily transfusable product affording the maximum level of factor to the individual. Next in the chronology of treatment products for hemophilia was clotting factor products. These freeze-dried products were developed in the early 1970s. The products were lyophilized and freeze dried and could be reconstituted and infused at home. This treatment offered the hemophilia population an independence that they had never previously experienced. Finally they were in control because they could self-infuse when necessary and provide themselves with prompt care when a bleeding episode developed. But a dark cloud loomed over the bleeding community. Approximately 80% to 90% of hemophilia A patients treated with factor concentrates became infected with the HIV virus. Factor concentrates were made from pooled plasma from a donor pool that was less than adequately screened. Additionally, manufacturing companies were less than stringent with sterilization methods and screening for HIV virus did not occur in blood banks until 1985. When each of these factors is brought to bear, the tragedy to the bleeding community is easily understood. According to the National Hemophilia Foundation,[2] there are 17,000 to 18,000 hemophilia patients (hemophilia A and B) in the United States. Of those, 4200 are infected with HIV/AIDS. There are no numbers available for wives or children who could have been secondarily infected. Recombinant products became available in 1989 and represent the highest purity product because they are not human derived. Recombinant technology uses genetic engineering to insert a clone of the factor VIII gene into mammalian cells, which express the gene characteristic. Production expenses for this product are unfortunately the most costly, and these costs are passed on to potential users.

Quality of Life Issues for Hemophilia A Patients

Having a child with severe hemophilia A or B presents special challenges to the parents and the family unit. The threat of hospitalizations, limited mobility, mainstreaming in schools, and the child's drive for independence present potentially stressful environments. Added to this is the cost of infusible factor, either recombinant or high purity products that could go as high as $50,000 if a patient has several bleeding episodes for which he needs to be hospitalized. Individuals with a chronic condition face many anxieties and may struggle with feelings of isolation, anger, and disappointment (Table 17.1). Fortunately, in the United States, there are hemophilia treatment centers that offer a network of needed services, and many states have local chapters of the National Hemophilia Foundation.[2] Prophylaxis with factor concentrates limits bleeding episodes, and the use of magnetic resonance imaging offers the physician a more effective means of evaluating joint damage.[3] Issues concerning medical insurance coverage continue to plague the hemophilia community.

The development of factor VIII inhibitors occurs in 15% to 20% of all hemophilia A individuals.[4] These inhibitors are autoantibodies against factor VIII that are time and temperature dependent and capable of neutralizing the coagulant portion of factor VIII. Treatment for patients who develop inhibitors is difficult and treatment protocols follow various paths. When the inhibitor is low titer or the individual is a low responder, physicians may infuse an appropriate level of factor VIII in an attempt to neutralize the inhibitor.[4] If this is not effective, patients must be treated with a factor sub-

Table 17.1 ⊙ Quality of Life Issues for Hemophilia A and B Patients

- Joint damage
- Reduced mobility
- Hemorrhage
- Fear
- Physical restrictions
- HIV/AIDS
- Hepatitis C
- Future insurability

stitute, usually **porcine** factor VIII or alternative therapies such as anti-inhibitor coagulant complex.[5] Gene therapy, as a treatment alternative, continues to provide hope for those suffering from hemophilia. The idea here is to insert a copy of the factor VIII or factor IX gene into a virus vector that will then lodge in the body and start producing normal amounts of circulating factor. Complications from rejection of the virus vector in humans have proved to be a delicate issue, yet there is optimism that gene therapy for hemophilia patients could eventually succeed.

Hemophilia B or Christmas Disease

Individuals with hemophilia B lack factor IX clotting factor. All of the conditions concerning inheritance, clinical symptoms, laboratory diagnosis, and complications are the same for severe hemophilia B individuals as for severe hemophilia A individuals. Hemophilia B accounts for only 10% of those with hemophilia. Patients with hemophilia B will have a prolonged aPTT and will have decreased factor assay activity. Treatment of hemophilia B consists of factor IX concentrates or prothrombin complex that is a mixture of factors II, VII, IX, and X.

Congenital Factor Deficiencies With Bleeding Manifestations

Patients having deficiencies of factors II, V, VII, and X are rare and are usually the result of consanguinity. Most of these disorders are autosomal recessive, affecting both males and females. Types of bleeding that may be observed are skin and mucous membrane bleeding. Joint and knee bleeding is unusual except for factor VII deficient patients. These patients may show joint hemorrhages and epistaxis. In a recent survey of the 225 hemophilia treatment centers in the United States, 7% of patients were identified with having a rare bleeding disorder.[6] Of these, factor VII was the most common. Abnormal preoperative screenings led to the diagnosis of most of these patients. When bleeding occurred in one half of these patients, no therapy was necessary.[6] Those individuals inheriting these deficiencies heterozygously tend to have few bleeding manifestations, since they will have one half of factor activity. Treatment of patients with inherited deficiencies of factors II, VII, and X consists of prothrombin complex concentrates. Factor VII clears rapidly from the plasma, and therefore booster doses are usually necessary to maintain clotting. Two new gene mutations, recently discovered, are especially pertinent to this discussion.

A prothrombin, factor II deficiency may occur as a result of a dysfunctional protein or as a result of diminished production of factor II. A structural defect in the protein is termed dysproteinemia and individuals with this particular deficiency may bleed. Additionally, a specific mutation in the prothrombin gene has been recognized since 1996. Located on chromosome 11, a single substitution of guanine to adenine at position 20210 of the prothrombin gene produces prothrombin G20210A. This mutation increases the prothrombin level and predisposes an individual to venous thrombosis.[7] Individuals should be screened for this mutation if any of the following are part of their patient history: a history of venous thrombosis at any age, venous thrombosis in unusual sites, a history of venous thrombosis during pregnancy, and a first episode of thrombosis before age 50.[8]

Another mutation recently discovered (1993) is factor V Leiden. This mutation is produced by substituting arginine with glutamine at position 506 of the factor V gene. The new gene product is factor V Leiden. In the normal coagulation scheme, once protein C is activated, it works to inactivate factors V and VIII, to inhibit the clotting mechanism. The mutated gene, factor V Leiden, impedes the degradation of factor V by protein C, causing activated protein C resistance. This condition accounts for increased clot formation with the subsequent development of deep vein thrombosis or other hypercoagulability conditions (see Chapter 19).

Congenital Factor Deficiencies Where Bleeding Is Mild or Absent

In this group of factor deficiencies are those concerned with contact activation and clot stabilization. Factors XI, XII, Fletcher, and Fitzgerald are each synthesized by the liver and are involved early in the coagulation cascade, in vitro. They become responsive when they contact surfaces such as glass in test tubes or ellagic acid in testing reagents. Factor XII deficiency is an autosomal recessive trait where there is a prolonged PTT in laboratory testing. Individuals with this deficiency do not bleed, however, and are more prone to pathologic clot formation. Factor XI deficiency or hemophilia C is an autosomal recessive trait with a high predominance in the Ashkenazi Jewish and Basque population in Southern France. The heterozygous frequency of this gene in this population group is 1:8.[9] Bleeding is unlikely, unless trauma or surgery occurs. There is little correlation between the level of factor XI activity and the severity of bleeding episodes. Fletcher factor or prekallikrein deficiency manifests itself as an autosomal dominant and recessive trait. Again patients experience thrombotic events such as myocardial infarction or pulmonary embolism. An interesting feature of this deficiency, in vitro, is that the initially prolonged aPTT will shorten upon prolonged incubation with kaolin reagents. Fitzgerald factor deficiency, also called high-molecular-weight kininogen deficiency, is a rare autosomal recessive trait. Deep vein thrombosis and pulmonary embolism are features of this disorder.[10]

Factor XIII Deficiency

Factor XIII is unique in that it is a transglutaminase rather than a protease as are most of the other coagulation factors. The role of this factor in coagulation is to provide stabilization to the fibrin clot through cross-linkage of fibrin polymers. Proper levels of factor XIII are essential for proper wound healing, hemostasis, and the maintenance of pregnancy. This factor is not tested for in the traditional coagulation tests such as PT, aPTT, thrombin time, or bleeding time. Therefore, in a patient with factor XIII disorder, the traditional coagulation screening test will be normal. Screening for factor XIII deficiency is accomplished through the 5 mol/L urea test, a primitive test which measures the stability or firmness of the clot after 24 hours in a 5 mol/L urea solution. If factor XIII is decreased, then the clot that is formed is stringy and loose, rather than the firm clot of stable hemostasis. Additionally, quantitative assays for factor XIII are available. Congenital deficiencies of factor XIII are rare autosomal recessive disorders. Deficiencies have been linked to poor wound healing, **keloid** formation, spontaneous abortion, and recurrent hematomas. Approximately, one half of patients have a family bleeding history, and large keloid scar formation appears to be a consistent finding in these patients.[11] Treatment of inherited disorders is through fresh frozen plasma or cryoprecipitate, a source of factor XIII. Acquired deficiencies of this factor may be associated with **Crohn's disease,** leukemias, DIC, and ulcerative colitis.

Bleeding Secondary to a Chronic Disease Process

Liver disease, renal disease, and autoimmune processes may lead to deficiencies in clotting factors that can cause bleeding. Because almost all of the procoagulants and inhibitors are synthesized by the liver, conditions such as alcoholic cirrhosis, biliary cancer, congenital liver defects, obstructive liver disease, and hepatitis can

each negatively affect clotting factor production and clotting factor function. Factors that have a short half-life such as factor VII and the vitamin K–dependent factors (II, VII, IX, and X) are particularly vulnerable. Liver disease brings a myriad of potential problems to coagulation capability. In addition to poor production and function of clotting factors, there is weak clearance of activated clotting factors and the accumulation of plasminogen activators. If plasmin is activated to a high degree, excessive clot lysis will be stimulated and DIC and hemorrhaging may result. Unexpectedly elevated prothrombin times in a previously well patient may signal the advent of liver disease and the patient should be carefully monitored. Patients with liver disease who are bleeding are treated with fresh frozen plasma, a source of all clotting factors and natural inhibitors. As little as 15 mL of plasma can increase the clotting factor activity by 15% to 25%.[12]

Renal disease, especially nephrotic syndrome, usually leads to poor renal filtration and the presence of low-molecular-weight coagulation proteins in the urine of about 25% of patients with these disorders. Impaired platelet function is a feature of renal disease, and patients with renal disorders are cautioned against taking aspirin or other platelet inhibitors.

The Role of Vitamin K in Hemostasis

Vitamin K is a fat-soluble vitamin necessary for the activation of factors II, VII, IX, and X. This vitamin is taken in through the diet in the form of green leafy vegetables, fish, and liver. It is also synthesized in small amounts by the intestinal bacteria *Bacteroides fragilis* and some strains of *Escherichia coli*. Newborns are usually vitamin K deficient because of the sterile environment of the small intestine, and therefore their levels of factors II, VII, IX, and X are low. Premature infants have levels of vitamin K–dependent factors as low as 20% to 30%.[13] As of the 1960s, all newborns are given vitamin K to avoid hemorrhagic disease of the newborn.

The vitamin K–dependent factors are low-molecular-weight proteins, with gamma-carboxyl residues at their terminal ends. To become activated and fully participate in the coagulation scheme, they must take on a second carboxyl group through the action of the enzyme gamma glutamyl carboxylase (Fig. 17.4). This reaction requires vitamin K. Once this reaction is accomplished, these factors can then bind to calcium and then to phospholipids for full participation in coagulation pathways.

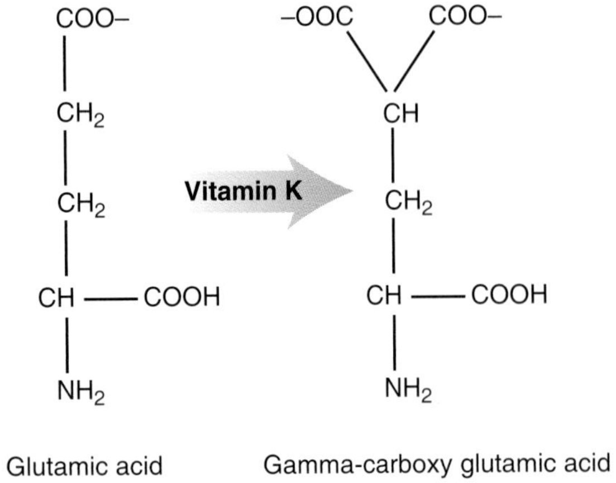

Figure 17.4 The carboxylation of the enzyme glutamic acid. This reaction requires vitamin K.

Table 17.2 ● Drugs That Cause a Deficiency of Vitamin K Clotting Factors

- Carbenicillin
- Moxalactam
- Cephamandole
- Cefoxitin
- Cefoperazone
- Tetracyclines
- Sulfonamides
- Aspirin

Vitamin K Deficiency and Subsequent Treatment

Vitamin K can be depleted through several mechanisms. Because body stores of vitamin K are extremely limited, dietary sources are important. In patients who have prolonged hospitalizations with only parenteral nutrition, dietary deficiency will likely develop and the patient may need to be supplemented. Long-term antibiotic therapy that disrupts normal flora, a source of vitamin K synthesis, may lead to vitamin K deficiency and subsequent bleeding. This is the case only if normal nutrition is also disrupted. Chronic diarrhea, biliary **atresia,** or other severe liver problems may lead to vitamin K synthesis, because bile salts are needed for proper absorption of vitamin K. Coumadin or warfarin oral anticoagulant therapy reacts because this substance is a vitamin K antagonist and therefore gamma carboxylation of factors II, VII, IX, and X is prevented. Patients on oral anticoagulant therapy need to be carefully monitored by anticoagulant clinics and diets need to be modified to compensate for the loss of vitamin K activity. Additionally, there is a long list of drugs that may interfere with vitamin K activity and subsequent hemostasis (Table 17.2).

If a patient is vitamin K depleted, the PT and aPTT will most likely be elevated but able to be corrected by normal plasma. Factor assays of the specific vitamin K factors will reveal a depressed activity. Factor VII with the shortest half-life will be depleted first within 2 days; the other factors will take between 3 and 10 days to reach low hemostatic levels. With mild bleeding, oral administration of vitamin K provides hemostatic recovery within a couple of hours. More emergent bleeding situations may result in parenteral administration of vitamin K, blood products, or infusion of prothrombin concentrate complex. An interesting side note is reports of patients who have used coumadin as an agent of suicide.[14]

Acquired inhibitors of coagulation will be discussed in Chapter 19.

CONDENSED CASE

A 7-year-old child had a fall from a piece of playground equipment. After 24 hours, he developed a deep hematoma in his right thigh and his parents brought him to the emergency department to be evaluated. His family history did not give any indication of any previous bleeding from birth or otherwise. **What tests should be ordered to rule out a coagulation defect?**

Answer

Although his family history does not indicate a clotting factor abnormality, preliminary clotting tests should include a bleeding time, PT, and aPTT. This patient has a normal PT but an aPTT of 50 seconds (reference range, 20 to 38 seconds). A factor assay was performed and indicated a mild factor VIII activity of 40% with a reference range of 50% to 150% activity. The patient was diagnosed with mild hemophilia A. This accident brought a previously undiagnosed condition to light. This is important information in this patient's personal and medical history. Future surgeries or traumas will need to be carefully monitored.

Summary Points

- Patients with recurrent bleeding episodes need to be evaluated for an inherited bleeding disorder.
- Bleeding comes under two main categories: open bleeds or closed bleeds.
- Plasma clotting factors need to maintain approximately 30% activity to achieve adequate clotting.
- The factor VIII molecule is carried into plasma by vWF.
- Hemophilias A and B are sex-linked recessive disorders.
- In hemophilia A, factor VIII is deficient; in hemophilia B, factor IX is deficient.
- Women are carriers of the defective hemophilia gene.
- Individuals with hemophilia experience prolonged bleeding from minor wounds.
- Individuals with hemophilia may experience many types of bleeding including joint bleeding leading to hemarthrosis, hematomas, umbilical cord bleeding, or mucosal bleeds.
- The bleeding time is normal in hemophilia A and B patients; the aPTT is elevated.
- Current treatment for hemophilia individuals consists of recombinant factor products.
- Most individuals with hemophilia in the United States use factor concentrates prophylactically.
- Prophylactic infusion of factor concentrates has minimized the physical disabilities that may have occurred from unexpected bleeding episodes.

- From 15% to 20% of all hemophilia A individuals develop factor VIII inhibitors.
- Individuals with factor II, V, VII, and X deficiencies may have minimal bleeding.
- Prothrombin complex concentrate is used to correct deficiencies of factors II, VII, IX, and X.
- Prothrombin G20210A is a mutation of the prothrombin molecule.
- Factor V Leiden is a genetic mutation of the factor V molecule that predisposes to clotting episodes.
- Deficiencies of factors XI, XII, Fletcher, and Fitzgerald usually lead to increased thrombotic events.
- Factor XIII is unique among clotting factors because it is a transglutaminase; the other clotting factors are proteases.
- An inherited deficiency of factor XIII may lead to poor wound healing and spontaneous abortions.
- Liver disease, renal disease, and autoimmune processes may lead to deficiencies in clotting factors that cause bleeding.
- Vitamin K is a fat-soluble vitamin necessary for the activation of factors II, VII, IX, and X.
- Vitamin K is available through the diet; small amounts are synthesized by normal intestinal flora.
- Newborns are vitamin K deficient and are given vitamin K at birth to avoid hemorrhagic disease of the newborn.
- If vitamin K is depleted, the PT and PTT will be prolonged.
- Coumadin, a therapeutic anticoagulant, is a vitamin K antagonist.

CASE STUDY

A 54-year-old woman was admitted to the hospital with hematuria, anemia, easy bruising, and progressive weakness. She gave no previous bleeding history or family history of bleeding even though she had multiple surgeries in the past. Her surgeries included knee replacement. During this admission, she is complaining of a deep bruise in her right upper thigh and hematuria. Her admitting laboratory data included the following:

WBC	6.0×10^9/L
Hgb	6.8 g/dL
Hct	20.2%
Platelets	321×10^9/L
PT	12.5 seconds (reference range, 10.5 to 12.4)
aPTT	67.6 seconds (reference range, <40)
Mixing studies: Immediate mixing and repeat PTT	39.6 seconds
aPTT after 1 hour	54.2 seconds
Factor VIII	4% (reference range, 50% to 150%)

What is your initial impression?

(continued on following page)

(Continued)

Insights to the Case Study

This patient's family history is helpful in eliminating a congenital hemostatic defect as a source of her hematuria. She has had successful surgery events in the past but now suffers with hematuria and deep bruising. An elevated aPTT value can be seen in anticoagulant therapy, particularly heparin, in clotting factor defects, and if a circulating inhibitor is present. Mixing studies in this patient show variable results with initial correction of the patient's aPTT and then subsequent prolongation upon incubation. A factor VIII inhibitor was considered as a likely explanation for the laboratory results and the low factor VIII assay value. Inhibitors or autoantibodies against factor VIII may develop in populations other than the hemophilia A population, where 10% to 30% develop these type of inhibitors. These inhibitors are directed against a portion of the factor VIII molecule and are time and temperature dependent. Once identified, the inhibitor should be quantitated using the Bethesda titer. In this procedure, equal volumes of pooled normal plasma that is platelet poor are mixed with patient platelet poor plasma at pH 7.4. The mixture is incubated for 2 hours and the PTT is repeated. If the patient plasma has anti–factor VIII activity, then some of the active factor VIII in the normal plasma will be affected. The level of inhibitor is seen as a percentage of the normal activity of the factor when compared to the control plasma. One Bethesda unit is equivalent to the inhibitor in which 50% factor activity will remain.

Review Questions

1. Which of the clotting factors is not a protease?
   a. Factor II
   b. Factor VII
   c. Factor XIII
   d. Factor IX

2. Why is the bleeding time normal in hemophilia A?
   a. Because of an increase in factor XIII
   b. Because the clotting problem is a factor VIII problem
   c. Because vWF is normal
   d. Because the clotting problem is a factor IX problem

3. The purest treatment product for hemophilia A patients is:

   a. cryoprecipitate.
   b. fresh frozen plasma.
   c. prothrombin complex concentrate.
   d. recombinant factor VIII.

4. One of the more fatal bleeds in a hemophilia patient involves:
   a. intracranial bleeding.
   b. mucosal bleeding.
   c. joint bleeding.
   d. epistaxis.

5. Which clotting factor deficiency is associated with poor wound healing?
   a. Factor II
   b. Factor X
   c. Factor XII
   d. Factor XIII

○ TROUBLESHOOTING

What Do I Do When Laboratory Results Are Not Consistent With the Patient's Physical Presentation?

A 74-year-old woman arrived in the emergency department with bruising over most of her extremities.

She gave no family or personal history of bleeding but did indicate that she had delivered eight children. Her bleeding time was slightly abnormal at 9 minutes (reference < 8 minutes), but her PT and aPTT were within normal range. Factor assays of factors VIII and IX were normal, and platelet aggregation studies were normal. What are the possibilities for the incongruities in this patient workup?

This patient presented a diagnostic dilemma. Quality control was verified at all levels on all pieces of equipment used. A repeat bleeding time, PT, and aPTT were performed and fell within ranges similar to the original. Factor assays were not repeated. These results stumped the coagulation staff. After careful consideration of exactly what was being tested for, the possibility of a factor XIII deficiency was considered. Factor XIII is necessary for clot stabilization and would healing. A 5 mol/L urea test was performed, and the results were abnormal. An inherited deficiency of factor XIII is the rarest of all of the bleeding disorders, presenting as autosomal recessive. Our patient has a history of multiple pregnancies and successful deliveries; therefore an inherited coagulation deficiency was not considered. A thorough medication check revealed that the patient was on cardiac medication, which potentially could have caused an inhibitory effect on factor XIII, because all other factor-related assays were normal. Cryoprecipitate was infused to prevent any future bleeding complication. The patient's cardiac medication was discontinued, and the patient was given an appropriate alternative medication for her cardiac condition.

(Many thanks to D. Castellone for the resource material for this case.)

WORD KEY

Atresia • As in biliary atresia, congenital closure, or absence of some or all of the major bile ducts

Crohn's disease • Inflammatory bowel disease marked by patchy areas of inflammation from the mouth to the anus

Hemarthrosis • Bloody effusion inside the joint

Hematoma • Swelling composed of a mass of clotted blood confined to an organ, tissue, or space or caused by a break in the blood vessel

Keloid • Scar that forms at the site of injury that appears to have a rubbery consistency and shiny surface

Porcine • Of or relating to swine (pigs)

References

1. Corriveau DM. Major elements of hemostasis. In: Corriveau DM, Fritsma GA, eds. Hemostasis and Thrombosis in the Clinical Laboratory. Philadelphia: JB Lippincott, 1988: 6.
2. www.hemophilia.org. Accessed June 14, 2005.
3. Berntrop E, Michiels JJ. A healthy hemophilic patient without arthropathy: From concept to clinical reality. Semin Thromb Hemost 29:5–10, 2003.
4. Fritsma G. Hemorrhagic coagulation disorders. In Rodak B, ed. Hematology: Clinical Principles and Applications, 2nd ed. Philadelphia: WB Saunders, 2002: 639–640.
5. Kleinman MB. Anti-inhibitor coagulant complex for the rescue therapy of acquired inhibitors to factor VIII: Case report and review of literature. Hemophilia 8:694–697, 2002.
6. Acharya SS, Coughlin A, Dimichele DM, et al. Rare Bleeding Disorder Registry: Deficiencies of II, V, X, fibrinogen and dysfibrinogenemia. J Thromb Hasemost 2:248–256, 2004.
7. Jensen R. Screening and molecular diagnosis in hemostasis. Clin Hemost Rev 13:12, 1999.
8. McGlennen RC, Key NS. Clinical laboratory management of the prothrombin G20210A mutation. Arch Pathol Lab Med 126:1319–1325, 2002.
9. Seligsohn U. High frequency of factor XI (PTA) deficiency in Ashkenazi Jews. Blood 51:1223, 1978.
10. Cheung PP, et al. Total kininogen deficiency (Williams trait) is due to an argstop mutation in exon 5 of the human kininogen gene. Blood 78:3919, 1991.
11. Al-Sharif FZ, Aljurf MD, Al-Momen AM, et al. Clinical and laboratory features of congenital F XIII deficiency. Saudi Med J 23:552–554, 2002.
12. Weiss AE. Acquired coagulation disorders. In: Corriveau DM, Fritsma GA, eds. Hemostasis and Thrombosis in the Clinical Laboratory. Philadelphia: JB Lippincott, 1988: 176.
13. Zipursky A, Desa D, Hsu E, et al. Clinical and laboratory diagnosis of hemostatic disorders in newborn infants. Am J Pediatr Hematol Oncol 1:217–226, 1979.
14. Fritsma GA. Hemorrhagic coagulation disorders. In: Rodak B, ed. Hematology: Clinical Principles and Applications. Philadelphia: WB Saunders, 2002: 173.

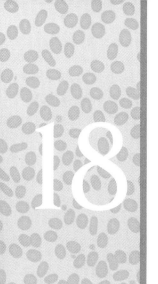
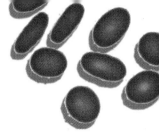

18

Fibrinogen, Thrombin, and the Fibrinolytic System

Betty Ciesla

The Role of Fibrinogen in Hemostasis

Disorders of Fibrinogen
Afibrinogenemia
Hypofibrinogenemia
Dysfibrinogenemia

The Unique Role of Thrombin in Hemostasis
Physiological Activators of Fibrinolysis
Naturally Occurring Inhibitors of Fibrinolysis
Measurable Products of the Fibrinolytic System

Disseminated Intravascular Coagulation
The Mechanism of Acute Disseminated Intravascular Coagulation
Clinical Symptoms and Laboratory Results in Acute Disseminated Intravascular Coagulation
Treatment in Acute Disseminated Intravascular Coagulation

Objectives

After completing this chapter, the student will be able to:

1. Identify the components of the fibrinolytic system.

2. Recall the role of fibrinogen in the coagulation and the fibrinolytic system.

3. Describe plasmin in terms of activation and inhibition.

4. Differentiate the role of thrombin in both the coagulation and fibrinolytic system.

5. Outline the inherited disorders of fibrinogen.

6. Describe the laboratory testing for fibrinolytic disorders.

7. Define conditions that may precipitate disseminated intravascular coagulation states.

8. Describe the laboratory testing and management of patients with disseminated intravascular coagulation event.

THE ROLE OF FIBRINOGEN IN HEMOSTASIS

Fibrinogen is the principal substrate of the coagulation and fibrinolytic system. This clotting factor has the highest molecular weight of all of the clotting factors, and it is the substrate upon which the coagulation system is centered. This factor is heat labile but stable in storage. When fibrinogen is transformed to fibrin under the influence of thrombin, it is the onset of solid clot formation. The formation of fibrin occurs within minutes due in part to a positive feedback mechanism within the hemostasis system. Once clotting factors are activated, they accelerate the activity of the next factor, pushing the reaction to conclusion. Negative feedback occurs when the activity of the reaction is delayed. This is the role played by naturally occurring inhibitors within the hemostatic system. With the assistance of factor XIII and thrombin, the fibrinogen molecule is stabilized by cross-linked fibrin. Within hours, the fibrinolytic system swoops in to dissolve the clots that have formed and to restore blood flow. The creation of cross-linked fibrin is an orderly process by which fibrinogen is cleaved into fibrinopeptides A and B by thrombin. Fibrinogen is composed of three pairs of polypeptide chains: alpha, beta, and gamma. When thrombin is generated, it cleaves small portions of the alpha and beta chains, creating fibrinopeptides A and B. The remaining portions of the alpha and beta chains stay attached to the fibrinogen molecule. With fibrinopeptides A and B cleaved, the fibrin monomer is created. These monomers spontaneously polymerize by hydrogen bonding to form a loose fibrin network, which is soluble. Trapped within the soluble clot are thrombin, antiplasmins, plasminogen, and tissue plasminogen activator (tPA). Because thrombin is now protected from its inhibitors, it activates factor XIII and calcium and then catalyzes the formation of peptide bonds between monomers, forming fibrin polymers that lead to an insoluble and resistant clot[1] (Fig. 18.1). Balance between the coagulation and fibrinolytic systems is critical for maintenance of circulation and injury repair. An imbalance in the coagulation system could cause excess clotting; an imbalance of the fibrinolytic system could cause hemorrhaging. Several other components may play a role in hemostatic balance. In early studies, it has been suggested that individuals with a high concentration of lipoprotein A may have reduced fibrinolytic activity due to decreased plasmin generation. Cholesterol and triglycerides are all fatty components of lipoproteins. It is conceivable that reduced plasmin generating activity in individuals with increased levels of lipoprotein will lead to less clot dissolution, leaving clots available for a pathological outcome.[2]

DISORDERS OF FIBRINOGEN

Appropriate levels of fibrinogen are necessary to maintain hemostasis and to cause platelets to aggregate. The reference range for fibrinogen is 200 to 400 mg/dL. Fibrinogen is an acute-phase reactant, meaning that there will be a transient increase in fibrinogen during inflammation, pregnancy, stress, and diabetes and when taking oral contraceptives. Therefore, a careful patient history is necessary when evaluating a problem involving fibrinogen. For the most part, decreases in fibrinogen result from acquired disorders such as acute liver disease, acute renal disease, or disseminated intravascular coagulation. Acquired increases in fibrinogen may be demonstrated in hepatitis patients, pregnant patients, or those with atherosclerosis.[3] The inherited disorders of fibrinogen are afibrinogenemia, hypofibrinogenemia, and dysfibrinogenemia. These conditions are rare and are marked by hematomas, hemorrhage, and ecchymoses depending upon severity.

Afibrinogenemia

The homozygous disorder, afibrinogenemia, is an autosomal recessive disorder that shows less than 10 mg/dL fibrinogen in the plasma. This small amount of fibrinogen is usually not demonstrable by traditional methods. Infants with afibrinogenemia will show bleeding from the umbilical stump; poor wound healing and spontaneous abortion are also features of this disorder. Laboratory results will show elevated PT, aPTT, **thrombin time (TT), reptilase time,** and abnormal platelet aggregation with most aggregating agents and elongated bleeding time. Cryoprecipitate and fresh frozen plasma are the replacement products used for medical management of bleeds for these patients.

Hypofibrinogenemia

Hypofibrinogenemia is the heterozygous form of afibrinogenemia. This disorder is autosomal recessive and patients show between 20 and 100 mg/dL fibrinogen in their plasma. Patients with this disorder may show mild spontaneous bleeding and severe postoperative bleeding. Results of laboratory testing, whether prolonged or normal, will depend on the amount of fibrinogen present.

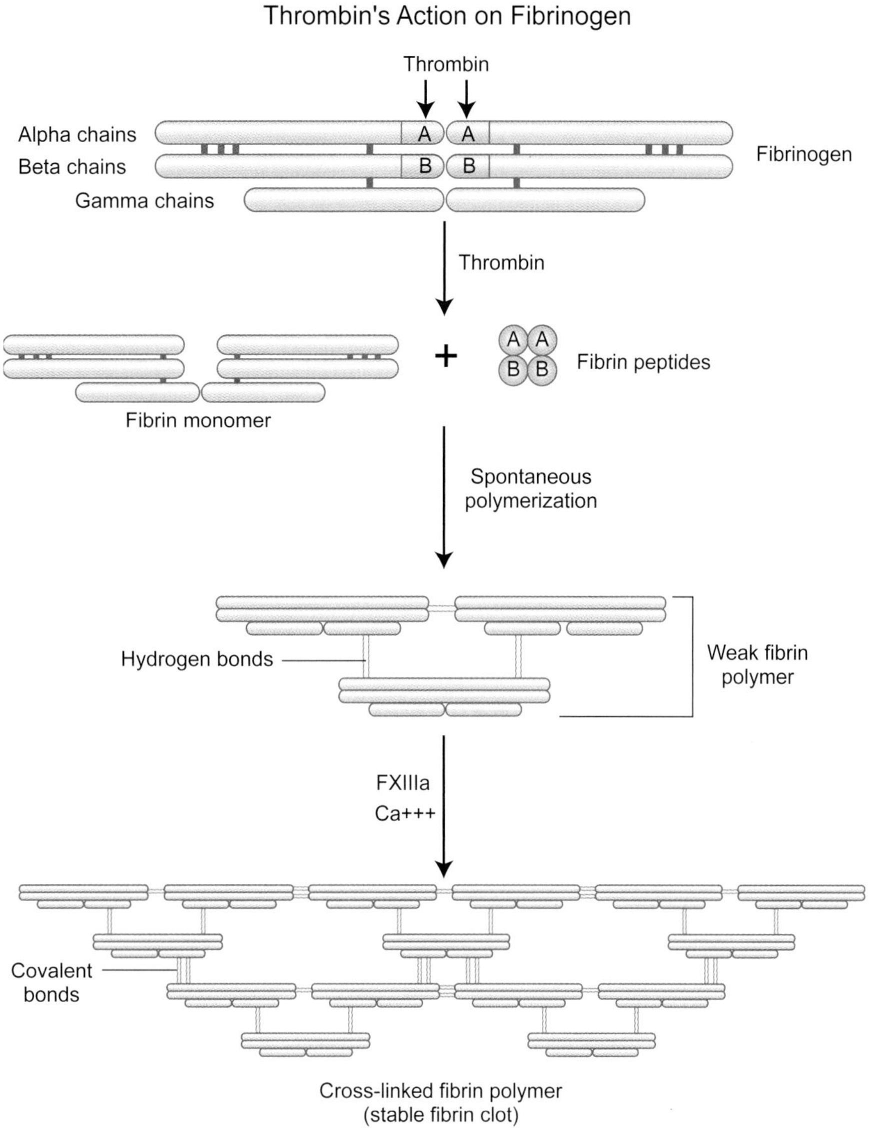

Thrombin's Action on Fibrinogen

Figure 18.1 Thrombin's activity on fibrinogen, from fibrin monomer to fibrin polymer.

Dysfibrinogenemia

These fibrinogen disorders are autosomal dominant and are inherited homozygously and heterozygously. They produce a qualitative disorder of fibrinogen in which an amino acid substitution produces a functionally abnormal fibrinogen molecule. Although these disorders are an academic curiosity, named for the city in which the patient was discovered, they are infrequently associated with a bleeding tendency. A few are associated with thrombosis.[4] Approximately 40 abnormal fibrinogens have been discovered. Because fibrin formation is affected by the abnormal fibrinogen molecule in dysfibrinogenemia, most of the normal laboratory assessments for fibrinogen will be abnormal. The PT, aPTT, TT, and reptilase time will be increased. An **immunologic assay** of fibrinogen that measures the antigenic level of fibrinogen is normal. The clottable assay for quantitative fibrinogen is abnormal as this assay is dependent on the proper amount and proper functioning fibrinogen.

THE UNIQUE ROLE OF THROMBIN IN HEMOSTASIS

Thrombin holds a respected place in the coagulation mechanism for its multiplicity of function and the numerous reactions it mediates. The impact of thrombin is far reaching from the initial activation of the platelet system to the initiation of the fibrinolytic system and subsequent tissue repair. Prothrombin is the precursor to thrombin and can only be converted by the action of factor X, factor V, platelet factor 3, and calcium. Thrombin is generated in small concentrations through injury to the endothelial cells and proceeds to initiate a more enhanced coagulation mechanism. Once generated, thrombin is involved in the platelet release reaction as well as platelet aggregation. Secondarily, thrombin stimulates platelets to produce the platelet inhibitor, prostacyclin, or PGI$_2$. With the coagulation system alerted, thrombin activates factors V and VIII, key cofactors in thrombus formation. Protein C, a naturally occurring inhibitor to coagulation, is also activated by thrombin. An additional product thrombomodulin which is secreted by endothelial cells amplifies protein C activity when complexed with thrombin.[5] With respect to the fibrinogen degradation, thrombin plays a key role in negative feedback by converting plasminogen to plasmin to digest the soluble fibrin clot. This interplay of thrombin disposition and thrombin initiation of clot disposal is part of the biologic control of hemostasis. Once the clot is dissolved, thrombin plays a role in repairing tissue and wounds (Fig. 18.2).

Physiological Activators of Fibrinolysis

A critical link in the chain of hemostasis is the dissolution of fibrin clots, which usually occurs several hours after the stable clot is formed. In this way, blood flow is restored at the local levels and tissue healing is precipitated. The body provides naturally occurring or physiological activators that initiate this process. The key component in this reaction is plasminogen, a plasma enzyme synthesized in the liver with a half-life of 48 hours. Plasminogen is converted to plasmin, chiefly through the action of tissue plasminogen activator (tPA), a substance released through the activity of endothelial cell damage and the production of thrombin. Additional plasminogen activators include factor

XIIa, kallikrein, and high-molecular-weight kininogen. Once produced, plasmin, a potent enzyme, does not distinguish between fibrin and fibrinogen and works to digest both. Additionally, plasmin also hydrolyzes factors V and VIII, and if circulating in the plasma as pathological free plasmin, the damage to the coagulation system is significant, as clots are dissolved indiscriminately. Of interest is the fact that tPA has been synthesized by **recombinant** technology and is presently used as a pharmaceutical product during stroke episodes for fibrinolytic therapy. As a "clot-busting" drug, it has been effective in thrombotic strokes and if injected within a small time-frame can spare the patient serious stroke side effects. Another plasminogen activator is urokinase, a protease present in the urine and produced by the kidney. The physiological effect of urokinase is minimal in clot dissolution; however, like tPA it is a valuable commercial product used in **thrombolytic therapy,** for patients with heart attacks, strokes, and other thrombotic episodes.[6] Streptokinase is an exogenous fibrinolytic agent, produced when a bacterial cell product forms a complex with plasminogen, a pairing that converts plasminogen to plasmin. This toxic product results from infection with beta-hemolytic streptococci and is a dangerous byproduct if this bacterial strain develops into a systemic infection. It has the most activity on fibrinogen.

Naturally Occurring Inhibitors of Fibrinolysis

The balance of hemostasis is aided by those products that restrain fibrinolytic activity. These products, plasminogen activator inhibitor 1 (PAI-1) and alpha-2-antiplasmin, act upon different substrates in the fibri-

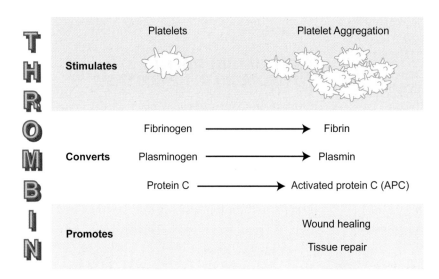

Figure 18.2 The multiple roles of thrombin in hemostasis.

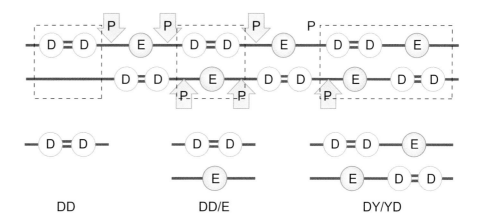

Figure 18.3 The formation of D-dimer and fibrin degradation products. P, plasmin; D, D domain; E, E domain.

P= Plasmin
D= D domain
E= E domain

nolytic system. PAI-1 is secreted by endothelial cells during injury and suppresses the function of tPA in the plasminogen-plasmin complex. Plasmin as a substrate is directly inhibited by alpha-2-antiplasmin in a 1:1 ratio at the target area. This inhibitor prevents plasmin binding to fibrin in an orderly fashion and claims the role as the most important inhibitor of the fibrinolytic system. Inherited deficiencies of this inhibitor invariably lead to hemorrhagic episodes. Secondary agents that can inhibit fibrinolysis are alpha-2-macroglobulin, C1 inactivator, and alpha-1-antitrypsin. These substances, as protease inhibitors, act upon thrombin formation. Because thrombin is one of the initiators of the generation of plasmin, the secondary effect on the fibrinolytic system is unavoidable.

Measurable Products of the Fibrinolytic System

Physiological fibrinolysis occurs in an orderly fashion, producing measurable products that can be captured by laboratory assays. Specifically, the byproducts of an orderly fibrinolytic system are fibrin split/degradation (FSP/FDP) products composed of fibrin fragments labeled as X, Y, D, and E and the D-dimers, D-D (Fig. 18.3).

The accurate and precise measurement of these products is the basis for therapeutic decisions once pathological clot forming and lysing has been initiated. FSPs/FDPs are formed from plasmin action on fibrin and fibrinogen. As plasmin degrades the fibrinogen molecule, different fragments are split leading to early and late degradation products. Normal levels of FDPs are eliminated through the RES system and usually measure

less than 40 µg/mL. Individuals with an intact and operational hemostatic system have normal FDPs. These products are measured semiquantitatively through direct latex agglutination of a thrombin clotted sample. Latex particles are coated with **monoclonal** antibodies to the human fibrinogen fragments D and E. The test is performed on serum using two dilutions, 1:15 and 1:20. It does not distinguish between fibrinogen and fibrin. Pathological levels of FDPs interfere with thrombin formation and platelet aggregation. Elevated levels may be seen in DIC, pulmonary embolism, obstetrical complications, and other conditions[7] (Table 18.1).

Once fibrin has been cross-linked and stabilized by factor XIII, a stable clot has been formed. When this clot is dissolved by plasmin, D-dimers are released. Therefore, D-dimers suggest a breakdown of fibrin clot

Table 18.1 ● Conditions That May Elevate Fibrin Degradation Products
• Disseminated intravascular coagulation
• Pulmonary embolism
• Abruptio placentae
• Preeclampsia
• Eclampsia
• Fetal death in utero
• Postpartum hemorrhage
• Polycystic disease
• Malignancies
• Lupus nephritis
• Thrombolytic therapy

and indirectly are an indication that clots have been formed at the site of injury, at the local level. Excess D-dimers are indicative of breakdown of fibrin products within the circulating blood. D-dimers can be assayed semiquantitatively and quantitatively. The semiquantitative assay uses monoclonal antibodies specific for this domain. A simple agglutination test, undiluted patient plasma is mixed with latex solution. Noticeable agglutination is a positive test and indicative of deep vein thrombosis (DVT), pulmonary embolism (PE), or disseminated intravascular coagulation (DIC). Quantitative D-dimer tests are automated and use an enzyme-linked immunosorbent assay (ELISA) procedure. The advantage of this procedure is its ability to detect low levels of D-dimer and to provide specific information as to whether pathological clotting as in DVT or PE has occurred. D-dimers assays have great utility in monitoring thrombolytic therapy.[8]

DISSEMINATED INTRAVASCULAR COAGULATION

The mere mention of the words "the patient has DIC" usually strikes fear into the hearts of attending physicians, laboratorians, and nursing staff. The acute DIC event is almost always unanticipated and dramatic. Fatal outcomes do occur. DIC is triggered by an underlying pathological circumstance occurring in the body (Fig. 18.4). As a result, the hemostatic system becomes unbalanced, hyperactivating the coagulation and/or the fibrinolytic system. This process is systemic, leading to excessive disposition of thrombi or excessive hemorrhage. Additionally, the process is consumptive, consuming clotting factors and platelets as soon as they are activated for coagulation. Usually the decrease in clotting factors is more overpowering than the increase in lysis. In broad terms, DIC is associated with obstetrical complications, malignancy, massive trauma, bacterial sepsis, asplenia, or necrotic tissue. Under each of these major headings are many other pathological possibilities for the initiation of a DIC event (see Table 18.2). Although most DIC occurs as acute, explosive episodes, there are conditions that may lead to a chronic compensated DIC state. These are much more difficult to diagnose because the bone marrow and liver perform an excellent job of maintaining equilibrium between the coagulation and the fibrinolytic system. Laboratory results may be minimally abnormal; yet once the underlying pathology intensifies, an acute DIC episode is likely.[9]

The Mechanism of Acute Disseminated Intravascular Coagulation

As is customary in normal hemostasis, both the coagulation and the fibrinolytic system are activated in parallel. What is missing in DIC is the negative feedback mechanism that holds the systems in balance. Table 18.2 is a composite of events in the DIC cycle:

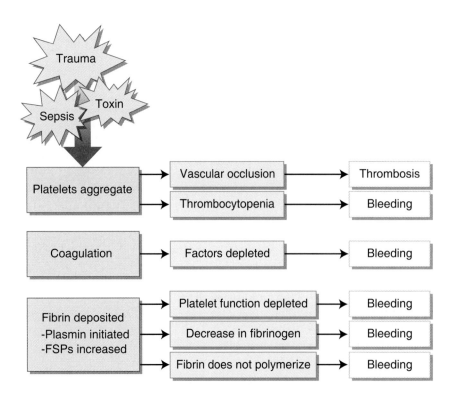

Figure 18.4 Conditions that may precipitate disseminated intravascular coagulation (DIC). Note the multiple pathways. FSPs, fibrin split products.

Table 18.2 ◉ Events Triggering Disseminated Intravascular Coagulation

Infections
- Gram-negative bacteria
- Gram-positive bacteria
- Malaria

Tissue Injury
- Crush injury
- Burns
- Massive head injury

Malignancy
- Acute promyelocytic leukemia
- Acute monoblastic or myeloblastic leukemia
- Microangiopathic disorders
- Thrombotic thrombo-cytopenia purpura
- Heat stroke

Gastrointestinal disorders
- Acute hepatitis

Obstetrical complications
- Maternal toxemia
- Abruptio placentae
- Hemolytic disease of the newborn
- Group B streptococcal infection
- Retained dead fetus

Other
- Snake bites
- Heparin-induced thrombosis
- Septic shock
- Hemolytic transfusion reaction
- Graft versus host disease

- Excessive generation of thrombin is triggered by thromboplastin release (endothelial cells, placenta, leukemic cells [promyelocytes or monoblasts], tumors).
- Simultaneous enzymatic conversion of fibrinogen to fibrin occurs.
- Plasmin generation simultaneously degrades fibrinogen/fibrin into FDPs; excess FDPs are formed.
- FDPs have affinity for fibrin monomers but fail to polymerize properly; excess FDPs have an anticoagulant effect.
- Plasmin causes inactivation of factors V, VIII, XI, and XII.
- Hemorrhage occurs as soluble fibrin monomers are formed; platelets are inactivated and clotting factors are inactivated as both are coated by the soluble monomers.
- Clots that are formed are not stable.

Although the body attempts to minimize damage once a DIC event occurs, the physiological inhibitors protein C, protein S, and thrombomodulin are each inactivated. A disorder related to DIC is primary fibrinolysis: activation of plasmin within the circulation by sources other than thrombin activation. In this rare condition, plasmin acts on fibrinogen and fibrin indiscriminately, therefore hemorrhage is inevitable. Since thrombin is bypassed, the platelet count is normal unlike the platelet count in DIC. Yet all other parts of the DIC coagulation profile are abnormal. There is controversy as to whether primary fibrinolysis is a disease entity unto itself or rather just a continuum in the vicious DIC cycle.

Clinical Symptoms and Laboratory Results in Acute Disseminated Intravascular Coagulation

In hemorrhagic episodes, most patients have extensive skin and mucous membrane bleeding, including ecchymosis, epistaxis, and petechiae. Areas of entry such as surgical incisions, catheters, or venipuncture sites may also ooze and must be carefully observed. In thrombotic episodes, patients may exhibit **acrocyanosis,** hypotension, or shock. Microthrombi may occur in the nose, genitalia or digits, or major organs such as kidney, liver, or brain.

Acute DIC is a medical emergency. The entire basic DIC coagulation profile is abnormal (Table 18.3). PT and PTT are prolonged, fibrinogen and platelets are decreased, and FDPs and D-dimers are dramatically increased. D-dimer results are an essential piece of data in emerging DIC patients; however, other pathologies such an inflammation, renal disease, or local clot may elevate the result.[10] For this reason, all laboratory data must be carefully reviewed in concert with clinical symptoms before reaching the diagnosis. It has been shown that not all patients in DIC have decreased fibrinogen levels. Indeed, recent studies have shown that for those patients exhibiting DIC but near normal fibrinogen, clinical outcomes were much poorer, resulting in severe organ failure.[11] Recovering patients should be monitored over time using the same initial profile for comparison and evaluation of their coagulation status. The patient will develop a microangiopathic hemolytic anemia due to microthrombi disposition in the small vessels. Schistocytes will be observed as a morphological marker for this process.

Table 18.3 ◉ Disseminated Intravascular Coagulation Laboratory Profile

- PT ↑
- aPTT ↑
- Platelets ↓
- Fibrinogen ↓
- D-dimer ↑

CONDENSED CASE

A 20-year-old woman came through the emergency department with unspecified complaints. A CBC was ordered and her platelet count was recorded as 17.0×10^9/L. A repeat sample was ordered from the emergency department, and with this run, the platelet count was recorded as 6.0×10^9/L. The patient failed to delta check with her CBC history, revealing an admission 3 weeks prior with a platelet count of 250×10^9/L. The technologist called the physician immediately with the report of the thrombocytopenia and inquired as to the patient history.

What additional steps should the technologist take to ensure the accuracy of this result?

Answer

The first step that comes to mind is to check the specimen for clots. Improperly mixed specimens are notorious for containing small clots. Emergency department personnel may not be aware that blue-top tubes need to be inverted at least five times for proper mixing. This was done and no clots were observed. Next the technologist queried the physician as to whether or not this was an expected result. Although the physician was less than cooperative, he did reveal that the patient has undergone a cardiac procedure and that the initial consensus was that the thrombocytopenia was medication induced. The patient was admitted and transfused with platelet concentrates, and the platelet count rose to 56×10^9/L. No additional history is known at this time.

Treatment in Acute Disseminated Intravascular Coagulation

If the precipitating event leading to the DIC is discovered, then successful treatment will involve resolution of this pathology. Surgery in the case of obstetrical complications or widespread use of antibiotics in the case of septicemia may stem the bleeding episode. However, because many clinicians are perplexed as to the root cause of the precipitating events, judicious use of blood products will stop the bleeding. Fresh frozen plasma is a source of all of the clotting factors; packed red cells will restore oxygen-carrying capacity; and platelet concentrates will enable clot formation. Heparin has been used in DIC cases when combined with antithrombin. Although controversial, this agent may provide needed antithrombotic activity to delay excessive coagulation.

Summary Points

- Fibrinogen is the key substrate of the coagulation and the fibrinolytic system.
- Fibrinogen has the highest molecular weight of all of the clotting factors.
- Thrombin acts upon fibrinogen to convert it to fibrin.
- Fibrin is stabilized by factor XIII and calcium to become an insoluble clot.
- Plasminogen is converted to plasmin primarily through tissue plasminogen activator and then proceeds to destroy the fibrin clot.

- Afibrinogenemia, hypofibrinogenemia, and dysfibrinogenemia are all inherited disorders of fibrinogen. Each of these may also be acquired disorders.
- Streptokinase is an exogenous fibrinolytic agent, produced when a bacterial cell product forms a complex with plasminogen.
- Naturally occurring inhibitors of fibrinolysis are plasminogen activator inhibitor 1 and alpha-2-antiplasmin.
- The byproducts of fibrinolysis are fibrin degradation products and D-dimers.
- Excess fibrin degradation products provide anticoagulant activity.
- D-dimers are produced from a cross-linked and stabilized fibrin clot.
- Excess D-dimers are an indication that clots have been formed and are being excessively lysed.
- Disseminated intravascular coagulation (DIC) is usually triggered by an underlying pathological event.
- In DIC patients will excessively clot or excessively bleed, or both.
- Laboratory results for a patient with acute DIC will show a prolonged PT and PTT, decreased fibrinogen and platelets, and increased fibrin degradation products and D-dimers.
- Treatment for DIC includes investigating and resolving the cause of the disorder and providing blood bank products as needed.

Review Questions

1. Which of the following is one of the key roles of thrombin with respect to fibrinogen?
   a. Changes fibrinogen into plasmin
   b. Releases fibrin split products
   c. Converts fibrinogen into fibrin
   d. Activates factors V and VIII

2. Which of the following laboratory assays will be *normal* in a patient with dysfibrinogenemia?
   a. Immunologic assay for fibrinogen
   b. Reptilase time
   c. Thrombin time
   d. PT and PTT

3. What is the primary purpose of the fibrinolytic system?
   a. To form a stable fibrin clot
   b. To activate the complement system

   c. To restore blood flow at the local level
   d. To inhibit coagulation

4. Which bacterial cell product will precipitate a DIC event?
   a. Neuraminidase
   b. Streptokinase
   c. Urokinase
   d. tPA

5. Which is the best possible treatment for a patient with DIC?
   a. Provide supporting blood products
   b. Give the patient tPA if there is excessive clotting
   c. Resolve the underlying cause of the DIC event
   d. Give the patient heparin therapy

CASE STUDY

A 27-year-old man was brought to the emergency department in serious condition. Earlier in the day, he was hiking and had been bitten on his leg by what he thought was probably a black snake. The leg was swollen, and the hiker was extremely lethargic and barely conscious. Additionally, he was bleeding from the site where he was bitten. When blood was drawn, the venipuncture site bled profusely. His lab results follow:

Platelets	27.0×10^9/L (Reference range, 150 to 450×10^9/L)
PFA	Not performed
PT	21.2 seconds (Reference range, 11.8 to 14.5)
PTT	53.7 seconds (Reference range, 23.0 to 35.0)
Fibrinogen	110 mg/dL (Reference range, 200 to 400)
D-dimer	3170 ng/mL D-Dimer units (Reference range, 0 to 200)

Given these laboratory results what is the most likely diagnosis? How can you account for his laboratory results?

Insights to the Case Study

Notice that the patient's basic coagulation profile was abnormal. His PT and PTT were markedly abnormal, his platelet count was markedly decreased, his fibrinogen was decreased, and his D-dimer was markedly prolonged. DIC was triggered by the snake bite. The venom of poisonous snakes will directly activate factor X or factor II. When this happens, clotting occurs within the vessels at an accelerated rate, consuming all of the clotting factors. Notice that the D-dimer result is extremely elevated. D-dimer is the smallest breakdown product of fibrin. When elevated, it is indicative of cross-linked fibrin within the circulating blood, rather than locally at the site of injury. The patient was given antivenin and supported by blood products until his condition stabilized.

[Case submitted by Wendy Sutula, MS, MT(ASCP), SH, Washington Hospital Center.]

○ TROUBLESHOOTING

What Do I Do When The Patient Is Scheduled for Surgery and the PTT Is Abnormal, But He Denies Any Bleeding Episodes?

A 24-year-old man had routine preoperative blood work done. Because of the results, he was referred to the hematology service. The young man denied any bleeding problems throughout his life and was taking no medications. None of his family members had any bleeding problems. A second sample reproduced the results of the first, which were as follows:

PT   13.9 seconds (Reference range, 11.8 to 14.5)

PTT   168.6 seconds (Reference range, 23.0 to 35.0)

The patient's PTT is extremely elevated. Three questions come to mind. Is the patient on heparin? Is there a circulating anticoagulant present? Does the patient have a congenital acquired factor deficiency? A thrombin time was performed in the unlikely event that the patient was somehow receiving heparin (most likely, low-molecular-weight heparin, which can be administered on an outpatient basis). The thrombin time was normal, so the hematologist then ordered a PTT mixing study.

Mixing study: Immediate 50:50 mix: PTT = 32.9

1-Hour incubated 50:50 mix: PTT = 34.3

Based on the mixing study results, one could conclude that the patient has a factor deficiency. Additionally, the incubated mixing study demonstrated that no slow-acting inhibitor is present. Because only the PTT is affected, the most likely factor would be one or more from the intrinsic pathway (factors XII, XI, IX, or VIII; HMWK; or prekallikrein). The hematologist then ordered factor assays, with the following results:

Factor VIII   109% activity (Reference range, 55% to 145%)

Factor IX   121% activity (Reference range, 61% to 140%)

Factor XI   86% activity (Reference range, 65% to 135%)

Factor XII   33% activity (Reference range, 50% to 150%)

As can be seen from the laboratory data, this patient was factor XII deficient. Unlike for factors VIII, IX, and XI, patients with a factor XII deficiency do not have bleeding problems. Factor XII–deficient patients tend to have very long PTTs, however, because the clotting time of a PTT is dependent on the in vitro activation of factor XII. Similar to HMWK and prekallikrein deficiency, factor XII–deficient patients may even have a tendency toward thrombosis. This young man had his surgery with no complications.

[Case submitted by Wendy Sutula, MS, MT(ASCP), SH, Washington Hospital Center.]

WORD KEY

Acrocyanosis • Blue or purple mottled discoloration of the extremities, especially the fingers, toes, and nose

Immunologic assay • Measuring the protein and protein-bound molecules that are concerned with the reaction of the antigen with its specific antibody

Monoclonal • Arising from a single cell

Recombinant • In genetic and molecular biology, pertaining to genetic material combined from different sources

Reptilase time • Coagulation procedure similar to thrombin time except that the clotting is initiated by reptilase, a snake venom; using reptilase, heparin will not affect the assay

Thrombin time • Using thrombin as a substrate, this assay measures the time it takes for fibrinogen to be converted to fibrin

Thrombolytic therapy • Using an agent that causes the breakup of clots

References

1. Loscalzo AD, Schafer AI. Thrombosis and Hemorrhage, 2nd ed. Baltimore: Williams and Wilkins, 1998: 1027–1063.
2. Falco C, Estelles A, Dalmau J, et al. Influence of lipoprotein A levels and isoforms on fibrinolytic activity: Study in families with high lipoprotein A levels. Thromb Haemost 79:818–823, 1998.
3. Liles DK, Knup CL. Disorders of plasma clotting factors. In: Harmening D, ed. Clinical Hematology and Fundamentals of Hemostasis. Philadelphia: FA Davis, 2002: 497.
4. Francis CW, Marder VJ. Physiologic regulation and pathologic disorders of fibrinolysis. In: Colman RW, et al, eds. Hemostasis and Thrombosis: Basic Principles and Clinical Practice, 3rd ed. Philadelphia: JB Lippincott, 1994: 1089.
5. Hosaka Y, Takahashi Y, Ishii H. Thrombomodulin in human plasma contributes to inhibit fibrinolysis through acceleration of thrombin dependent activation of plasma carboxypeptidase. Thromb Haemost 79:371, 1998.

6. Fritsma G. Normal hemostasis and coagulation. In: Rodak B, ed. Hematology: Clinical Principles and Applications, 2nd ed. Philadelphia, WB Saunders, 2002: 625.

7. Jensen R. The diagnostic use of fibrin breakdown products. Clin Hemost Rev 12:1–2, 1998.

8. Janssen MC, Sollershein H, Verbruggen B, et al. Rapid D-dimer assay to exclude deep vein thrombosis and pulmonary embolism: Current status and new developments. Semin Thromb Hemost 24:393–400, 1998.

9. Cunningham VL. A review of disseminated intravascular coagulation: Presentation, laboratory diagnosis and treatment. M L O July:48, 1999.

10. Bick RL, Baker WF. Diagnostic efficacy of the D-dimer assay in disseminated intravascular coagulation (DIC). Thromb Res 65:785–790, 1992.

11. Wada H, Mori Y, Okabayashi K, et al. High plasma fibrinogen levels is associated with poor clinical outcome in DIC patients. Am J Hematol 72:1–7, 2003.

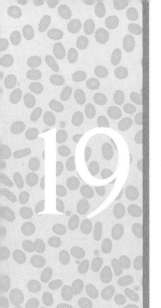
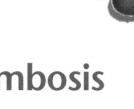

19

Introduction to Thrombosis and Anticoagulant Therapy

Mitra Taghizadeh

Physiological and Pathological Thrombosis

Pathogenesis of Thrombosis

    Vascular Injury

    Platelet Abnormalities

    Coagulation Abnormalities

    Fibrinolytic Abnormalities

    Antithrombotic Factors (Coagulation Inhibitors)

Thrombotic Disorders

    Inherited Thrombotic Disorders

    Acquired Thrombotic Disorders

Laboratory Diagnosis for
Thrombotic Disorders

Anticoagulant Therapy

    Antiplatelet Drugs

    Anticoagulant Drugs

    Thrombolytic Drugs

Objectives

After completing this chapter, the student will be able to:

1. Define thrombophilia and thrombosis.

2. Indicate risk factors associated with inherited and acquired thrombosis.

3. List hemostatic changes responsible for pathological thrombosis.

4. Describe antithrombin, protein C, and protein S with regard to properties, mode of action, factors affected, and complications associated with their deficiencies.

5. List inherited risk factors for thrombosis and their frequency of occurrence.

6. List the most common acquired risk factors associated with thrombosis.

7. Describe activated protein C resistance with regard to pathophysiology, mode of action, and associated complications.

8. Describe heparin-induced thrombocytopenia in regard to the cause, patient's clinical manifestations, and pathophysiology of the disease.

9. Name the laboratory tests used for the diagnosis of factor V Leiden and heparin-induced thrombocytopenia.

10. List the types of anticoagulant drugs used for the treatment of thrombotic disorders.

11. Explain the mechanism of action of each anticoagulant drug commonly used for the treatment of thrombotic disorders.

12. Name the most common laboratory test used for monitoring of heparin therapy.

13. Name the most common laboratory test used for monitoring of Coumadin therapy.

Hypercoagulability refers to environmental, inherited, and acquired conditions that predispose an individual to thrombosis. Thrombosis is the formation of a blood clot in the vasculature. Two types of thrombosis are known: arterial and venous thrombosis. Arterial thrombosis is mainly composed of platelets with small amounts of red cells and white cells whereas venous thrombosis is composed of fibrin clot and red cells. Thrombosis may result from vascular injury, platelet activation, coagulation activation, defects in the fibrinolytic system, and defects in physiological inhibitors. Arterial and venous thrombosis along with complicating thromboembolism is the most important cause of death in the developed countries. More than 800,000 people die annually from myocardial infarction (MI) and thrombotic stroke in the United States.[1] It has also been reported that venous thromboembolic disease is the most common vascular disease after atherosclerotic heart disease and stroke.[1]

This chapter will focus on the physiology and pathology of thrombosis, thrombotic disorders, laboratory diagnosis, and anticoagulant therapy.

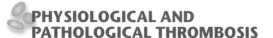 PHYSIOLOGICAL AND PATHOLOGICAL THROMBOSIS

Normal hemostasis refers to the body's physiological response to vascular injury. Normal clot formation and clot dissolution is accomplished by interaction among five major components: vascular system, platelets, coagulation system, fibrinolytic system, and inhibitors. These components must be in the functional state for normal hemostasis to occur. Imbalance in any of the above components will tilt the hemostatic scale in favor of bleeding or thrombosis. There are two systems of hemostasis: the primary and secondary hemostatic systems. Primary hemostasis refers to the process by which the platelet plug is formed at the site of injury, while secondary hemostasis is defined as the interaction of coagulation factors to generate a cross-linked fibrin clot to stabilize the platelet plug to form physiological thrombosis.

Physiological thrombosis results from the body's natural response to vascular injury. It is localized and is formed to prevent excess blood loss. Pathological thrombosis includes deep venous thrombosis, arterial thrombosis, and pulmonary embolism. Pathological thrombosis may be caused by acquired or inherited conditions. Arterial thrombosis is primarily composed of platelets with small amounts of fibrin and red and white cells. This clot may be also referred to as the "white clot." Complications associated with arterial thrombosis are occlusions of the vascular system leading to infarction of tissues.[1] Factors causing arterial thrombosis are hypertension, hyper viscosity, qualitative platelet abnormalities, and **atherosclerosis.**

Venous thrombosis is composed of large amounts of fibrin and red cells resembling the blood clot formed in the test tube. Venous thrombosis is associated with slow blood flow, activation of coagulation, impairment of the fibrinolytic system, and deficiency of physiological inhibitors. The most serious complication associated with venous thrombosis is demobilization of the clot. This occurs when a clot is dislodged from the site of origin and filtered out in the pulmonary circulation.

PATHOGENESIS OF THROMBOSIS

Hemostatic changes that are important in the pathogenesis of thrombosis are vascular injury due to the toxic effect of chemotherapy; platelet abnormalities (more important in arterial thrombosis); coagulation abnormalities, fibrinolytic defects, and deficiencies of the antithrombotic factors.

Vascular Injury

Vascular injuries play an important role in arterial thrombosis. Vascular injury initiates platelet adhesion to exposed subendothelium. The adherent platelets release the contents of alpha and dense granules such as ADP, calcium, and serotonin, causing platelet aggregation and platelet plug formation. In addition, blood coagulation is initiated by tissue factor released from the damaged endothelial cells. The fibrin clot formed would then stabilize the platelet plug. The vascular endothelial injury may occur by endothelial cell injury, atherosclerosis, hyperhomocysteinemia, or other disorders that may interfere with arterial blood flow. In cancer patients, vascular endothelial cell injury may occur as a result of the toxic effect of chemotherapeutic drugs.

Platelet Abnormalities

Platelets are the main components of arterial thrombosis. As platelets interact with the injured vessels, platelet adhesion and aggregation occur. In normal hemostasis, excess platelet activation is prevented by antiplatelet activities of endothelial cells such as generation of prostacyclin. In the disease state, excess platelet activation can reflect thromboembolic disease or exacerbation of thrombotic episodes.[1]

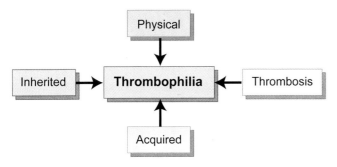

Figure 19.1   Risk factors for thrombosis.

Coagulation Abnormalities

Risk factors associated with hypercoagulability can be divided into environmental, acquired, or inherited factors[1,2] (Fig. 19.1) .

Environmental factors are linked to transient conditions that may result from surgery, immobilization, and pregnancy or therapeutic complications associated with oral contraceptives, hormone replacement therapy, chemotherapy, and heparin treatment.

Acquired risk factors are associated with conditions that hinder normal hemostasis such as cancer, nephrotic syndrome, **vasculitis,** antiphospholipid antibodies, myeloproliferative disease, hyperviscosity syndrome, and others[1] (Table 19.1). Inherited risk factors are associated with genetic mutations that result in deficiency of naturally occurring inhibitors such as protein C, protein S, or antithrombin (AT); accumulation of procoagulant factor as in prothrombin G20210A[1,3]; or clotting factor resistance to anticoagulant activities of physiological inhibitors as in activated protein C resistance (APCR) (Table 19.2). These conditions disturb the

Table 19.1 ◎ Conditions Associated With Acquired Thrombosis

• Cancer
• Surgery (especially orthopedic surgery)
• Liver disease
• Immobility
• Nephritic syndrome
• DIC
• Pregnancy
• Antiphospholipid antibodies
• Drugs
• Others

Table 19.2 ◎ Conditions Associated With Inherited Thrombosis

• Protein C deficiency
• Protein S deficiency
• Antithrombin deficiency
• Prothrombin G20210A
• APCR
• Hyperhomocysteinemia
• Elevated factor VIII
• Factor XII deficiency

hemostatic regulation in favor of increased risk of thrombosis.

Fibrinolytic Abnormalities

The function of the fibrinolytic system is the breakdown of fibrin clots. As in the coagulation system, the fibrinolytic system is controlled by a specific group of inhibitors. Plasmin is an activated form of plasminogen and has a primary role in fibrin breakdown. Plasmin is inhibited by alpha-2-antiplasmin (the main inhibitor of plasmin), alpha-2-macroglobulin, alpha-1-antitrypsin, AT, and C1 esterase. Plasminogen activation is also inhibited by proteins such as plasminogen activator inhibitors I, II, and 3 (PAI-1, PAI-2, and PAI-3).[3] A decrease in fibrinolytic activities, in particular decreased levels of tissue plasminogen activator (tPA) and elevated levels of PAI-1, results in impairment of fibrinolysis in vivo, resulting in arterial and venous thrombosis.[1]

Antithrombotic Factors (Coagulation Inhibitors)

Antithrombotic factors are plasma proteins that interfere with the clotting factors and therefore prevent thrombin formation and thrombosis. Three types of naturally occurring inhibitors are AT, prothrombin cofactor II, and protein C.

Antithrombin

AT is a plasma protein made in the liver. AT neutralizes the activities of thrombin (IIa), IXa, Xa, XIa, and XIIa. The inhibitory action of AT against clotting factors is slow; however, its activity is markedly increased when AT binds to heparin (Fig. 19.2). AT deficiency is associated with thrombosis.[1,2,4]

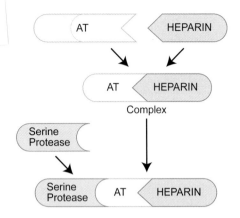

Figure 19.2 Effect of antithrombin on serine proteases.

Heparin Cofactor II

Heparin cofactor II is another coagulation inhibitor. It acts against thrombin, and it is heparin dependent. Heparin cofactor deficiency alone is not associated with thrombosis.[1]

Protein C and Protein S

Protein C is a vitamin K–dependent protein made in the liver. Protein C circulates in the form of zymogen. Protein C should be activated to a serine protease (activated protein C) in order to exert its inhibitory effects against the clotting factors. Protein C is activated by the action of thrombin-thrombomodulin complex and protein S as a cofactor[1,2,4] (Fig. 19.3).

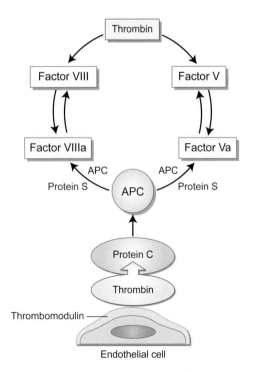

Figure 19.3 Protein C pathway.

Protein S is a vitamin K–dependent protein made in the liver that is necessary for activation of protein C. Once protein C is activated, it will deactivate cofactors Va and VIIIa. Deficiencies of proteins C and S are associated with thrombosis.

THROMBOTIC DISORDERS
Inherited Thrombotic Disorders

Inherited thrombotic disorders are associated with genetic mutations that result in deficiencies of one or more of the naturally occurring inhibitors such as AT, heparin cofactor II, protein C, and protein S. Increased procoagulant factor such as in prothrombin G20210A mutation is associated with thrombosis. Other causes for inherited thrombotic disorders are AT, proteins C and S deficiencies, factor V Leiden, or an inherited form of hyperhomocysteinemia caused by an enzyme deficiency (see Table 19.2).

Antithrombin Deficiency

AT deficiency was first discovered in 1965.[1] This disorder is inherited as an autosomal dominant disorder. It has been reported that 1 in 600 people have AT deficiency.[1] There are two types of AT deficiencies: type I and type II. Type I is a quantitative disorder in which there is a reduction in the concentration of AT. Type II is a qualitative disorder in which the concentration of AT is normal but the molecule is functionally abnormal. Deficiency of AT is associated with recurrent venous thrombosis, which may include almost every vein site.[1] The thrombotic event may be primary (in the absence of triggering factors) or may be followed by another risk factor such as pregnancy, surgery, or any other acquired factors. Acquired AT deficiency may be associated with DIC, liver disease, nephrotic syndrome, oral contraceptives, and pregnancy.[1]

Heparin Cofactor II Deficiency

Heparin cofactor II was first discovered in 1974.[3] Heparin cofactor II is inherited as an autosomal dominant trait. It is a heparin-dependent factor whose inhibitory effect is primarily against thrombin. Many studies have shown the heparin cofactor deficiency alone is not associated with thrombosis.[1]

Protein C Deficiency

Protein C deficiency is inherited as an autosomal dominant trait. Similar to AT deficiency, there are two types of protein C deficiencies: type I (quantitative deficiency) and type II (qualitative deficiency). Type I deficiency is the most common form and is associated with both reduction of immunologic and functional activity of protein C to 50% of normal. Type II is characterized by a normal amount of an abnormal protein.[4] More than 160 different protein C mutations has been reported between the two types.[1,4] Most of the mutations are missense or nonsense mutations. The most common complications associated with protein C deficiency are venous thromboembolism in heterozygous adults. Other reported complications are arterial thrombosis, neonatal **purpura fulminans** in homozygous newborns, and warfarin-induced skin **necrosis**.[1]

Many studies show that most patients with protein C deficiency alone are asymptomatic.[1] This finding indicates that thrombotic episodes may be provoked by some additional inherited or acquired risk factors in these patients. Acquired protein C deficiency may be associated with vitamin K deficiency, liver disease, malnutrition, DIC, and warfarin therapy.[1]

Protein S Deficiency

Protein S deficiency was discovered in 1984.[1] It is inherited in an autosomal dominant fashion. Protein S circulates in plasma in two forms: free (40%) and bound to C4b-binding protein (60%). The cofactor activity of protein S is carried primarily by free protein S. As with AT and protein C, protein S deficiency is divided into two types. Type I is a quantitative disorder in which total protein S (free and bound), free protein S, and protein S activity levels are reduced to about 50% of normal.[1] Type II protein S is a qualitative disorder deficiency and is divided into type IIa and type IIb. In type IIa protein S deficiency, free protein S is reduced while total protein S is normal. In type IIb, both free and total protein S levels are normal .[1] Type IIb protein S deficiency has been reported in patients with factor V Leiden. Similar to protein C deficiency, many patients with thrombosis have additional inherited or acquired risk factors.[1] Most patients with protein S deficiency may experience venous thrombosis. However, arterial thrombosis has been reported in 25% of patients with protein S deficiency.[1] Acquired protein S deficiency may be associated with vitamin K deficiency, liver disease, and DIC.

Activated Protein C Resistance (Factor V Leiden)

APCR is an autosomal dominant disorder discovered in 1993.[1,4] APCR was found in 20% to 60% of patients with recurrent thrombosis with no previously recognized inherited thrombotic disorder. The majority of cases (92%) are inherited and caused by mutation of

factor V, Arg506Gln, referred to as factor V Leiden.[1] Factor V Leiden is the most common inherited cause for thrombosis in the white population of northern and western Europe. In the United States, factor V Leiden is seen in 6% of whites.[1] The homozygous form of factor V Leiden has a 80-fold increased risk of thrombosis, while heterozygous carriers have a 2- to 10-fold increase in thrombosis.[1] Recall that factors V and VIII are inactivated by the protein C–protein S complex. Mutated factor V, factor V Leiden, is not inactivated and leads to excessive clot formation. The thrombotic risks are further increased if other inherited or acquired risk factors coexist. The thrombotic complications associated with factor V Leiden are venous thromboembolism (VTE). Another reported complication is recurrent miscarriage. Factor V Leiden has also been reported as a risk factor for myocardial infarction. Smoking increases the risk of thrombosis to 30-fold in individuals who have factor V Leiden.[1] Other causes of activated protein C (8%) are related to pregnancy, oral contraceptives, cancer, and other acquired disorders (Fig. 19.4).

Laboratory Diagnosis of APCR

APCR may be evaluated by coagulation assays, which include a two-part aPTT test. The principle of the test is the inhibition of factor Va by APC, which will cause prolongation of aPTT. Therefore, the aPTT is performed on patient plasma with and without APC. The results are expressed in a ratio.[1]

$$\frac{\text{Patient aPTT + APC}}{\text{Patient aPTT − APC}}$$

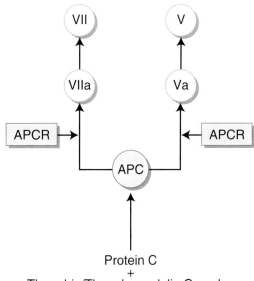

Figure 19.4 Activated protein C resistance pathway.

Reference ranges vary from lab to lab but in general the normal ratio is 2 or greater. A range of <2 is diagnostic.

aPTT is decreased when is APC is added to the normal plasma. Plasma from patients with APCR has a lower ratio than the reference ranges established for normal patients. A DNA test is available to confirm the specific point mutation in patients with factor V Leiden.

Prothrombin Mutations

Prothrombin mutation (G20210A) is the second most prevalent cause of an inherited form of hypercoagulability. It is caused by a single point mutation. It is an autosomal dominant disorder that causes an increase in concentration of plasma prothrombin. The risk of venous thromboembolism increases as the plasma prothrombin level increases to a level greater than 115 IU/dL.[1] As with factor V Leiden, prothrombin mutation tends to follow a geographic and ethnic distribution with the highest prevalence in whites from southern Europe. About half of the cases are reported in northern Europe.[1]

Similar to factor V Leiden, the thrombotic episodes develop early before the age of 40.[1]

Other Inherited Thrombotic Disorders

Elevated activity levels of factor VIII are associated with VTE. It has been reported that if factor VIII activity is greater than 150%, the risk for VTE increases to 3-fold, and if the activity is greater than 200%, the thrombotic risk increases to 11-fold.[1] Factor XII deficiency is also associated with thrombosis.

Factor XII is a contact factor that initiates the intrinsic pathway activation. Patients with factor XII deficiency will have a prolonged aPTT but no bleeding problem. Factor XII plays a major role in the fibrinolytic system and in activation of plasminogen to plasmin. Therefore, patients with factor XII deficiency would have an impaired fibrinolysis and are prone to thrombosis.[3]

Dysfibrinogenemia is an inherited abnormality of the fibrinogen molecule with variable clinical presentation. Twenty percent of cases may present arterial or venous thrombosis. Bleeding has been reported in 20% of cases, and 60% of patients may be asymptomatic.[3]

Tissue factor pathway inhibitor (TFPI) deficiency is another marker for thrombosis. TFPI plays an important role in prevention of clot formation. It inhibits factor Xa and factor VIIa–TF complex.[3] The deficiency of this inhibitor is associated with thromboembolic disorder.

Hyperhomocysteinemia can be inherited or acquired. Homocysteine is an amino acid formed during the conversion of methionine to cysteine. Hyperhomocysteinemia results from either deficiencies of the enzymes necessary for production of homocysteine (inherited form) or deficiencies of vitamin cofactors (B_6, B_{12}, and folate) in an acquired form. Increased levels of homocysteine in the blood are reported to be a risk factor for stroke, MI, and thrombotic disorder.[1,3]

Disorders of the fibrinolytic system such as plasminogen deficiency, tPA deficiency, and increased plasminogen activator inhibitor are associated with thrombotic disease.[1]

Acquired Thrombotic Disorders

There are many situations that may lead to acquired thrombotic disorders. They may be associated with underlying diseases such as cancer, surgery, liver disease, nephrotic syndrome, DIC, pregnancy, and vitamin K deficiency. Drugs such as oral contraceptives or hormone replacement therapy may predispose to thrombosis.

Lupus Anticoagulant/Antiphospholipid Syndrome

The antiphospholipid (aPL) syndrome is an acquired disorder in which patients produce antibodies to phospholipids binding protein known as beta-2-glycoprotein I (β_2GPI) or apolipoprotein (aPL).[5] Clinical manifestations of aPL antibodies are associated with thrombosis and fetal losses. The IgG2 subtype of aPL is usually associated with thrombosis. Thrombotic episodes include venous and arterial thrombosis and thromboembolism. The usual age at the time of thrombosis is generally about 35 to 45. Men and women are equally affected.[5] Thrombosis may occur spontaneously or may be associated with other predisposing factors such as hormone replacement therapy, oral contraceptives, surgery, or trauma. A small number of patients with aPL antibodies may manifest bleeding if there is a concurrent thrombocytopenia or coagulopathy such as hypoprothrombinemia.[5]

The most common form of aPL antibodies are lupus anticoagulant (LA) and anticardiolipin (ACA). The thrombotic manifestations may be primary (independent autoimmune disorder) or secondary (associated with other autoimmune disorders such as systemic lupus erythematosus [SLE]). In vitro, LA acts against phospholipid-dependent coagulation assays such as aPTT, which was not corrected with 1:1 mix with normal plasma.[4,5] This will be explained in the next section. Patients with aPL antibodies may present with thrombosis and fetal loss. Bleeding is uncommon, unless the patient has thrombocytopenia or decreased prothrombin as well.

Laboratory Assays for Antiphospholipid Antibodies

Common tests used to detect lupus anticoagulants are aPTT, Kaolin clotting time (KCCT), dilute Russell viper venom test (DRVVT), and dilute PT. For both a prolonged aPTT and DRVVT, a mixing study should be performed. In a mixing study, the patient plasma is mixed with normal plasma and the test is repeated. In the presence of lupus anticoagulant the mixing study does not correct to normal. Lupus anticoagulant is confirmed by the addition of excess platelets (platelet neutralization test or hexagonal phase phospholipids [DVV Confirm]).[4,6.] The International Society of Hemostasis and Thrombosis has recommended four criteria for the diagnosis of lupus anticoagulants: (1) prolongation of a phospholipid-dependent test, (2) evidence for the presence of an inhibitor (mixing study), (3) evidence that the inhibitor is directed against phospholipids (confirmatory test), and (4) lack of any other specific inhibitor (Table 19.3). Other factors that are helpful in the diagnosis of lupus anticoagulants are the clinical presentation since these patients lack bleeding. Lupus anticoagulant may coexist with anticardiolipin antibodies in patients presenting with an acquired thrombosis and fetal loss. Therefore, the test for ACLA is recommended as well. ACLAs are detected by the ELISA method.[6] Other detectable antibodies are anti–β_2GPI.[6]

Heparin-Induced Thrombocytopenia

HIT is an immune-mediated complication associated with heparin therapy. HIT may develop in 3% to 5% of patients receiving unfractionated heparin.[1] HIT usually develops between 5 and 14 days after heparin ther-

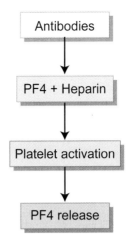

Figure 19.5 Pathophysiology of HIT.

apy. About 36% to 50% of patients with HIT develop life-threatening thrombosis. The thrombotic tendency can last for at least 30 days.[1] Venous thrombosis (extremity venous thrombosis) is more common than arterial thrombosis. Other complications of HIT include thrombocytopenia, heparin-induced skin lesions (10% to 20% of patients), and heparin resistance.[1] The pathogenesis of HIT is that antibodies are produced against heparin–platelet factor 4 complex. This immune complex binds to platelet FC receptors, causing platelet activation, formation of platelet microparticles, thrombocytopenia, and hypercoagulable state (Fig. 19.5).

HIT is independent of dosage or route of administration of heparin. This condition should be suspected in any patient whose platelet count falls below 50% of the baseline value after 5 days of heparin treatment[1] and in patients who develop thrombosis with or without thrombocytopenia during heparin therapy.[1]

Laboratory Diagnosis of HIT

Laboratory diagnosis of HIT includes functional assays or immunoassays. Functional assays measure platelet activation or aggregation in the presence of HIT serum and heparin. Functional assays include heparin-induced platelet aggregation, heparin-induced platelet adenosine triphosphate (ATP) release by lumiaggregometry, [14C]-serotonin release assay ([14C]-SRA) release by ELISA, and platelet microparticle formation by flow cytometry. Heparin-platelet factor 4 antibodies are detected by ELISA. When HIT is suspected, heparin should be stopped immediately and be replaced by alternative anticoagulant drugs (danaparoid, argatroban). Warfarin should be avoided in the acute phase of thrombosis because it may cause venous limb **gangrene**.[1] Patients receiving heparin **should** have a base-

---

Table 19.3 ● Criteria for the Diagnosis of Lupus Anticoagulant

- Prolongation of at least one phospholipid-dependent tests
- Lack of correction of mixing studies
- Correction of the abnormal result with the addition of excess phospholipids
- Lack of any other specific inhibitor

line platelet count and platelet monitoring every third day between 5 and 14 days.[1]

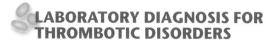

LABORATORY DIAGNOSIS FOR THROMBOTIC DISORDERS

The availability of a wide range of assays to evaluate the hypercoagulable state has enhanced the diagnosis of inherited and acquired thrombotic events. However, the assays are expensive and time consuming. These laboratory tests should be considered for patients in whom the test results will impact the choice, intensity, and duration of anticoagulant therapy, family planning, and prognosis.[1]

The clinical events that justify laboratory evaluation of hypercoagulable states are listed in Table 19.4. Patients who lack a positive family history should be evaluated for an acquired form of thrombosis such as malignancy, myeloproliferative disorders, and aPL antibodies.[1,7] Laboratory assays should not be done at the time of acute thrombosis or when the patient is receiving any anticoagulant therapy because it may affect the results of the assays.[1] Levels of fibrin degradation products and (D-dimer) are increased in patients with acute venous thromboembolism. Lack of elevated D-dimer in patients evaluated for acute DVT or PE has an excellent negative predictive value for thrombosis.[1]

Functional tests are preferred over immunologic assays. The screening laboratory tests used for evaluation of patients suspected of having a hypercoagulable state are summarized in Table 19.5.

ANTICOAGULANT THERAPY

Thromboembolic diseases are treated by antithrombotic drugs. Antithrombotic agents include antiplatelet drugs, anticoagulant drugs, and thrombolytic drugs. Antiplatelet drugs prevent platelet activation and aggregation and are most effective in the treatment of the arterial diseases. Anticoagulant drugs inhibit thrombin and fibrin formation and are used commonly for the treatment of venous thrombosis. Thrombolytic drugs are used to break down fibrin clots, to restore vascular function, and to prevent loss of tissues and organs.

Antiplatelet Drugs

There are numerous agents used against platelets. Aspirin (acetylsalicylic acid) is an antiplatelet drug that irreversibly affects platelet function by inhibiting the cyclooxygenase (COX) enzyme and thereby the formation of thromboxane A_2 (TXA_2). TXA_2 is a potent platelet-activating substance released from the activated platelets. Aspirin is rapidly absorbed from the gastrointestinal tract and the plasma concentration is at peak 1 hour after aspirin ingestion.[1] The effect of aspirin on platelets starts 1 hour after ingestion and lasts for the entire platelet life span (approximately 1 week).[1] Aspirin is effective in the treatment of **angina**, acute MI, transient ischemic attack, stroke, arterial **fibrillation**, and prostatic heart valve. The minimum effective dosage for these conditions is 75 to 325 mg/day.[1] Aspirin toxicity includes gastrointestinal discomfort, blood loss, and the risk of systemic bleeding. A low dose of aspirin (30 to 75 mg/day) has shown to have an antithrombotic effect.[1] Some patients may develop aspirin resistance. Patients who become resistant to aspirin have a higher rate of heart attacks and strokes. Aspirin resistance can be evaluated by platelet aggregation tests.

Other antiplatelet drugs include dipyridamole, thienopyridines, ticlopidine, and clopidogrel.[1]

Table 19.4 ● Conditions That Require Evaluation for Hypercoagulable States

- Recurrent thrombosis in patients <45 years old
- Patients with a positive family history
- Recurrent spontaneous thromboses
- Thrombosis in unusual sites
- Heparin resistance
- Proteins C and S deficiency
- Thrombosis associated with pregnancy and estrogen therapy
- Unexplained recurrent pregnancy loss

Table 19.5 ● Screening Laboratory Tests for Hypercoagulable State

- Activated protein C resistance
- Functional assays for antithrombin, protein C, and protein S
- Prothrombin G20210A by polymerase chain reaction
- APTT, DRVVT, mixing studies, and confirmatory test for lupus anticoagulant
- Enzyme-linked immunosorbent assays for anticardiolipin antibody
- Factor VIII activity

Anticoagulant Drugs

Anticoagulant drugs are used for the prevention and treatment of thromboembolic disorders. Short-term anticoagulant drugs such as heparin are administered by intravenous infusion or subcutaneous injection. Long-term anticoagulant drugs such as Coumadin are orally administered.

Heparin

Heparin is present in human tissue as naturally occurring highly sulfated glycosaminoglycan. Commercially unfractionated heparin (UFH) is isolated from bovine lung or porcine intestine. It contains a mixture of polysaccharide chains with a molecular weight of 4000 to 30,000 daltons.[1] Heparin sulfate is a heparin-like substance made by the vascular endothelium. The anticoagulant activity of heparin is enhanced by binding to AT. Heparin–AT complex inactivates thrombin and factor Xa (see Fig. 19.2).

The half-life of heparin is dose dependent. Heparin is cleared from the circulation by the reticuloendothelial system and metabolized by the liver.[1] Heparin is given in a weight-adjusted dosage with an initial bolus (high dose) followed by continuous infusion (lower dose).

Heparin dosage is monitored by aPTT value to range from 1.5 to 2.5 times the mean of the laboratory normal ranges. This level of aPTT is equivalent to heparin levels of 0.3 to 0.7 U/mL that can be measured by factor Xa activity assay.[1,8]

The adverse effects of heparin include bleeding, HIT, and heparin resistance. Heparin resistance may occur as a result of nonspecific binding of heparin to plasma proteins, platelets, and endothelial cells or as a result of AT deficiency.

Low-Molecular-Weight Heparin

Low-molecular-weight heparin (LMWH) is derived from the UFH via enzymatic digestion to produce smaller and low-molecular-weight glycosaminoglycan molecules. The mean weight of LMWH is about 5000 daltons.[1] LMWH has a higher half-life and has low affinity to bind to plasma proteins and endothelial cells.[1,9] The half-life of the drug is not dose dependent. LMWH is administered subcutaneously, once or twice daily based on the body's weight, and does not require monitoring.[1] LMWH has a higher inhibitory effect on factor Xa than on factor IIa.[9] LMWH is cleared by the kidney. The adverse reaction of LMWH includes bleeding, HIT, or sensitivity to LMWH. The LMWH drugs available in the United States, which are approved by FDA, are heparinoids, Lepirudin (recombinant hirudin), Fon daparinux (pentasaccharides), Argatroban, and Bivalirudin.

Coumadin

Coumadin is a vitamin K antagonist drug that inhibits the vitamin K–dependent coagulation factors. Warfarin is a Coumadin derivative that is widely used in the United States as an oral anticoagulant drug. Warfarin inhibits carboxylation of the vitamin K–dependent factors (II, VII, IX, X) as well as vitamin K–dependent anticoagulant proteins such as protein C and protein S. The half-life of warfarin is about 36 hours.[1] Warfarin is given orally as a long-term anticoagulant. Warfarin dosage varies from patient to patient and depends on dietary stores of vitamin K, liver function, preexisting medical conditions, and concurrent medications. Warfarin therapy is monitored by PT/international normalized ratio (INR).

The INR is a method to standardize PT assays against differences in commercial thromboplastin reagent.[10] The INR was established by the World Health Organization (WHO).[1] Each thromboplastin reagent is calibrated against a WHO reference preparation. The INR is calculated using the following formula: INR = (PT ratio)^{ISI}, where ISI refers to the international sensitivity index, which is calculated for each thromboplastin reagent against a reference thromboplastin reagent.[1]

According to the American College of Chest Physicians' consensus panel, the therapeutic range of INR is 2.0 to 3.0 for the treatment of venous thromboembolism. For prosthetic mechanical heart valves and prevention of recurrent MI, a higher dose of warfarin is required to attain an INR of 2.5 to 3.5.[1]

The most common adverse effect of Coumadin therapy is bleeding, which is directly dose related.[10] Patients with an INR of greater than 3.0 are at the higher risk of bleeding. Warfarin crosses the placenta and therefore should be avoided during pregnancy. Another rare but devastating complication of warfarin therapy is skin necrosis. This phenomenon mostly occurs in patients who receive high doses of warfarin and may have heterozygous protein C deficiency.[1] Skin necrosis is caused by the rapid drop in protein C in patients who have preexisting protein C deficiency resulting in a thrombotic state.[1]

Thrombolytic Drugs

Thrombolytic drugs are commonly used in acute arterial thrombosis for immediate thrombolysis, restoration of vascular integrity, and prevention of tissue and organ damage. Most fibrinolytic drugs are made by recombinant techniques and are fashioned after tPA and urokinase. Urokinase is not fibrin specific and causes hypofibrinogenemia by the breakdown of fibrinogen. Urokinase can be used for the treatment of venous thromboembolism, MI, and thrombolysis of clotted catheters.[1] Streptokinase is a thrombolytic agent obtained from beta-hemolytic streptococci. Streptoki-nase is not fibrin specific, and because it is antigenic, it may cause allergic reactions.

Bleeding is the most common complication associated with thrombolytic drugs. Thrombolytic therapy does not require monitoring, however, prior screening tests such as PT, aPTT, TT, fibrinogen, and platelet count may be helpful to predict patients who are at high risk of bleeding.[3]

CONDENSED CASE

A technical representative for a reference laboratory experienced severe pain behind his left knee 1 day after a visit to one of his laboratory accounts. He tried to pass it off as muscle pain because of a recent basketball game, but walking became difficult for him. Over the next 24 hours, he noticed that the area of pain became swollen, red, and even more sensitive. **What is your clinical impression?**

Answer

This patient may be experiencing deep vein thrombosis. Upon further questioning, it was discovered that the patient had done significant highway driving during the week; most of the time keeping his left knee in a bent position. He eventually went to the emergency department, where the thrombosis was diagnosed. His PT and aPTT results were normal, but his D-dimer results were higher than the normal range. A **venogram** demonstrated a clot behind the left knee. The patient was treated appropriately and started on a regimen of Coumadin with careful outpatient monitoring.

Summary Points

- Hypercoagulability refers to conditions that predispose an individual to thrombosis.

- Risk factors associated with hypercoagulability can be divided into those that are environmental, acquired, or inherited.

- Thrombosis is the formation of blood clots in the vasculature. Thrombosis can be arterial or venous.

- Arterial thrombosis is mainly composed of platelets with small amount of red cells and white cells, whereas venous thrombosis is composed of fibrin clot and red cells

- Thrombosis may result from vascular injury, platelet activation, coagulation activation, defect in fibrinolytic system, and defect in physiological inhibitors.

- Physiological thrombosis results from the body's natural response to vascular injury. It is localized and is formed to prevent excess blood loss.

- Pathological thrombosis includes deep venous thrombosis, arterial thrombosis, and pulmonary embolism. Pathological thrombosis may be caused by acquired or inherited conditions.

- Thromboembolism is formed when clot is dislodged from the origination site and filtered out in the pulmonary circulation.

- Physiological anticoagulant is plasma protein and includes antithrombin, heparin cofactor II, protein C, and protein S.

- Antithrombin is made in the liver. It inhibits factors IIa, IXa, Xa, XIa, and XIIa. Heparin increases the inhibitory action of antithrombin.

- Protein C is a vitamin K–dependent protein made in the liver. Protein C is activated by thrombin-thrombomodulin complex. Protein S is a cofactor for activation of protein C. Activated protein C deactivates factors Va and VIIIa.

- Inherited risk factors are associated with genetic mutations that result in deficiency of naturally occurring inhibitors such as protein C, protein S, or antithrombin; accumulation of procoagulant factors as in prothrombin G20210A; or clotting factor resistance to anticoagulant activities of physiological inhibitors as in activated protein C resistance.

- The majority (92%) of activated protein C resistance cases are inherited and are caused by mutation of factor V Arg506Gln, referred to as factor V Leiden.

- Acquired thrombotic disorders are associated with underlying diseases or drugs.

- Antiphospholipid syndrome is caused by antibodies against phospholipid-dependent coagulation assays such as aPTT, which was not corrected with 1:1 mix with normal plasma. The most common form of aPL antibodies are lupus anticoagulant (LA) and anticardiolipin (ACA).

- Laboratory tests for LA include aPTT or dRRVT; mixing studies, and confirmatory studies. Anticardiolipin antibodies are tested by ELISA.

- Heparin-induced thrombocytopenia (HIT) is an immune-mediated thrombotic complication associated with heparin therapy. The antibody is produced against heparin–platelet factor 4 complexes.

- Diagnostic tests for HIT include heparin-dependent platelet activation assays and detection of the antibody by ELISA.

- Antithrombotic drugs include antiplatelet drugs, anticoagulant drugs, and thrombolytic drugs.

- Aspirin is an antiplatelet drug that inhibits the cyclooxygenase (COX) enzyme and therefore prevents formation of thromboxane A_2 (TXA_2). TXA_2 is a potent platelet-activating substance released from the activated platelets.

- Heparin is a short-term anticoagulant drug. It is administered intravenously or intramuscularly.

- Heparin dosage is monitored by aPTT value to range from 1.5 to 2.5 times the mean of the laboratory control.

- Coumadin is a vitamin K antagonist drug that inhibits the vitamin K–dependent coagulation factors (II, VII, IX, and X).

- Coumadin is an oral anticoagulant that is administered as a long-term anticoagulant. It is monitored by PT/INR.

- Thrombolytic drugs include tPA, urokinase, and streptokinase.

CASE STUDY

A 30-year-old woman was referred to the hospital for evaluation. She presented with a history of multiple spontaneous abortions. She is currently complaining of pain and swelling in her left thigh. Her family history and her past medical history were unremarkable. The patient is currently on oral contraceptives. The patient's laboratory results were as follows:

WBC	8.0×10^9/L (Reference range, 4.4 to 11.0)
RBC	4.7×10^{12}/L (Reference range, 4.1 to 5.1)
Hgb	14.0 g/dL (Reference range, 12.3 to 15.3)
Hct	43% (Reference range, 36 to 450)
Platelets	250×10^9/L (Reference range, 150 to 4000)
PT	13.5 seconds (Reference range, 10.9 to 12.0)
aPTT	52 seconds (Reference range, 34 to 38)
dRVVT	Prolonged
aPTT 1:1 mixing study	Not corrected immediately and after 2 hours' incubation
dRVV confirm	Corrected
ACA	Present

Insights to the Case Study

The diagnosis of lupus anticoagulant was made based on the physical findings, patient's history, and the laboratory results. Physical finding reveals that the patient had had multiple fetal losses and had pain and swelling in her thigh at the time of medical evaluation. The lack of a positive family history with thrombosis ruled out any inherited thrombotic disorder. Platelet count was normal, indicating that the thrombotic episodes are not related to any cause of platelet activation.

aPTT and dRVVT were both prolonged; however, the patient did not have any bleeding problems. A prolonged aPTT and dRVVT in the absence of bleeding ruled out any clotting factor deficiency. Mixing study with normal plasma differentiates factor deficiency from an inhibitor. Lack of bleeding rules out factor VIII inhibitor. Lupus anticoagulant is

(continued on following page)

(Continued)

against in vitro phospholipid-dependent tests. In dRVVT confirmatory tests, excess phospholipids are added to the test system to neutralize the lupus antibodies and therefore correct the prolonged dRVVT initially done. The platelet neutralization test is another confirmatory test used for confirmation of lupus anticoagulant. This test is used for correction of a prolonged aPTT in patients with lupus anticoagulant. Lupus anticoagulant belongs to a group of antibodies called antiphospholipid antibodies (ACA), which include lupus anticoagulant and anticardiolipin antibodies. Lupus anticoagulant may coexist with ACA in some patients. Therefore, it is important to test for both antibodies when lupus anticoagulant is suspected. The ACA antibody can be detected by ELISA and was positive in this patient. This patient was put on Coumadin treatment and was monitored by INR.

Review Questions

1. The primary inhibitor of the fibrinolytic system is:
   a. antiplasmin.
   b. protein S.
   c. antithrombin.
   d. protein C.

2. Dilute Russell's Viper Venom test (dRVVT) is helpful in the diagnosis of:
   a. HIT.
   b. factor VIII inhibitor.
   c. lupus anticoagulant.
   d. ACA.

3. The lupus anticoagulant is directed against:
   a. phospholipid-dependent coagulation tests.
   b. factor VIII.
   c. fibrinogen.
   d. vitamin K–dependent clotting factors.

4. Which statement is correct regarding Coumadin?
   a. It is used for the treatment of bleeding disorders.
   b. It acts on factors XII, XI, IX, and X.
   c. It is used for a short-term therapy.
   d. It acts on vitamin K–dependent clotting factors.

5. Which statement is correct regarding protein C?
   a. It is a cofactor to protein S.
   b. Its activity is inhibited by heparin.
   c. It forms a complex with antithrombin.
   d. It is a physiological inhibitor of coagulation.

6. Activated protein C resistance is associated with:
   a. mutation of factor VIII.
   b. deletion of factor VI.
   c. mutation of factor V.
   d. deletion of factor VIII.

7. Thrombin-thrombomodulin complex is necessary for:
   a. activation of protein C.
   b. activation of antithrombin.
   c. activation of protein S.
   d. activation of factors V and VIII.

8. Heparin-induced thrombocytopenia is caused by:
   a. antibody to platelet factor 4.
   b. antibody to heparin–platelet factor 4 complex.
   c. lupus anticoagulant.
   d. antibody to heparin.

9. Which of the following drugs would put an individual at risk for thrombosis?
   a. Aspirin
   b. Dipyridamole
   c. Streptokinase
   d. Oral contraceptives

10. Which of the following results are correct regarding lupus inhibitors?
    a. Prolonged aPTT on undiluted plasma and 1:1 mix of patient plasma with normal plasma
    b. Corrected aPTT on a 1:1 mix of patient plasma with normal plasma after 2 hours' incubation
    c. Normal undiluted aPTT and prolonged aPTT on a 1:1 mix of patient plasma with normal plasma
    d. Normal undiluted aPTT and 1:1 mix of patient plasma with normal plasma

○ TROUBLESHOOTING

What Do I Do When the Lab Results Indicate That the Patient Is Not Responding to Heparin?

A coagulation sample from the intensive care unit was given to the laboratory on the evening shift. The patient had experienced multiple trauma due to an automobile accident. He had multiple fractures and internal injuries. His condition was grave. Heparin therapy was initiated as a result of the multiple trauma. The patient's admitting PT and aPTT was in the normal range: PT = 12.0 seconds (11 to 14 seconds) and PTT = 26 seconds (24 to 36 seconds). The most recent coagulation sample, 2 days from the patient's admission, shows a PTT of 32 seconds. The intensive care unit asked for the sample to be repeated since the patient had been on heparin for 48 hours.

This case illustrates some of the difficulties with heparin therapy. Heparin was discovered in 1916 as a polysaccharide found in the liver. It binds to antithrombin forming a complex that inhibits the activity of clotting factors II, IX, X, XI and XII.

The therapeutic anticoagulant is usually administered intravenously, but it can be given subcutaneously. Patients clear heparin individually at their own rate, and there is no dose-dependent relationship. The half-life of heparin is 90 minutes, and most of the time heparin is given in a bolus dose of 5000 to 10,000 units, depending on the weight of the patient. Heparin may be monitored by the PTT and the factor Xa–activity curve. If monitored by PTT, the general therapeutic range is 1.5 to 2.5 times the mean of the normal range set by the institution. In the case study, the patient's PTT is virtually unchanged even after 48 hours of heparin therapy. There are several possibilities for this scenario. The first possibility that comes to mind is to check the sample for small clots; although most automated coagulation instruments have a clot-sensing device. There were no clots in this sample. An additional possibility is that the patient has an antithrombin deficiency in which case heparin as an anticoagulant would not be effective. However, patients with an antithrombin deficiency are usually prone to clot formation, and there were no indications of this in the patient's history. Next is the possibility of heparin-induced thrombocytopenia, a condition in which unfractionated heparin forms a complex with platelet factor IV, causing thrombocytopenia, thrombosis, and heparin resistance. This is a significant complication of heparin therapy that can lead to death. The technologist in this case inquired as to the patient's admitting platelet count and referred the information to the pathologist. In follow-up, it was discovered that the patient's platelet count had plummeted from the admitting count of 160,000 to 60,000 in 3 days. All unfractionated heparin was discontinued including heparin flush of intravenous sites. The patient was started in a heparin alternative therapy and continued to make slow progress until an eventual recovery.

WORD KEY

Angina • Oppressive pain or pressure in the chest caused by inadequate blood flow and oxygenation to the heart muscle

Atherosclerosis • Cholesterol-lipid-calcium deposits in the walls of arteries

Fibrillation • Usually refers to a cardiac fluttering due to faulty electric supply to the heart

Gangrene • Death of tissue usually resulting from deficient or absent blood supply

Necrosis • Death of cells, tissue, or organs

Purpura fulminans • Rapidly progressing form of purpura occurring principally in children; of short duration and frequently fatal

Vasculitis • Inflammation of the blood vessels.

Venogram • Radiograph of the veins

References

1. Deitcher SR, Rodgers GM. Thrombosis and antithrombotic therapy. In: Greer JP, et al, eds. Wintrobe's Clinical Hematology, 11th ed, Vol 2. Philadelphia: Lippincott Williams and Wilkins, 2004: 1714–1750.
2. Goodnight SH, Griffin JH. Hereditary thrombophilia. In: Williams WJ, et al, eds. Hematology, 6th ed. New York: McGraw-Hill, 2001: 1697–1706.
3. Ehsan A, Plumley JA. Introduction to thrombosis and anticoagulant therapy. In: Harmening D, ed. Clinical Hematology and Fundamentals of Hemostasis, 4th ed. Philadelphia: FA Davis, 2002: 535–558.
4. Bauer KA. Inherited disorders of thrombosis and fibrinolysis. In: Nathan DG, et al, eds. Hematology of Infancy and Childhood, 6th ed, Vol 2. Philadelphia: WB Saunders, 2003: 1583–1659.
5. Rand JH. Lupus anticoagulant and related disorders. In: Williams WJ, et al, eds. Hematology, 6th ed. New York: McGraw-Hill, 2001: 1715–1727.
6. Konkle BA, Palermo C. Laboratory evaluation of the hypercoagulable state. In: Spandofer J, Konkle BA, Merli

GJ, eds. Management and Prevention of Thrombosis in Primary Care. New York: Oxford University Press, 2001: 16–25.

7. Bauer KA. Approach to thrombosis. In: Loscalzo J, Schafer AI, eds. Thrombosis and Hemostasis, 3rd ed. Philadelphia: Lippincott Williams and Wilkins, 2003: 330–340.

8. Haire WD. Deep venous thrombosis and pulmonary embolus. In: Kitchens CS, Alving BM, Kessler CM, eds. Consultative Hemostasis and Thrombosis. Philadelphia: WB Saunders, 2002: 197–221.

9. Merli G. Prophylaxis for deep vein thrombosis and pulmonary embolism in the surgical and medical patient. In: Spandofer J, Konkle BA, Merli GJ, eds. Management and Prevention of Thrombosis in Primary Care. New York: Oxford University Press, 2001: 135–147.

10. Schulman. Oral anticoagulation. In: Williams WJ, et al, eds. Hematology, 6th ed. New York: McGraw-Hill, 2001: 1777–1786.

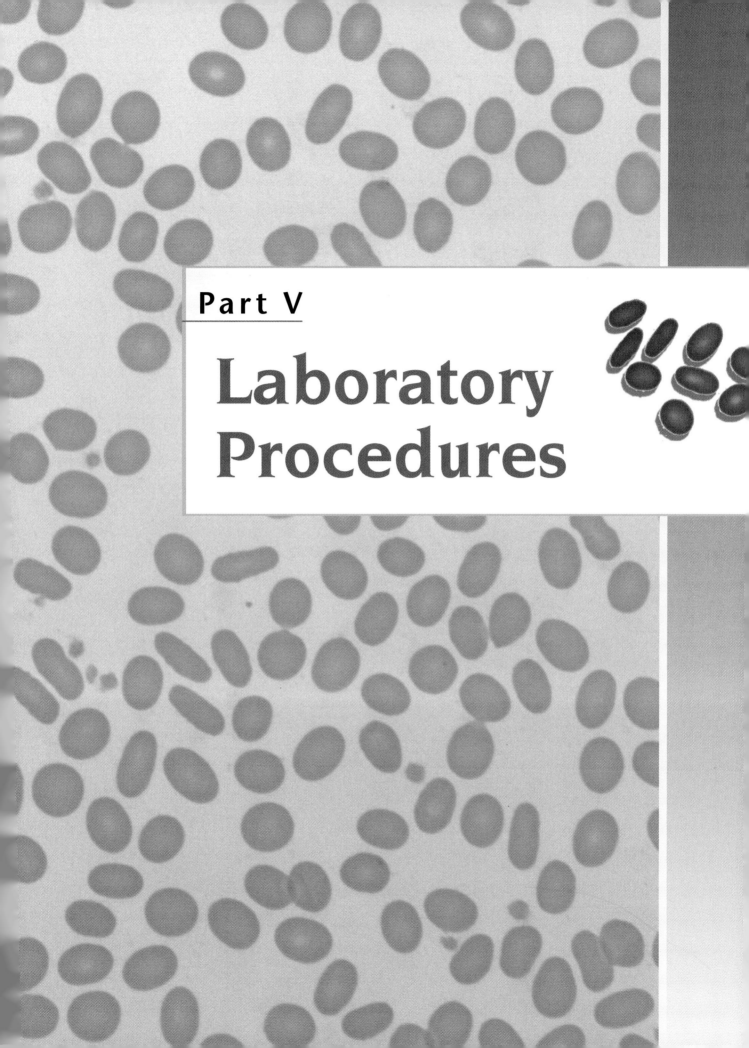

Part V

Laboratory Procedures

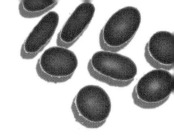

20

Basic Procedures in a Hematology Laboratory

Lori Lentowski and Betty Ciesla

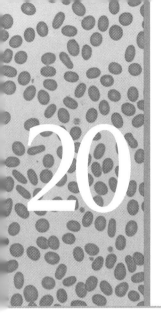

Microhematocrit
  Principle
  Reagents and Equipment
  Specimen Collection and Storage
  Quality Control
  Procedure
  Interpretation

Calculating Red Blood Cell Indices
  Normal Average Values

Modified Westergren Sedimentation Rate
  Principle
  Reagents and Equipment
  Specimen Collection and Storage
  Quality Control
  Procedure
  Normal Ranges
  Limitations
  Conditions Associated With…

Manual Reticulocyte Procedure
  Principle
  Reagents and Equipment
  Specimen Collection and Storage
  Quality Control
  Procedure
  Normal Values
  Conditions Associated With…
  Limitations

Reticulocyte Procedure With Miller Eye Disc
  Principle
  Reagents and Equipment
  Specimen Collection and Storage
  Quality Control

Procedure
  Normal Values
  Conditions Associated With…
  Limitations

Peripheral Smear Procedure
  Principle
  Reagents and Equipment
  Specimen Collection and Storage
  Quality Control
  Procedure
  Limitations

Performing a Manual Differential and Assessing Red Blood Cell Morphology
  Principle
  Reagents and Equipment
  Specimen Collection and Storage
  Quality Control
  Procedure

Unopette White Blood Cell/Platelet Count
  Principle
  Reagents and Equipment
  Specimen Collection and Storage
  Quality Control
  Procedure
  Cell Counts and Calculations
  Normal Values
  Limitations

Sickle Cell Procedure
  Principle
  Reagents and Equipment
  Specimen Collection and Storage
  Quality Control

Procedure

Interpretation of Results and Result Reporting

Limitations

Cerebrospinal Fluid/Body Fluid Cell Count and Differential

Principle

Reagents and Equipment

Specimen Collection and Storage

Quality Control

Procedure

Prothrombin Time and Activated Partial Thromboplastin Time: Automated Procedure

Principle

Reagents and Equipment

Specimen Collection and Storage

Quality Control

Procedure

Results

Limitations

Qualitative D-Dimer Test

Principle

Reagents and Equipment

Specimen Collection and Storage

Quality Control

Procedure

Interpretation

Results

Limitations

An Approach to Interpreting Automated Hematology Data

Principle

Instruments

Flow Cytometry: The Basics in Hematology Interpretation

Overview

Principles

Data Interpretation: One Role for the Medical Technologist

Flow Cytometry Case Studies

The following procedures are representative of *basic methods* employed in hematology laboratories and have been written in Standard Operating Procedure (SOP) format.

We hope they will provide a ready reference and give students the opportunity to preview how a procedure would be introduced into the clinical setting. In addition to the SOPs, specific manufacturer's instructions on instrumentation and reagents would be strictly followed in a working clinical laboratory.

Information on scatterplots and flow cytometry is presented at the end of this chapter. This information is fairly basic and serves only to kindle the interest of the student and expose them to this subject matter. No attempt has been made to create comprehensive coverage of these areas.

MICROHEMATOCRIT

Principle

The hematocrit or packed cell volume measures the concentration of red blood cells (RBCs) in a given volume of whole blood in a capillary tube. This volume is measured after appropriate centrifugation time and is expressed as a percentage of the total blood sample volume. A whole blood sample in an anticoagulated tube is centrifuged at 10,000 to 13,000 rpm for 5 minutes. Erythrocytes are packed at the bottom of the capillary tube and the hematocrit is expressed as a measurement of this level compared to the plasma level. The interface between plasma and red cells is marked by a buffy coat that is composed of leukocytes and platelets. The hematocrit percentage is read below the buffy coat layer. A microhematocrit value can assist in evaluating fluid status, in clarifying various degrees of anemia, and in monitoring acute hemorrhagic conditions. The hematocrit value is also useful in calculating indices, which in turn can help determine the morphological classification of anemias.

Reagents and Equipment

1. Microhematocrit centrifuge (Fig. 20.1)
2. Microhematocrit reader disk
3. Capillary tubes (Fig. 20.2)
   a. Plain-blue tip (for EDTA [ethylenediaminetetraacetic acid] tubes)
   b. Heparinized-red tip (for Microtainer specimens)
   Note: both types of tubes contain self-sealing clay
4. Mechanical rocker

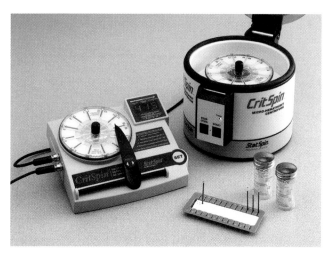

Figure 20.1   Standard microhematocrit centrifuge. Maximum packing time is dependent on a calibrated centrifuge.

Specimen Collection and Storage

1. Fresh whole blood collected in EDTA in which the patient tube is at least half full.
2. Capillary blood collected in an EDTA Microtainer.

Quality Control

Hematocrits are run in duplicate and must agree within ±1%.

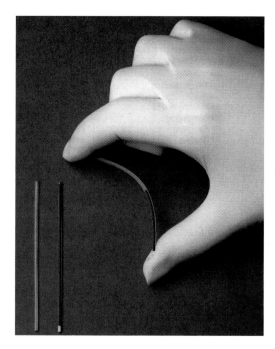

Figure 20.2   Standard and flexible capillary tubes.

Procedure

1. Mix EDTA tube by placing on a mechanical rocker for 3 minutes.
2. After adequate mixing, fill the self-sealing capillary tubes two thirds to three fourths full. Prepare the tubes in duplicate.
3. Wipe the outside of the capillary tubes with lint-free wipe or gauze.
4. Invert the tube so that the blood runs to sealed end.
5. Place the tubes directly across from each other in the microhematocrit centrifuge, with the sealed ends away from the center of centrifuge.
6. Record the identification and the position number of each patient specimen.
7. Place the head cover and hand-tighten only. Close the outer lid.
8. Centrifuge for 5 minutes, for maximum packing.
9. Remove the tubes from the centrifuge and place in the microhematocrit reader. Read the hematocrit according to the manufacturer's instructions. The results are recorded in percent. The tubes should match within ±1%.

Interpretation

The spun capillary tube should have three visible sections: RBCs, buffy coat (contains leukocytes and platelets), and plasma. Read the hematocrit results by placing the centrifuged capillary tube in the groove of the plastic indicator reader. The bottom of the red cell column should meet with the black line on the plastic indicator (Fig. 20.3).

1. Rotate the bottom plate so the 100% line is directly beneath the red line on the plastic indicator and hold the bottom plate in this position. With use of the finger hole, rotate the top plate so that the spiral line intersects the capillary tube at the plasma air space.
2. Rotate both discs together until the spiral line intersects the capillary tube at the white cell–red cell line.
3. The volume of red cell is read in percentage from the point on the scale directly beneath the red line of the plastic indicator. The hematocrit percentage is read between the red cell column and the clear plasma column.

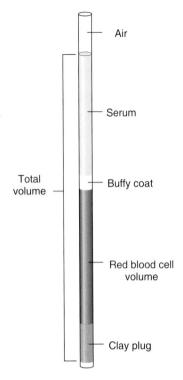

Air

Serum

Total
volume

Buffy coat

Red blood cell
volume

Clay plug

Figure 20.3 Capillary tubes. Note the distinct layers once blood sample has been spun.

CALCULATING RED BLOOD CELL INDICES

The morphological classification of anemias is based upon the size and hemoglobin content of the red cell. The values derived as red cell indices give important clues as to the differential diagnosis of the anemia. The hematocrit value is an important parameter used in calculating these indices. See calculations below:

a. Mean corpuscular volume (MCV)

$$MCV = \frac{\text{Hematocrit } \% \times 10}{\text{Erythrocyte count}} = fL$$

$$\text{Example: } \frac{35\% \times 10}{4.0} = 87.5 \text{ fL}$$

b. Mean corpuscular hemoglobin (MCH)

$$MCH = \frac{\text{Hemoglobin} \times 10}{\text{Erythrocyte count}} = pg$$

$$\text{Example: } \frac{14.0 \times 10}{4.0} = 35 \text{ pg}$$

c. Mean corpuscular hemoglobin concentration (MCHC)

$$MCHC = \frac{\text{Hemoglobin} \times 100}{\text{Hematocrit}} = \%$$

$$\text{Example: } \frac{14 \times 100}{42} = 33.3\%$$

Normal Average Values

Hematocrit

Newborn (1 to 7 days)	56 ± 2%
Adult (female)	42 ± 2%
Adult (male)	47 ± 2%

Normal Erythrocyte Indices Values

MCV 80 to 96 fL
MCH 27 to 32 pg
MCHC 32% to 36%

Notes

- Buffy coats are not included as part of the red cell column.
- Repeat procedure if specimen has leaked in the centrifuge.
- Repeat procedure if centrifuge has been stopped manually.

MODIFIED WESTERGREN SEDIMENTATION RATE

Principle

The erythrocyte sedimentation rate (ESR) is a nonspecific screening test indicative of inflammation. It is used as an initial screening tool and also as a follow-up test to monitor therapy and progression or remission of disease. This test measures the distance that RBCs will fall in a vertical tube over a given time period. The ESR is directly proportional to red cell mass and inversely proportional to its surface area. The ESR is reported in millimeters. Any condition that will increase rouleaux formation will usually increase the settling of red cells. Factors affecting the ESR are as follows:

- Red cell shape and size: Specimens containing sickle cells, acanthocytes, or spherocytes will settle slowly and give a decreased ESR
- Plasma fibrinogen and globulin levels: Increased fibrinogen or globulin levels

will cause increased settling and give an increased ESR
- Mechanical and technical conditions: Surfaces that are not level will influence red cell settling. Specimens that are not properly anticoagulated will also affect red cell settling. EDTA is the recommended anticoagulant.

Reagents and Equipment

1. Sediplast Autozero Westergren ESR system (Fig. 20.4)
   a. Fixed bore pipettes
   b. Sedivials filled with 0.2 mL of 3.8% sodium citrate
   c. Vial holder (rack)
2. Disposable plastic pipettes
3. Rotator/mixer
4. Timer

Specimen Collection and Storage

Specimens are collected in EDTA. Tubes must be at least half full, well mixed, and free of clots and/or fibrin. ESR can be set up on specimens at room temperature up to 4 hours old. Refrigerated specimens (2 to 8°C) can be set up until 24 hours old.

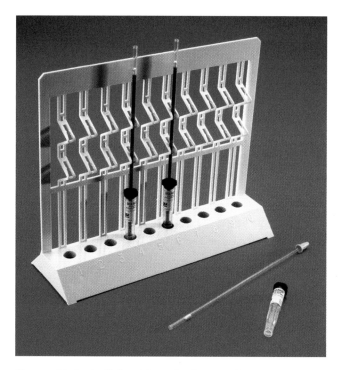

Figure 20.4 Sediplast ESR rack. The sample must be placed on a level surface with no vibration.

Quality Control

Commercially prepared controls stored at 2 to 8°C are valid until expiration date. Controls are prepared like patients' specimens. Controls are run once daily prior to setting up patient tests. Do not report out patient results unless controls are in reference range.

Procedure

1. Mix the EDTA tube on the rotator/mixer for a minimum of 5 minutes. If the sample has been refrigerated, allow 30 minutes for the sample to come to room temperature before proceeding.
2. Remove the top of the Sediplast vial, which contains 3.8% sodium citrate. Using a disposable pipette, add blood to the indicated line, return the top, and mix thoroughly.
3. Insert Westergren tube into Sediplast vial with a slight twist, allowing the blood to rise to the zero mark.
4. Place the vial in the rack on a level surface.
5. Set a timer for one hour and read at the end of the hour.
6. Record the ESR in millimeters per hour.

Normal Ranges

Men   0 to 15 mm/hr
Women 0 to 20 mm/hr

Limitations

1. Tubes not filled properly will yield erroneous results.
2. Refrigerated specimens must come to room temperature for 30 minutes prior to testing.
3. The ESR rack must be on a level surface and free of vibration. Vibration can cause a falsely increased ESR.
4. Cold agglutinins can cause a falsely elevated ESR. An ESR can be performed at 37°C (incubator) for 60 minutes with no ill effects.
5. Cell size and shape affect ESR, usually resulting in a decreased ESR result.
6. Increased rouleaux formation, excessive globulin, or increased fibrinogen will increase the ESR.
7. Specimen must be free of clots and/or fibrin.
8. A tilted ESR tube gives erroneous results.
9. Hemolyzed samples are not acceptable.
10. Specimens older than 24 hours are not acceptable.

Conditions Associated With...

Increased ESR

1. Kidney disease
2. Pregnancy
3. Rheumatic fever
4. Rheumatoid arthritis
5. Anemia
6. Syphilis
7. Systemic lupus erythematosus
8. Thyroid disease
9. Elevated room temperature

Decreased ESR

1. Congestive heart failure
2. Hyperviscosity
3. Decreased fibrinogen levels
4. Polycythemia
5. Sickle cell anemia

Note: A rapid ESR method (ESR Stat Plus) is now available, which gives a result in 3 minutes.

MANUAL RETICULOCYTE PROCEDURE

Principle

The reticulocyte count is an index of bone marrow red cell production. The reticulocyte is the cell stage immediately before the mature erythrocyte. This cell spends 2 to 3 days maturing in the bone marrow before it is released into the peripheral circulation, where it spends an additional day of maturation. The reticulocyte count is the most effective measure of erythropoietic activity. Reticulocytes contain RNA and can be observed using supravital stains such as New Methylene Blue or Brilliant Cresyl Blue. Low reticulocyte counts indicate decreased erythropoietic activity. Increased reticulocyte counts indicate increased erythropoietic activity usually as the bone marrow compensates in response to anemic stress. Therefore, reticulocyte counts are a reflection of bone marrow health or injury. These counts assist physicians in diagnosis, treatment, or monitoring of patients with various anemias.

Reagents and Equipment

1. New Methylene Blue (Supravital Stain)
2. Test tubes
3. Microscope slides with a frosted end
4. Microscope with ×100 (oil immersion objective)
5. Transfer pipettes

Specimen Collection and Storage

1. One EDTA tube or EDTA Microtainer
2. Specimens can be stored at room temperature for 8 hours or refrigerated at 2 to 8°C for 24 hours.

Quality Control

Commercially prepared controls are performed each day when reticulocytes are reported manually. Controls are prepared like the patient specimens and follow the procedure below for counting reticulocytes. Do not report out patient results until quality control results fall within the acceptable reference range.

Procedure

1. Mix 4 drops of New Methylene Blue with 4 drops of patient's blood. If the specimen is a small amount (such as a Microtainer), add an equal amount of stain to the Microtainer after the CBC has been completed.

    complete blood count

2. Let the specimen mix for 10 to 15 minutes. Make a wedge smear and let it air dry. Label the smears with the patient's name, specimen number, and the date.
3. Allow the smear to completely dry and read under the microscope using ×100 oil immersion.
    a. Count the number of reticulocytes in 1000 cells.
    b. Use the following formula to calculate the percentage of reticulocytes

$$\text{Number of reticulocytes} = \frac{\text{number of reticulocytes counted per 1000 cells} \times 100}{1000}$$

$$\text{Example: } \frac{35 \times 100}{1000} = 3.5\%$$

Normal Values

Adults: 0.5% to 2.0%
Infants: 2.5% to 6.5%

Conditions Associated With...

Decreased Reticulocyte Count

1. Aplastic anemia
2. Exposure to radiation or radiation therapy
3. Chronic infection

4. Medications such as azathioprine, chloramphenicol, dactinomycin, methotrexate, and other chemotherapy medications
5. Untreated pernicious anemia/megaloblastic anemia

Increased Reticulocyte Count

1. Rapid blood loss
2. High elevation
3. Hemolytic anemias
4. Medications such as levodopa, malarial medications, corticotrophin, and fever-reducing medications
5. Pregnancy

Limitations

1. Recent blood transfusion can interfere with accurate reticulocyte results.
2. Mishandling, contamination, or inadequate refrigeration of the sample can interfere and cause inaccurate test results.
3. Red cell inclusions such as Heinz bodies, siderocytes, and Howell-Jolly bodies can be mistaken for reticulocytes. If these are counted as reticulocytes, they will falsely increase the reticulocyte count. Inclusions should be confirmed with Wright's stain.

RETICULOCYTE PROCEDURE WITH MILLER EYE DISC

Principle

A Miller Eye Disc is placed inside the microscope eyepiece as an aid to counting reticulocytes. This reticule is a large square inside a small square and provides the technologist the ability to isolate the reticulocytes while counting.

Reagents and Equipment

1. New Methylene Blue (Supravital Stain)
2. Test tubes
3. Slides
4. Microscope with Miller ocular eye disc
5. Transfer pipettes

Specimen Collection and Storage

1. One EDTA tube or EDTA Microtainer
2. Specimens can be stored at room temperature for 8 hours or refrigerated at 2 to 8°C for 24 hours.

Quality Control

Commercially prepared controls are performed each day when reticulocytes are reported. Controls are prepared like the patient specimen and follow the procedure below for counting reticulocytes. Do not report out patient results until quality control results are acceptable.

Procedure

1. Mix 4 drops of new methylene blue with 4 drops of patient blood in a test tube. If the specimen is a small amount (such as a Microtainer), add an equal amount of stain to the Microtainer after the CBC has been completed.
2. Let the specimen mix for 10 to 15 minutes. Make an appropriate smear with feather edges. Label the slides with the patient's name, specimen number, and date.
3. Allow the smear to completely dry and read the slides under the microscope with oil immersion using the Miller Eye Disc (Fig. 20.5).
   a. The Miller Eye Disc is a counting aid that provides a standardized area in which to count RBCs. There are two squares that make up the disc. Square 1 is nine times the area of square 2.
   b. To use the disc, all reticulocytes are counted in the large (1) and the small (2) square. The RBCs are counted only in the small square.
   c. Count the number of reticulocytes in 111 red cells in the small square. At this time, the counting is concluded and the number of reticulocytes is reported.
   d. Use this formula for calculating reticulocytes in percentage. See example.

$$\% \text{ Reticulocytes} = \frac{\text{Total number of reticulocytes counted in large square} \times 100}{\text{Total RBCs in small square} \times 9}$$

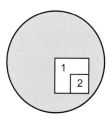

Figure 20.5 Miller Eye Disc. Count RBCs only in the small square; reticulocytes are counted in both squares.

Example: $\dfrac{40 \times 100}{900 \times 9} = 4.0\%$

Normal Values

Adults: 0.5% to 2.0%
Infants: 2.5% to 6.5%

Conditions Associated With...

Decreased reticulocyte count

1. Aplastic anemia
2. Exposure to radiation or radiation therapy
3. Chronic infection
4. Medications such as azathioprine, chloramphenicol, dactinomycin, methotrexate, and other chemotherapy medications
5. Untreated pernicious anemia and megaloblastic anemia

Increased reticulocyte count

1. Rapid blood loss
2. High elevation
3. Hemolytic anemias
4. Medications such as levodopa, malarial medications, corticotrophin, and fever-reducing medications
5. Pregnancy

Limitations

1. Recent blood transfusion can interfere with accurate reticulocyte results.
2. Mishandling, contamination, or inadequate refrigeration of the sample can interfere and cause inaccurate test results.
3. Red cell inclusions such as Heinz bodies, siderocytes, and Howell-Jolly bodies may be mistaken for reticulocytes. Counting these inclusions may cause a falsely elevated reticulocyte count. Inclusions must be confirmed with Wright's stain.

See automated reticulocyte information on page 326.

PERIPHERAL SMEAR PROCEDURE

Principle

When automated differentials do not meet specified criteria programmed into the automated hematology instrument, the technologist/technician must perform a manual differential count from a prepared smear. There are two types of blood smears: the wedge smear and the spun smear. The wedge smear will be discussed in this procedure. Smears are prepared by placing a drop of blood on a clean glass slide and spreading the drop using another glass slide at an angle. The slide is then stained and observed microscopically. A well-stained peripheral smear will show the red cell background as red orange. White cells will appear with blue purple nuclei with red purple granules throughout the cytoplasm. A well made, well distributed peripheral smear will have a counting area at the thin portion of the wedge smear which is approximately 200 red cells not touching. A good counting area is an essential ingredient in a peripheral smear for evaluating the numbers of and types of white cells present and evaluating red cell and platelet morphology.

Reagents and Equipment

1. Glass slides (frosted)
2. Wooden applicator sticks
3. DIFF-SAFE (an apparatus designed to avoid removing the tube top)

Specimen Collection and Storage

1. EDTA specimen or EDTA Microtainer
2. Smears are made from EDTA
   a. Microtainers within 1 hour of collection
   b. EDTA blood within 2 to 3 hours
   c. Check all Microtainers for clots with applicator sticks

Quality Control

A random slide is picked after it has been stained and a technologist/technician checks the quality of the stain for the WBCs and RBCs, platelets, and the distribution of cells (see Principle)

Procedure

1. Insert the DIFF-SAFE dispenser through the stopper of the tube held in an upright position.
2. Turn the tube upside down and apply pressure at the frosted end of the slide. When the drop of blood appears, discontinue pressure.
3. Using a second slide (spreader slide), place the edge of the second slide against the surface of the slide at an angle between 30 and 45 degrees (Fig. 20.6).
4. Bring the spreader slide back into the blood drop until contact is made with the drop of blood.

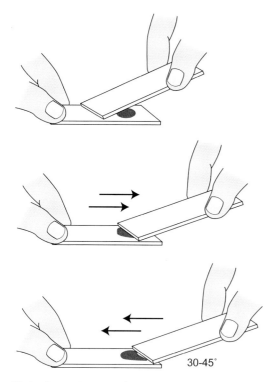

Figure 20.6 Preparing a wedge-type smear. Size of drop and angle of spread are important features.

5. Move the spreader slide forward on the slide, so a smear is made approximately 3 to 4 cm in length. The smear should be half the size of the slide, with no ridges, and a "feather edge" should be toward the end of the smear.
6. Label the frosted end of the slide with the patient's last name and first initial, specimen number, and the date.
7. Allow the smear to air dry completely.
8. Proceed with staining. Manual Wright staining is not found often in the clinical laboratory setting. Most clinical laboratories have an automated staining instrument attached to their automated CBC analyzer. If there is no automated stainer attached to the analyzer, there still is a separate staining instrument.

Limitations

1. The angle between the slides is dependent upon the size of the blood drop and viscosity of the blood. The optimal angle is 45 degrees.
2. The larger the drop of blood and lower the hematocrit, the higher the angle needs to be so the blood smear is not too long.
3. Blood with a higher hematocrit needs to have a lower angle so the smear is not too short and thick.

4. Glass slides must be clean; otherwise, this results in imperfect distribution of cells and improper staining.
5. Once the drop of blood has contact on the slide, the smear needs to be made immediately. Otherwise, the blood will clump and dry, again resulting in uneven distribution of WBC and platelets.

PERFORMING A MANUAL DIFFERENTIAL AND ASSESSING RED BLOOD CELL MORPHOLOGY

Principle

When blood samples are evaluated by the use of automated hematology analyzers, this analysis includes automated differentials. Specific criteria pertaining to normal, abnormal, and critical values have been programmed into the analyzers by the institution, and if the differentials do not meet these criteria, verification is necessary. This is done by performing manual differentials and further evaluating the peripheral smear. First, a differential white blood cell (WBC) count is performed to determine the relative number of each type of white cell present. Technologists/technicians must recognize and properly record the type(s) of white cell observed. Simultaneously, red cell, white cell, and platelet morphology is noted and recorded. Also, a rough estimate of platelets and WBC counts is made to determine if these numbers generally correlate with the automated hematology analyzer. Technologists/technicians must be proficient at recognizing red and white cell abnormalities, identifying them correctly, and quantifying them.

Reagents and Equipment

1. Microscope
2. Immersion oil
3. Differential cell counter

Specimen Collection and Storage

Well-made stained blood smear obtained from a capillary puncture or an EDTA tube at least three-fourths full.

Quality Control

The slide should have three zones: head, body, and tail (Fig. 20.7). In the tail area, neutrophils and monocytes predominate, while red cells lie singly. In the body area, lymphocytes predominate, and red cells overlap each other to some extent.

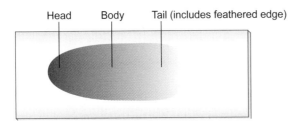

Figure 20.7 Three zones of wedge preparation.

1. WBCs should contain a blue nucleus along with a lighter staining cytoplasm.
2. RBCs should have good quality of color ranging from buff pink to orange.
3. Platelets should be blue with granules and no nucleus.

Procedure

Observations Under ×10

1. Place a well-stained slide on the stage of the microscope, smear side up, and focus using the low-power objective (×10).
2. Check to see if there are good counting areas available free of ragged edges and cell clumps.
3. Check the WBC distribution over the smear.
4. Check that the slide is properly stained.
5. Check for the presence of large platelets, platelet clumps, and fibrin strands.

Observations Under ×40 x-: WBC Estimates

1. Place a drop of immersion oil on the slide and change the objective to ×50 oil. (In cases where no ×50 is available, use the ×40 high dry with no oil.)
2. Choose a portion of the peripheral smear where there is only slight overlapping of the RBCs. Count 10 fields, take the total number of white cells and divide by 10, and refer to Table 20.1 to determine the WBC estimate.

Table 20.1 ○ Estimated WBC Count From Peripheral Smear	
WBC/High-Power Field	Estimated WBC Count
2 to 4	4.0 to 7.0 × 10⁹/L
4 to 6	7.0 to 10.0 × 10⁹/L
6 to 10	10.0 to 13.0 × 10⁹/L
10 to 20	13.0 to 18.0 × 10⁹/L

Table 20.2 ○ Platelet Estimate From Peripheral Smear	
Average No. of Platelets per ×100 Field	Platelet Count Estimate
0 to 1	<20,000
1 to 4	20,000 to 80,000
5 to 8	100,000 to 160,000
10 to 15	200,000 to 300,000
16 to 20	320,000 to 400,000
>21	>420,000

3. An alternative technique is to do a WBC estimate by taking the average number of white cells and multiplying by 2000.

Observations Under ×100: Platelet Estimates

1. Platelet estimates are done under ×100 with the RBCs barely touching, approximately 200 RBCs. This takes place under the ×100 objective (oil). On average there are 8 to 20 platelets per field. See Table 20.2.
2. Ten fields are counted using the zigzag method. This method of counting is done by going back and forth lengthwise or sidewise (Fig. 20.8).

   Platelets per oil immersion field (OIF)

   <8 platelets/OIF = decreased

   8 to 20 platelets/OIF = adequate

   >20 platelets/OIF = increased

3. After the 10 fields are counted, the number of platelets is divided by 10 to get the average. The average number is now multiplied by a factor of 20,000 for wedge preparations. For monolayer preparations, use a factor of 15,000.

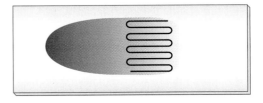

Figure 20.8 Zigzag method of performing differential.

Example: 120 platelets/10 fields =
12 platelets per field

12 × 20,000 = 240,000 platelets

Manual Differential Counts

1. These counts are done in the same area as WBC and platelet estimates with the red cells barely touching.
2. This takes place under ×100 (oil) using the zigzag method previously described in the platelet estimate (see Fig. 20.8).
3. Count 100 WBCs including all cell lines from immature to mature. Normal values for WBCs can be found in Table 20.3.

Observing and Recording Nucleated Red Blood Cells (nRBCs)

1. If nRBCs are observed while performing the differential, they need to be reported. These elements in a peripheral smear are indicative of increased erythropoietic activity and usually a pathologic condition. Additionally, the presence of nRBCs per 100 white cells will falsely elevate the white count and is clinically significant.
2. Correct the WBC count if the nRBC count is greater than 5 nRBCs/100. The following formula is applied for correcting NRBCs:

WBC × 100/NRBC + 100

Example : If WBC = 5000 and 10
NRBCs have been counted

Table 20.3 ● Normal Differential Results in Adults and Infants

WBC Type	Adult	Infant
Segmented neutrophils	50% to 70%	37% to 67%
Bands	1% to 10%	4% to 14%
Lymphocytes	20% to 44%	18% to 38%
Monocytes	4% to 10%	1% to 12%
Eosinophils	0% to 4%	1% to 4%
Basophils	0% to 2%	0% to 2%

Then

5,000 × 100/110 = 4545.50

The corrected white count is 4545.50.

Recording RBC Morphology

1. Scan area using ×100 (oil immersion).
2. Observe 10 fields.
3. Red cells are observed for size, color, hemoglobin content or pallor, and shape.
4. Normal morphology
   a. Normocytic: normal cell size and shape
   b. Normochromic: normal hemoglobin content and color
5. Abnormal morphology: Red cell morphology is assessed according to size, shape, hemoglobin content, and the presence or absence of inclusions. See the following sample grading system. Note that red cell morphology must be scanned in a good counting area. Two questions should be asked, *Is the morphology seen in every field? Is the morphology pathologic and not artificially induced?* Table 20.4 represents a system derived to determine a quantitative scale.
   a. Report RBC **size** (see Table 20.5 for a composite list of red cell morphologies matched to clinical conditions). *Anisocytosis* is a term meaning variation in the size of the RBCs. The average size of an RBC is 7.2 μm with a range of 6.8 to 7.5 μm.
      - Normocyte: normal size of RBC
      - Macrocyte: larger than the normal RBC (>8.2 μm) and is the result of a defect in nuclear maturation or stimulated erythropoiesis
      - Microcytic: smaller than the normal RBC, <7.2 μm, and is associated with a decrease in hemoglobin synthesis
   b. **Shape.** *Poikilocytosis* is the general term for mature erythrocytes that have a shape other than the round, biconcave disk. Poikilocytes can be seen in many shapes.
      - Acanthocyte: thorny projections that are irregularly distributed around the red cell and lack an area of a central pallor.
      - Burr cell (echinocyte): short and spike-like projections that are evenly distributed around the cell membrane.
      - Ovalocyte (elliptocyte): an elongated oval cell. They are a result of a membrane defect.

- Schistocyte: red cell fragments that are irregular in shape and size. They are usually half the size of the normal RBC; therefore, they have a deeper red color.
- Sickle cells: crescent shaped with usually one end pointed. They can vary in size but are usually smaller than the normal RBC. These occur due to a decrease in oxygen and decrease in pH.
- Spherocyte: red cells that lack the central pallor or the biconcave disk. Usually they are smaller (<6 μm) and appear darker from the red cell background. They can appear as artifacts if the slide is examined in too thin of an area.
- Stomatocyte: Red cell with a slit-like central pallor that resembles a mouth. These are the result of increased sodium ions and decreased potassium ion concentration within the cytoplasm of RBCs.
- Target cell: Red cell with a "target" or bull's-eye appearance. The cell appears with a central bull's eye that is surrounded by a clear ring and then an outer red ring.
- Teardrop: resembles a tear and usually smaller than the normal RBC.

c. Variation in erythrocyte color. A normal erythrocyte has a pinkish-red color with a slightly lighter-colored center (central pallor) when stained with a blood stain, such as Wright. The color of the erythrocyte is representative of hemoglobin concentration in the cell. Under normal conditions, when the color, central pallor, and hemoglobin are proportional, the erythrocyte is referred to as normochromic. To grade color variations, use the method described in Table 20.5.

- Hypochromia: increased central pallor and decreased hemoglobin concentration.
- Polychromasia: is used to describe erythrocytes that have a faint blue-orange color and those that are slightly larger than normal red cells.

d. **Inclusions**. There are several inclusions that can be seen in erythrocytes and/or white cells. Use Table 20.6 for grading inclusions. Inclusions are listed in alphabetical order.

- Auer rods are aggregates of fused lysosomes, appearing as red needle-like inclusions. They are found in WBCs and are pathological.
- Basophilic stippling is tiny round granules that stain deep blue with Wright's stain. They are evenly distributed throughout the red cell and are composed of ribosomes and RNA. They do not occur in vivo but only on the smear.
- Cabot rings are delicate thread-like inclusions in the RBC. They can take on a variety of shapes such as a ring, figure-of-eight, or twisted.
- Döhle bodies are light blue-staining inclusions found in Wright-stained blood smears. They are usually observed in the periphery of the cytoplasm of neutrophils. Döhle bodies are aggregates of rough endoplasmic reticulum (RNA).
- Hemoglobin C crystals are found in blood smears that are normochromic and normocytic with at least 50% target cells. The shape of the C crystal is usually oblong in homozygous conditions. In hemoglobin SC disease, the hemoglobin C crystal is shaped like a gloved hand.
- Heinz body inclusions can either be round or irregularly shaped. They are made of denatured hemoglobin. These inclusions tend to lie close to the periphery of the cell. Observation of these inclusions is seen with supravital stains such as Brilliant Cresyl Blue or Crystal Violet. They are NOT observed on Wright's stain.
- Howell-Jolly bodies are round, dark-staining nuclear remnants of DNA. When present, there is only one or two per red cell.
- Pappenheimer bodies (siderocytes) are seen as small dark-blue or purple dots in clusters along the periphery of the red cells in Wright stain. They are a result of a defect of iron and aggregated with mitochondria and ribosomes. Proof of these inclusions is done with a Prussian blue stain. See Table 20.7 for a composite of inclusions matched to disease states.
- Toxic granulation is an increased number of primary granules with intensified coloring. These can be found in segmented neutrophils and band forms.

Table 20.4 ⊙ Qualitative Grading of RBC Morphology	
	Grade Degree of Abnormalities
1 to 5 cells/10 fields	Slight
6 to 15 cells/10 fields	Moderate
>15 cells/10 fields	Marked

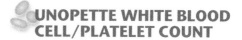

UNOPETTE WHITE BLOOD CELL/PLATELET COUNT

Principle

The Unopette system is a system of prefilled blood dilution vials containing solutions that will preserve certain cell types while lysing others. Capillary pipettes are available to draw up different volumes of blood. The dilution is determined by the type of capillary used. The diluted blood is added to a hematocytometer chamber,

Table 20.5 ⊙ Red Cell Morphologies Matched to Clinical Conditions

RBC Morphology	Relative Clinical Conditions	RBC Morphology	Relative Clinical Conditions
Anisocytosis	Severe anemias	Schistocytes	Hemolytic anemias related to burns and prosthetic implants
Microcytes	Iron deficiency		Renal transplant patients
	Hemoglobinopathies		Disseminated intravascular coagulation (DIC)
Macrocytes	Megaloblastic anemias (vitamin B_{12} deficiency and folic acid deficiency)		Hemolytic uremic syndrome (HUS)
	Pernicious anemia		Thrombotic thrombocytopenic purpura (TTP)
	Folic acid deficiency	Sickle cells	Sickle cell anemia
Acanthocytes	Abetalipoproteinemia	Spherocytes	ABO incompatibility
	Neonatal hepatitis		DIC
	Postsplenectomy		Bacterial toxins
	Heparin administration		Hemolytic anemias
	Cirrhosis of liver with associated hemolytic anemia		Blood transfusion reactions
			Congential spherocytosis
Burr cells	Variety of anemias	Stomatocyte	Alcoholism
	Gastric carcinoma		Hereditary spherocytosis
	Peptic ulcers		Infectious mononucleosis
	Renal insufficiency		Lead poisoning
	Uremia		Liver disease including cirrhosis
	Pyruvate kinase deficiency		Malignancies
Ovalocytes	Hemoglobin C disease		Thalassemia minor
	Hemolytic anemias	Target cells	Hemoglobinopathies: HbC disease, S-C, S-S
	Hereditary ovalocytosis		Sickle cell thalassemia
	Iron deficiency anemia		Hemolytic anemias
	Megaloblastic anemia		Iron deficiency
	Pernicious anemia		Liver disease including cirrhosis
	Sickle cell trait		Postsplenectomy
	Thalassemia	Teardrops	Myeloproliferative syndromes
			Severe anemias

Table 20.6 ⊙ Grading Inclusions	
Rare	0 to 1/hpf
Few	1 to 2/hpf
Mod	2 to 4 /hpf
Many	> 5/hpf

hpf, high-power field.

and cells are counted in a specified area. For this procedure, whole blood is added to ammonium oxalate diluent, which lyses the red cells while preserving platelets, leukocytes, and reticulocytes.

Table 20.7 ⊙ Inclusion Matched to Disease	
RBC/WBC Inclusion	**Disease Association**
Auer rods	Acute myeloid leukemias
Basophilic stippling	Lead poisoning
	Arsenic poisoning
	Severe anemias
	Sideroblastic anemia
	Hemolytic anemia
	Unstable hemoglobin
	Pyrimidine 5'-nucleotidase deficiency
Cabot rings	Lead poisoning
	Pernicious anemia
Döhle bodies	Infection
	Burn patients
Hemoglobin C	Hemoglobin C disease
Heinz bodies	G6PD deficiency
Howell-Jolly bodies	Hemolytic anemias
	Sickle cell anemia
	Pernicious anemia
	Postsplenectomy
	Megaloblastic anemia
	Lead poisoning
Pappenheimer bodies	Iron loading anemias
	Sideroblastic anemia
	Postsplenectomy
	Lead poisoning
	Thalassemia
Toxic granulation	Infections
	Burn patients
	Drug therapy

Reagents and Equipment

1. Unopette reservoirs containing ammonium oxalate diluent. Check expiration dates and do not use expired Unopettes. Protect from sunlight. Storage temperature is 1 to 30°C.
2. Unopette capillary pipette, 20 μL.
3. Hematocytometer: improved Neubauer ruling
4. Hematocytometer coverslips
5. Petri dish lined with filter paper that has been moistened and two applicator sticks to hold the hematocytometer
6. Microscope with phase
7. Hand counter

Quality Control

1. All WBC and platelet counts are done in duplicate. WBC counts should agree ±20%. Platelet counts must agree ±10%. If they do not agree, repeat counts.
2. A visual estimate of the white count and the platelets can be done on the peripheral smear. Refer to charts.
3. Laboratory professionals are trained and tested for proficiency. Results are documented in their training file.

Specimen Collection and Storage

Specimen of choice is a Microtainer EDTA or EDTA tube, which should be at least half full.

Procedure

1. Specimen should be well mixed and left on a rocker for at least 5 minutes before using.
2. Check Unopettes for clarity and contents. If the Unopette chambers appear cloudy or the amount of reagent looks questionable, do not use.
3. With the reservoir on a flat surface, puncture the diaphragm of the reservoir using the protective shield of the capillary pipette.
   a. Using a twist action, remove protective shield from the pipette assembly.
   b. Holding the pipette and the tube of blood almost horizontally, touch the tip of the pipette to the blood. The pipette will fill by capillary action and will stop automatically when the blood reaches the end of the capillary bore in the neck of the pipette.
   c. Wipe the excess blood from the outside of the capillary pipette. Be careful not to touch

the tip of the capillary when wiping off excess blood.

    d. Before entering the reservoir, it is necessary to force some air out of the reservoir. Do not expel any liquid and maintain pressure on reservoir.

    e. Place an index finger over opening of overflow chamber and position pipette into reservoir neck.

    f. Release pressure on reservoir and then remove finger. The negative pressure will draw blood into pipette.

    g. Rinse the capillary pipette with the diluent by squeezing the reservoir gently two or three times. This forces diluent up into, but not out of, the overflow chamber and releases pressure each time to ensure the mixture returns to the reservoir.

    h. Return protective shield over upper opening and gently invert several times to mix blood adequately.

    i. Allow the Unopette to stand for 10 minutes to allow RBCs to hemolyze. Leukocyte counts should be performed within 3 hours.

4. Charge hematocytometer

    a. Mix the dilution by inversion and convert the Unopette to the dropper assembly.

    b. Gently squeeze Unopette and discard first 3 or 4 drops. This allows proper mixing, with no excess diluent in the tip of the capillary.

    c. Carefully charge hematocytometer with the diluted blood, gently squeezing the reservoir to release contents until chamber is properly filled. Be sure to charge both sides and not to overfill chambers.

5. Place the hematocytometer in the premoistened Petri dish and leave for 15 minutes. This allows the sample to settle evenly.

Cell Counts and Calculations

A WBC count is performed with a Neubauer hematocytometer.

1. Using the ×10 microscope magnification, WBC are counted using all nine squares of the counting chamber. Count both sides of the chamber and average the count. Refer to diagram below.

2. When counting, the cells that touch the extreme lower and the extreme left lines are not included in the count.

3. Use the following formulas to calculate the WBC.

$$\text{Cells/mm}^3 = \frac{\text{average No. of cells} \times \text{depth factor (10)} \times \text{dilution factor (100)}}{\text{Area}}$$

Example: side 1 = 85 cells
Side 2 = 95 cells
90 cells average/all 9 squares counted

$$\frac{90 \times 10 \times 100}{9} = 10,000 \text{ WBCs}$$

Normal Values

WBC/mm^3
Adult: 4000 to 10,000
Newborn: 10,000 to 30,000

1. Platelet counts are performed with a Neubauer hematocytometer (Fig. 20.9).

    a. Counting is done using ×40 dry phase contrast objective. Platelets will have a faint halo. The middle square of the hemacytometer chamber is counted. It contains 25 small squares.

    b. Count 5 of the 25 squares if the platelet count is >100,000. Take the average of both sides. Refer to diagram below.

    c. To calculate platelets, use the following formula
      • If 5 squares of middle square counted

Multiply No. of platelets × 5000
= No. of platelets/mm^3

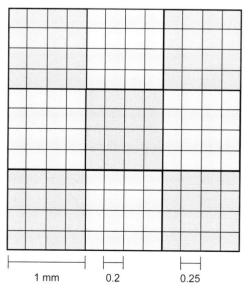

1 mm   0.2   0.25

Figure 20.9 Neubauer hemocytometer counting chamber. Note the difference in depth depending on area examined.

- If 25 squares of middle square are counted (if the platelet count is <100,000, count all 25 squares of the middle square):

Multiply No. of platelets × 1000 = No. of platelets/mm^3

Platelets
150,000 to 410,000 platelets/mm^3

Limitations

1. Specimen should be properly mixed and have sufficient volume of blood so there is no dilution of anticoagulant.
2. The capillary tube must be filled completely and be free of any air bubbles.
3. After the hematocytometer is charged, it should be placed in a premoistened Petri dish to prevent evaporation while the cells are settling out.
4. The light adjustment is critical. It is important for both WBCs and especially platelets. If the condenser is not in the correct position, it will fade out platelets.
5. Debris and bacteria can be mistaken for platelets.
6. Clumped platelets cannot be counted properly; the specimen must be recollected. The anticoagulant of choice is EDTA for preventing platelet clumping.
7. Avoiding overloading of hemacytometer chamber.

SICKLE CELL PROCEDURE

Principle

The sickle screen kit provides a procedure based on differential solubility. Hemoglobin S is insoluble when combined with a buffer and a reducing agent. This occurs when the blood is mixed with the buffer and sodium hydrosulfate solution. Specimens containing hemoglobin S are insoluble and show a turbid cloudy solution. Normal adult hemoglobin A is soluble and produces a transparent solution. The presence of hemoglobin S in either the heterozygous or homozygous state will produce a cloudy solution. Because this is a qualitative screening procedure, all positives need to be followed up with hemoglobin electrophoresis at alkaline or acid pH or isoelectric focusing.

Reagents and Equipment

1. Sickle cell kit
   a. Phosphate buffer/sodium hydrosulfite solution. Prepare by pouring entire contents of sodium hydrosulfite vial into one phosphate buffer bottle. Cap and mix for 1 to 2 minutes. Reagent, once reconstituted is good for 5 days when stored at 2 to 8°C.
   b. Unmixed reagents are good until expiration date on package when stored at 2 to 8°C.
2. 12 × 75-mm test tubes
3. Test tube caps or parafilm
4. 50-μL pipette and tips
5. Reading rack

Specimen Collection and Storage

1. Whole blood obtained in EDTA, heparin, or sodium citrate.
2. Specimens can be refrigerated at 2 to 8°C for up to 2 weeks before testing.

Quality Control

Commercially prepared negative and positive controls are run along with the patient's blood. Control results must be correct to report patient results.

Procedure

1. Pipette 4 mL of the phosphate buffer/sodium hydrosulfite solution to each test tube, (one for each test and each control).
2. Add 50 μL of well-mixed whole blood or control to each labeled tube.
3. Cover each tube with a cap or parafilm, invert to mix three or four times.
4. Place each tube in the reading rack at room temperature and let them incubate for 10 to 20 minutes.

Interpretation of Results and Result Reporting

Positive: If hemoglobin S is present (or any other sickling hemoglobin [hemoglobin C Harlem]), the solution will be turbid and the lines on the reading rack are not visible.

Negative: If no sickling hemoglobin is present, the lines on the reading rack will be visible through the solution (Fig. 20.10).

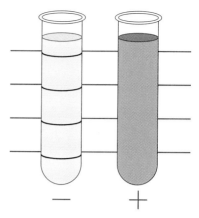

Figure 20.10 Tube solubility screen for hemoglobin S. The procedure simply gives an indication of the presence of hemoglobin S and should be followed up with electrophoresis.

Limitations

1. Severe anemias can cause false negatives. Therefore, if the hemoglobin is less than 8 g%, the sample volume should be doubled (100 μL).
2. False negatives can occur with infants under 6 months, because hemoglobin F is insoluble in the test solution. Therefore, testing on infants up to 6 months should not be done.
3. Patients with multiple myeloma, cryoglobulinemia, and other dysglobulinemias may give false-positive results, because the high protein level may affect the test.
4. Some rare hemoglobin variants such as hemoglobin C Harlem or C Georgetown may give false-positive results. These are sickling hemoglobins but do not contain hemoglobin S.
5. Patients who have been recently transfused may give false-positive or false-negative results.
6. Patients who have sickle trait give positive results. Confirm these with hemoglobin electrophoresis.
7. Positive results and/or questionable results should be confirmed with hemoglobin electrophoresis.

CEREBROSPINAL FLUID/BODY FLUID CELL COUNT AND DIFFERENTIAL

Principle

The examination of the cellular component of body fluids is an important part of total body fluid testing. Cell counts are performed in a counting chamber. Cerebrospinal fluid (CSF), synovial fluids, and serous fluids

of the pleural, pericardial, and peritoneal cavities all have characteristic cellular elements, which often change with disease in predictable patterns. Cell counts and cell morphology are key elements in identifying abnormalities within each of these systems. The methods outlined here present a *unique method and calculation reference* for performing fluid counts. For the standard cell counting formula, refer to the Unopette method for manual cell counts on page 311.

Reagents and Equipment

1. Saline
2. Slide stainer
3. Phase microscope
4. Neubauer hemacytometer with coverslip
5. Petri dish
6. Pipettes
   a. 0.2 MLA
   b. 0.1 MLA
   c. 1.0 volumetric
   d. 10.0 volumetric
7. 12 × 75-mm plastic tubes
8. Cytospin
9. Disposable Cytofunnels with white filter attached
10. Bovine albumin, 22%
11. Hyaluronidase
12. Plain microhematocrit tubes
13. Crystal violet diluent

Specimen Collection and Storage

Cerebrospinal Fluid

1. Collected in the sterile plastic tubes from the spinal tray. The laboratory accepts tubes 1 and/or 4.
2. Tube 4 is the preferred tube because it is least likely to be contaminated with blood.
3. CSF cell counts should be performed within **1 hour** of receipt in the laboratory because cells lyse on prolonged standing and accurate counts become impossible.

Synovial and Serous Fluids (Pleural, Pericardial, and Peritoneal)

1. Fluids should be collected in a heparinized tube or EDTA tube.
2. Perform testing within 4 hours.
3. The addition of hyaluronidase to the fluid may reduce the viscosity of synovial fluid.

Quality Control

The College of American Pathologists has removed daily quality control for all body fluids. Each laboratory receives proficiency testing at least two times a year from their proficiency program.

Procedure

Cell Counting Method

1. Based on the gross appearance of the fluid, dilute the specimen by one of the following methods:
   a. METHOD A (clear or slightly cloudy fluid) Dilute 1:2 with crystal violet diluent (0.2 mL specimen + 0.2 mL diluent)
   b. METHOD B (moderately cloudy fluid) Dilute 1:11 with saline (0.1 mL specimen + 1.0 mL saline) using a volumetric pipette. Then dilute 1:2 with crystal violet diluent (0.2 mL of 1:11 dilution + 0.2 mL diluent)
   c. METHOD C (very cloudy or bloody fluid) Dilute 1:101 with saline (0.1 mL specimen + 10.0 mL saline) using a volumetric pipette. Then dilute 1:2 with crystal violet diluent (0.2 mL of 1:101 dilution + 0.2 diluent)
2. Using a plain microhematocrit tube, fill each side of the hemacytometer with the dilution. Place the hemacytometer in a premoistened Petri dish. Allow the cells to settle for 3 to 5 minutes in the Petri dish.
   a. Place the hematocytometer in the phase microscope. Determining the number of squares to be counted depends on the initial viewing of the fluid on the hematocytometer chamber under the microscope. This is the judgment of the technologist/technician.
   b. Using the ×20 or ×40 objective, count the WBCs and RBCs on each side. Now enter the WBC and RBC of each dilution in the CSF/body fluid worksheet (see Table 20.9).
   c. Combine the two totals and take the average for the WBC and RBC counts, which must agree within 20%. If this criterion is not met, reload the chamber and redo the counts.
   d. The gross appearance of non-CSF fluid will determine whether an RBC dilution is needed. If the fluid is cloudy and bloody, then the red cells are too numerous to count; report RBCs as "TNTC."
   e. Tables 20.8 and 20.9 offer a unique calculation reference for fluids. Once a dilution is determined and counts are performed for various fluids, then data can be plugged into these ready reference tables for a quick calculation of a final result. For example:

	Dilution (A, B, or C)	No. of Squares Counted	No. of Cells Count 1	Count 2	Average No. of Cells	Calculation	Result
WBC	A	9	90	100	95	95 × 2.2 = 209	209/µL
RBC	A	9	26	30	28	28 × 2.2 = 61.6	62/µL

Differential Using the Cytospin Method

Figures 20.11, 20.12, and 20.13 represent a variety of cells in body fluids.

1. Prepare slide for the cytospin by first labeling the slide with the patient's name, specimen number, and date.
2. Attach slide for cytospin with the cytocup by the Cytoclip.
3. Add 1 drop of 22% albumin to the bottom of the cytocup.
   a. Clear to slightly cloudy to moderately cloudy fluid, add 200 µL of specimen.
   b. Very cloudy or bloody fluid, add 50 to 100 µL of specimen.
4. Place assembled slide/cytocup into a position of the head with a balance in the position opposite to its location.
5. Cover cytospin head with lid and lock in place by pushing center down on the base.
6. Program the cytospin for 10 minutes at 700 rpm.
   a. "Hi" acceleration for serous and synovial fluids.
   b. "Lo" acceleration for CSF.
7. Start the unit. Upon cycle completion, remove the sealed head. Remove the clip assembly and hold it in a horizontal position with the funnel facing down.

Table 20.8 ⊙ Reference Factors for Fluid Calculations

Total No. of Squares Counted	Multiplication Factors		
	Method A	Method B	Method C
1	×20	×220	×2020
2	×10	×110	×1010
3	×6.7	×73.3	×673.3
4	×5.0	×55	×505
5	×4.0	×44	×404
6	×3.3	×36.7	×336.7
7	×2.9	×31.4	×288.6
8	×2.5	×27.5	×252.5
9	×2.2	×24.4	×224.4
10 Small center	×100	×1100	×10,100
11 Small center	×50	×550	×5050

8. Release the tension clip and remove the sample chamber and filter card. Remove the slide from the clip and allow to fully air-dry.
9. Stain the slides in the stainer and allow to completely dry.
10. Perform a differential count on the stained smear. See Table 20.10 for normal results.
   a. Identify the cells as segmented neutrophils, lymphocytes, monocytes, eosinophils, and others. The others include mesothelial, macrophages, and tumor cells. For a chart including abnormal cells in CSF, see Table 20.11.
   b. Upon completion of the differential, any abnormal cells should be reviewed by a pathologist. For abnormal cells in serous fluids, see Table 20.12. For synovial fluids, see Table 20.13. For color and appearance for CSF, see Table 20.14. (see page 318.)

PROTHROMBIN TIME AND ACTIVATED PARTIAL THROMBOPLASTIN TIME: AUTOMATED PROCEDURE

Principle

Presently, coagulation instruments are fully automated to analyze large volume of samples with a high degree of accuracy. Many of the instruments have the capability to analyze samples using clotting, chromogenic, or immunoassay methods. The clot method of photodetection is described here. This method uses light transmission (optical detection method) to determine prothrombin (PT) and activated partial thromboplastin time (aPTT) times. The optical detection method detects the change in absorbance as a light-emitting diode recognized fibrin or clot formation. A sensor picks up the light beam and converts into an electrical signal. The electrical power is signaled and calculated by a microcomputer to determine the coagulation time. Some automated coagulation testing now identifies variables such as lipemia and hemolysis and are still able to present accurate clotting times.

Reagents and Equipment

1. Automated coagulation analyzer that uses optical detection
2. Volumetric pipettes: 1 mL and 10 mL
3. Centrifuge
4. Thromboplastin
   a. Reconstitute with 10 mL of reagent grade deionized water.
   b. Immediately, recap and mix until contents are completely dissolved.
   c. Allow reagent to stand for 15 minutes.
   d. Check package insert for stability, once reconstituted.

Table 20.9 ⊙ Fluid Worksheet

	Dilution A, B, or C	No. of Squares Counted	No. of Cells Count 1 Count 2	Average No. of Cells	Calculation	Result
WBC					____ × ____ = __	/μL
RBC					____ × ____ = __	/μL

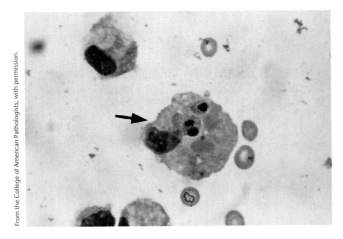

From the College of American Pathologists, with permission.

Figure 20.11   Histiocyte in peritoneal fluid.

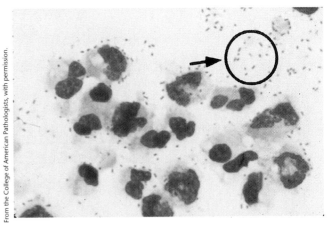

From the College of American Pathologists, with permission.

Figure 20.13   Bacteria in CSF.

5. Coagulation controls, two levels: reconstitute according to manufacturer's instructions.
6. Deionized water
7. Calcium chloride solution
8. aPTT reagent

Specimen Collection and Storage

1. Collect whole blood into vacuum tube with 3.2% sodium citrate. There needs to be a 9:1 dilution of blood to anticoagulant.
   a. 4.5 mL of blood with 0.5 mL of anticoagulant or
   b. 2.7 mL of blood with 0.3 mL of anticoagulant
2. Specimens with hematocrits greater than 60%, see Limitations.
3. Specimens should not be obtained through a heparin lock or any other heparinized line.
4. Specimens are spun down for 5 minutes at 3000 rpm to be platelet poor.

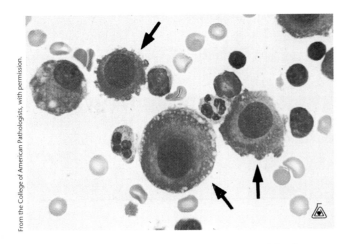

From the College of American Pathologists, with permission.

Figure 20.12   Mesothelial cell in pleural fluid.

5. Coagulation samples are good for 24 hours at room temperature or refrigerated.

Quality Control

1. Coagulation controls are of the laboratory's choice. Follow manufacturer's instructions for reconstitution and stability.
2. Coagulation controls are run at the beginning of each shift.
3. If quality control is out, repeat if necessary. If still out, troubleshoot and/or notify supervisor.

Procedure

PT

1. Prepare reagents and controls.
2. Place reagents and control inside analyzer.
3. Replenish any other materials.
4. Run quality control.
5. Verify quality control; repeat any controls if necessary and document any abnormal controls.
6. Load centrifuged specimen onto instrument with cap removed.
7. Press "Start."
8. The instrument places 50 µL of the patient's plasma into a cup, incubates the sample for 3 minutes, and 100 µL of thromboplastin is added (Fig. 20.14).

aPTT

1. Follow steps 1 through 7 in the PT procedure.
2. The instrument places 50 µL of the patients plasma into a cup, incubates for 1 minute,

Table 20.10 ● Normal Fluid Results

Normal Results	CSF Adult	CSF Neonate	Serous (Pleural, Pericardial, Peritoneal)	Synovial
Appearance	Clear and colorless	Clear and colorless	Pale yellow and clear	Pale yellow and clear
RBC	0 to 1/mm^3	0 to 3/mm^3	0 to 1/mm^3	0 to 1/mm^3
WBC	0 to 5/mm^3	0 to 30/mm^3	0 to 200/mm^3	0 to 200/mm^3
Neutrophils (includes bands)	2% to 6%	0% to 8%	<25%	<25%
Lymphs	40% to 80%	5% to 35%	<25%	<25%
Monocytes	5% to 45%	50% to 90%	Included with others	Included with others
Others (includes)	Rare	Rare	Monocytes and macrophages 65% to 75%	Monocytes and macrophages 65% to 75%

See Figures 20.11, 20.12, and 20.13 for fluid cells.

adds 50 μL of aPTT reagent, continuing with another incubation for 3 minutes, and finally adds 50 μL of calcium chloride to the specimen (Fig. 20.15).

Results

1. Reference range: PT 9.8 to 11.7 seconds INR 2.0 to 3.0
2. Reference range: aPTT 25.0 to 31.0 seconds

3. Critical results
   a. PT >50.00 seconds
   b. INR >4.9
   c. aPTT >100.00 seconds

Limitations

1. Specimens with hematocrits greater than 60% will affect clotting times, with a clotting time that is falsely prolonged.

Table 20.11 ● Causes of Abnormal Cells in CSF

Abnormal Results	CSF	Abnormal Results	CSF
Increased neutrophils	Acute inflammation Early viral meningitis Bacterial meningitis (see Fig. 20.13)	Increased monocytes	Newborn infants Recovery phase of meningitis
Increased lymphocytes	Neurosyphilis Viral, fungal, and tubular meningitis Alzheimer's disease Multiple sclerosis Tumors Lymphocytic leukemias and lymphomas Reactive lymphocytes to include plasma cells in most of the above diseases, particularly in multiple sclerosis and viral meningitis	Increased macrophages	Siderophages present, indicating a CNS hemorrhage in past 48 hours Erythrophages present, indicating an active CNS bleed and if siderophages are also present Lipophages present in brain abscesses and cerebral infarctions
		Increased eosinophils	Parasitic infections Postmyelogram specimens
		Tumor/malignant cells	Acute and chronic leukemias Primary neurologic tumors
		Others	Choroid plexus and ependymal cells seen in post pneumoencephalogram specimens

Table 20.12 ⊙ Abnormal Cells in Serous Fluids	
Abnormal Results	**Serous Fluids (Pleural, Pericardial, and Peritoneal)**
↑RBC	Traumatic Hemorrhage Malignancy of infarctions
↑WBC >1000/mm³	Infections Malignancies Inflammatory conditions
>50% Neutrophils	Acute inflammatory conditions Infectious processes
>50% Lymphocytes	Tuberculosis Carcinomas Lymphoproliferative diseases
Increased reactive lymphs and plasma cells	Multiple myeloma Malignancy and tuberculous effusions
Malignant cells	Diagnostically significant if found on the differential Solid tumors and hematology malignancies shed into these types of fluids are caused by metastatic adenocarcinoma
<1% Mesothelial	Tuberculous effusions

Table 20.13 ⊙ Abnormal Cells in Synovial Fluids	
Abnormal Results	**Synovial Fluids**
>80% Neutrophils	Septic arthritis Later stages of rheumatoid arthritis
Lymphocytes	Early stages of rheumatoid arthritis
Reactive lymphocytes/ plasma	Early stages of rheumatoid arthritis
Monocytes	Viral infections: Hepatitis and rubella arthritis associated with serum sickness
Eosinophilia	Chronic urticaria and angioedema Rheumatic fever Parasitic infections Metastatic disease Rheumatoid arthritis

Table 20.14 ⊙ Color and Appearance in CSF	
Color/appearance	**CSF**
Colorless	Normal
Cloudy	Infections
Straw	Excess protein
Yellow	Xanthochromia
Bloody	Traumatic tap CNS hemorrhage

2. Specimens with hematocrits greater than 60% will need to be drawn differently than ordinary samples. Either the amount of anticoagulant will need to be adjusted, or the amount of whole blood delivered to the sample will need to be adjusted. Formulas are provided for both circumstances.

a. Anticoagulant adjustment

Volume of blood × (100 − hematocrit) × 0.00185 = amount of anticoagulant to be added

b. Volume of blood adjustment

Volume of blood × (60/100) − hematocrit = mL of whole blood to be added

QUALITATIVE D-DIMER TEST

Principle

D-dimer is a fibrin fragment that results when plasmin acts on cross-linked fibrin in the presence of factor XIII.

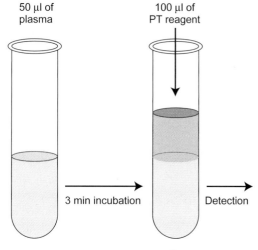

50 µl of plasma   100 µl of PT reagent

3 min incubation   Detection

Figure 20.14 Prothrombin time procedure.

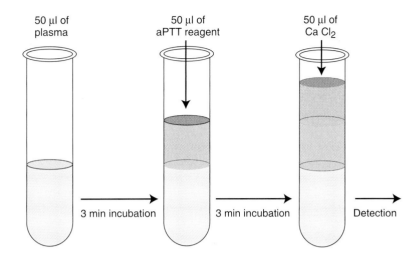

50 µl of
plasma

50 µl of
aPTT reagent

50 µl of
Ca Cl₂

3 min incubation   3 min incubation   Detection

Figure 20.15 Activated partial thromboplastin time procedure.

Therefore, D-dimers are formed from an insoluble fibrin clot. This semiquantitative assay, available since the 1990s, provides evidence of normal or abnormal levels of D-dimer. Latex particles are coated with mouse anti–D-dimer monoclonal antibodies. When mixed with plasma containing D-dimers, agglutination will occur. The test plays an important role in detecting and monitoring patients suspected of thrombotic disorders. Its clinical uses are for detecting deep vein thrombosis (DVT), pulmonary embolism (PE), and, in patients with disseminated intravascular coagulation (DIC), postoperative complications or septicemia. Quantitative D-dimer procedures are available, using latex-enhanced turbidimetric methods. The qualitative test, however, has widespread use in most coagulation laboratories as a screening test for D-dimers.

Reagents and Equipment

1. D-dimer kit containing reagents (stored at 2 to 8°C), good until expiration date on the kit.
   a. Test reagent solution containing red cell anti–XL-FDP antibody conjugate
   b. Negative control solution containing 0.9% saline solution
   c. Positive control solution containing purified D-dimer fragment
2. Plastic agglutination trays
3. White plastic stirrers
4. Timer
5. Pipette 10 µL with disposable tips

Specimen Collection and Storage

1. Collect venous whole blood into a vacuum tube with 3.2% sodium citrate. There needs to be a 9:1 dilution of blood to anticoagulant.

   a. 4.5 mL of blood with 0.5 mL of anticoagulant OR
   b. 2.7 mL of blood with 0.3 mL of anticoagulant
2. Collection of venous blood into heparin is acceptable.
3. Store specimens at 18 to 24°C. Specimens should be tested within 4 hours from the time of specimen collection. If testing will take place after 4 hours, specimens must be refrigerated at 2 to 8°C and are good up to 24 hours.

Quality Control

1. Quality control is performed under several conditions
   a. Daily
   b. When opening a new kit
   c. When receiving a new shipment
   d. When a new lot number is put into use
2. A whole blood sample that has a negative D-dimer result is used for the quality control.
3. Quality control method
   a. Follow directions in the procedure to do the quality control, steps 1 through 5.
   b. Now add 1 drop of positive control to the test well, and proceed with steps 6 through 8b.

Procedure

1. Allow reagents to come to room temperature for at least 20 minutes before use.
2. Specimen should be thoroughly mixed; do not allow cells to settle out.
3. For each sample, pipette 10 µL of whole blood into each reaction well; the first labeled (nega-

tive control well) and (test well) on a plastic agglutination tray.

4. Add 1 drop of the negative control to the negative control well.

5. Add 1 drop of the test reagent to the test well.

6. With a plastic stirrer, mix the contents of each well thoroughly for 3 to 5 seconds, using a different stirrer for each well and spreading the reagent across the entire well surface.

7. To promote agglutination, mix by gentle rocking of the plastic agglutination tray for 2 minutes.

8. At the end of the 2 minutes, observe for the presence of agglutination.

   a. Positive results: agglutination is present in the test well compared to no agglutination in the negative well.

   b. If the negative control well agglutinates, the test is invalid.

   c. If the test result is negative, add 1 drop of positive control to the test well and rock the plastic tray. Agglutination should occur within 15 seconds. If agglutination does not occur with the addition of the positive control, the test is invalid.

Interpretation

1. Positive: Agglutination seen in the test well and no agglutination seen in the negative control well.

2. Negative: No agglutination seen in the test well and the negative control well. This would be confirmed by adding the positive control to the test well and agglutination occurs.

3. Invalid

   a. Agglutination occurs in the negative control well.

   b. No agglutination occurs with the positive control.

Results

Negative: No agglutination seen in negative agglutination well (<0.5 mg/L)

Positive: Agglutination seen in undiluted sample (0.5 to 4.0 mg/L)

Positive samples can be diluted 1:8 or 1:64 to provide more specific data on the amount of D-dimer present.

Limitations

The presence of cold agglutinins in patient samples can cause agglutinations in patient's blood. This may cause agglutination of the negative control, thereby invalidating the test results.

AN APPROACH TO INTERPRETING AUTOMATED HEMATOLOGY DATA

Automated hematology has totally changed the landscape of the hematology laboratory. Fewer manual techniques are required, as more operations become automated. Work patterns have shifted as hematology professionals are expected to maintain quality and morphologic acuity and adjust to increasingly complex instrumentation. Operators of automated instruments (technologists) are expected to have a variety of interpretive skills. Additionally, most of the white cell differentials that *are* reviewed are usually abnormal. Accurate and discriminating cell identification skills are essential.[†]

As students are trained in their clinical rotations, they become familiar with the instrumentation provided by their clinical site. Yet few students have the luxury of having been trained on automated instrumentation during the didactic portion of their training. Most universities are only able to offer information rather then actual practice on automated equipment. What is needed for the entry-level practitioner is a way to **approach** interpreting the visual automated data. This skill is not necessarily practiced at university programs, since owning and operating automated equipment are usually cost prohibitive. Training students on multiparameter instruments is primarily left to clinical rotations. This section will attempt to give students a thoughtful approach to bridging the divide between the classroom and the clinical training ground with respect to automated principles and data interpretation. It will NOT be comprehensive and all inclusive. This presentation will cover basic concepts.

Presently, there is an entire menu of services that automated instrumentation provides including

- Embedded quality control programs
- Delta checks
- Flagging systems when data fall out of range
- Preparation, examination, and reporting of white cell differentials
- Automatic maintenance in some instruments

Most hematology instruments operate under several basic principles, and these will be outlined.

[†]The author wishes to acknowledge Joyce Feinberg MT (ASCP) of Beckman-Coulter and Kathy Finnegan MS, MT (ASCP) SH of the MT Program at Stony Brook NY for their assistance with this section.

Principles

The Coulter Principle

Using this technology, cells are sized and counted by detecting and measuring changes in electrical resistance when a particle passes through a small aperture. This is called the electrical impedance principle of counting cells. A blood sample is diluted in saline, a good conductor of electrical current, and the cells are pulled through an aperture by creating a vacuum. Two electrodes establish an electrical current. The external electrode is located in the blood cell suspension. The second electrode is the internal electrode and is located in the glass hollow tube, which contains the aperture. Low-frequency electrical current is applied to the external electrode and the internal electrode. DC current is applied between the two electrodes. Electrical resistance or impedance occurs as the cells pass through the aperture causing a change in voltage. This change in voltage generates a pulse (Fig. 20.16). The number of pulses is proportional to the number of cells counted. The size of the voltage pulse is also directly proportional to the volume or size of the cell.[1]

Radiofrequency

Radiofrequency (RF) resistance is a high-voltage electromagnetic current flowing between the electrodes to detect the size of cells based on the cellular density. RF is a high-frequency pulsating sine wave. Conductivity or RF measurements provide information about the internal characteristics of the cell. The cell wall acts as a conductor when exposed to high-frequency current. As the current passes through the cell, measurable changes are detected. The cell interior density or nuclear volume is directly proportional to pulse size or a change in RF resistance. The nuclear to cytoplasmic ratio, nuclear density, and cytoplasmic granulation are determined.[1]

Optical Scatter

A sample of blood is diluted with an isotonic diluent and then hydrodynamically focused through a quartz flow cell. Cells pass through a flow cell on which a beam of light is focused. The light source is a laser light that is light amplification by stimulated emission of radiation. Laser light or monochromatic light is emitted as a single wavelength. As the cell passes through the sensing zone, light is scattered in all directions. Photodetectors sense and collect the scattered rays at different angles. These data are then converted to an electric pulse. The number of pulses generated is directly proportional to the number of cells passing through the sensing zone. The patterns of light are measured at various angles: forward light scatter at 180 degrees and right angle scatter at 90 degrees. Cell counts, size, cell structure, shape, and reflectivity are determined by the analysis of the scatter light data. Forward angle light scatter (0 degree) is diffracted light which relates to volume. Forward low-angle light scatter (2 to 3 degrees) relates to cell size or volume. Forward high-angle scatter (5 to 15 degrees) relates to the internal complexity or refractive index of cellular components. Orthogonal light scatter (90 degrees) or side scatter is a combination of reflection and refraction and relates to internal components.[1]

VCS Technology (Volume, Conductivity, and Scatter)

Low-frequency current measures volume, while high-frequency current measures changes in conductivity, and light from the laser bouncing off white cells characterizes the surface shape and reflectivity of each cell. This technology differentiates white cell characteristics.

Hydrodynamic Focusing

This is a technique that narrows the stream of cells to single file, eliminating data above and below the focus points. Hydrodynamic focusing allows greater accuracy and resolution of blood cells. Diluted cells are surrounded by a sheath fluid, which lines up the cells in a single file while passing through the detection aperture. After passing through the aperture, the cells are then directed away from the back of the aperture. This process eliminates the recirculation of cells and the counting of cells twice.

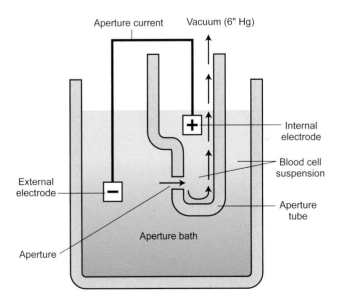

Figure 20.16 Coulter principle of electric impedance.

Use of Flow Cells

Flow cells are composed of quartz rather than glass and provide a better atmosphere in which to measure cellular qualities. Light does not bend and UV light can pass through the flow cell. Cell characteristics are then measured. The flow cells measure cell volume, internal content, and cell surface, shape, and reflectivity.

Multiple Angle Polarized Scatter Separation

Each cell is analyzed through a flow cytometry cell as it is subjected to a variety of angled light scatter. Five subpopulations of cells are identified.

Instruments

Basic automated hematology analyzers provide an electronic measured red cell count (RBC), white cell count (WBC), platelet count (Plt), mean platelet volume (MPV), hemoglobin concentration (Hb), and the mean red cell volume (MCV). From these measured quantities, the hematocrit (Hct), mean cell hemoglobin (MCH), mean cell hemoglobin concentration, and the red cell distribution width (RDW) are calculated. The newer analyzers include white cell differential counts, relative or percent and absolute number, and reticulocyte analysis. The differential may be a three-part differential that includes granulocytes, lymphocytes, and monocytes or a five-part differential that includes neutrophils, lymphocytes, monocytes, eosinophils, and basophils. The new generation of analyzers now offers a sixth parameter, which is the enumeration of nucleated RBCs (nRBCs). Hematology instruments also include verification systems. The verification system uses review of past results or delta checks and instrument flagging that includes R flags, population flags, suspect flags, and definitive or quantitative flags.[1]

How Data Are Reported

In most automated systems, the complete blood count is numerically reported. The differential is numerically recorded and then graphically displayed. These displays include scatterplots, scattergrams, and histograms. The basic principles behind the graphic displays of these data are fairly universal. Scatterplots and scattergrams place a specific cell on a grid identification system while histograms measure size thresholds of white cells, red cells, and platelets compared to the normal data for each of these cell groups.

Scatterplots and scattergrams provide colorful imaging of normal and abnormal cells. An operator can

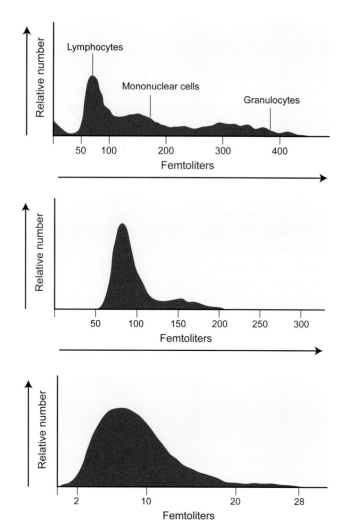

Figure 20.17 Coulter scatterplots of (A) leukocytes, (B) red cells, and (C) platelets.

immediately notice a particular deviation in numbers of and distribution of a particular cell line by analyzing scatterplots (Fig. 20.17).

Beckman-Coulter Instrumentation

Coulter STKS, Coulter GEN S, and Coulter LH 750 series (http://www.beckmancoulter.com) use VCS technology, which is an acronym for volume (V), conductivity (C), and laser light scatter (S). The simultaneous measurement of cell volume, conductivity, and light scatter provides high statistical accuracy. The cell volume is measured by electrical impedance using low-frequency direct current. To ensure accuracy, Coulter has incorporated pulse editing and sweep flow technology. This technology allows the cells that are being counted to line up in a single file to ensure size measurement integrity and to prevent cells from being counted twice. The RBC, WBC, and platelet counts are obtained by analyzing the number of pulses generated. The RBC, WBC, and platelet data are then plotted in the form of a histogram. The cell number is plotted on the y-axis, and the cell size is plotted on the x-axis. The MCV and RDW are derived from the RBC histogram. The MPV is derived from the platelet histogram. The HCT, MCH, and MCHC are calculated. Hemoglobin is measured by the cyanmethemoglobin method.

Conductivity is measured by using high-frequency electromagnetic current for nuclear and granular constituents. Conductivity is influenced by the internal structures of the cell such as the nuclear-to-cytoplasm ratio and the cytoplasmic granular content. A monochromatic helium:neon laser is the light source to measure light scatter for surface structure, shape, and granularity. Forward angle light scatter is affected by cell shape, surface characteristics, and cytoplasmic granular content. The enumeration of relative percentage and the absolute number of each five cells are displayed in a scatterplot.[1]

What Knowledge Is Necessary for the Operator of an Automated Instrument?

Operating automated cell counting instrumentation requires many skills. The operator must:

1. Know normal reference ranges.
2. Be familiar with normal scatterplots and histograms for the particular piece of equipment.
3. Be familiar with the flagging criteria determined by the particular laboratory information system (LIS).
   - Reference ranges will be preset according to the LIS; specimens that fall out of the reference range are *flagged*.
4. Be familiar with delta checks.
   - Delta checks are historical checks of test results from the patient's previous samples.
5. Be familiar with reflex testing.
   - Reflex testing represents additional testing such as manual slide reviews, etc., which must be accomplished before test results can be released. Operators make decisions on which reflex tests to perform.
6. Notify the appropriate personnel of critical results.
   - Critical results are those results that exceed or are markedly decreased from the reference range or the patient history of results.
7. Be familiar with daily maintenance procedures.

8. Be familiar with specimen handling and requirements.

A Sample Case Using Coulter VCS Technology

An approach to verifying and sending these results (this approach can be used for each automated system explained in this section).

1. The CBC results look normal (Fig. 20.18).
2. When we preview the results, we can see that the eosinophil count is extremely high on the differential report.
3. We also notice that the eosinophil area on the scatterplot is particularly bright.
4. The eosinophil result on the differential is flagged.
5. Delta check revealed that the patient sample had been run on the instrument 4 days before with normal results in all categories.
6. Since the abnormal results have been flagged, reflex testing demands that the best course of action is to do a manual smear review and verify the large number of eosinophils.
7. Once this is accomplished, then the results can be verified.

A Preview of Other Automated Cell Counting Instrumentation

This section will present the Sysmex and Cell-Dyne instrumentation. The Sysmex instrument uses hydrodynamic focusing, while the Cell-Dyne instrument uses optical scatter and impedance.

Sysmex Instrumentation

Sysmex (Roche Diagnostics Corporation) manufactures a full line of hematology analyzers that include the K-4500, which provides a WBC, RBC, platelet, and three-part differential. The SE series and SF-3000 perform a CBC with a five-part differential. The newest analyzer added to the line is the XE-2100, which provides a CBC, five-part differential, and a fully automated reticulocyte count.

The SE series measures WBC, RBC, and platelets using direct current electrical impedance for counting and sizing of cells, hydrodynamic focusing, and automatic discrimination for accuracy and precision. The SE series generates the standard hematology parameters and the added parameters of RDW-SD (red cell distribution width by standard deviation), RDW-CV (red cell distribution width by coefficient), and MPV (mean platelet volume). Hemoglobin values are determined by

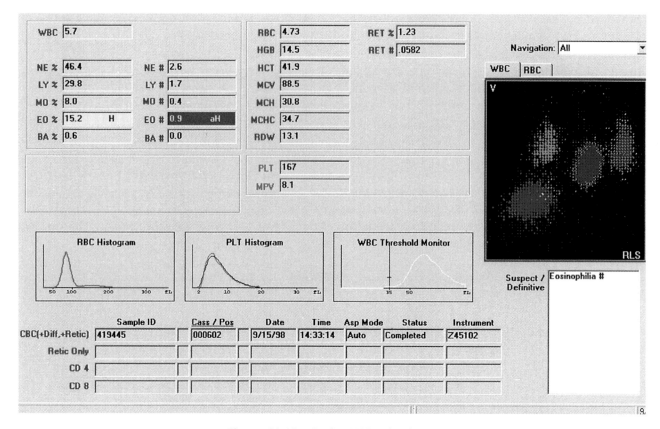

Figure 20.18 Coulter VCS technology.

the use of a cyanide-free, nontoxic reagent and are measured at 555 nm. The white cell count uses a separate channel and utilizes DC electrical impedance.

The principle for the white cell five-part differential includes simultaneous measurements of RF and DC detection methods for separating the white cell popula-tions. There are four separate detection channels for the determination of each white cell type. A plot of low-frequency DC impedance plotted on the *x*-axis, and high-frequency current RF on the *y*-axis determines lymphocytes, monocytes, and granulocytes. This chan-nel is called the DIFF channel (Fig. 20.19). The second

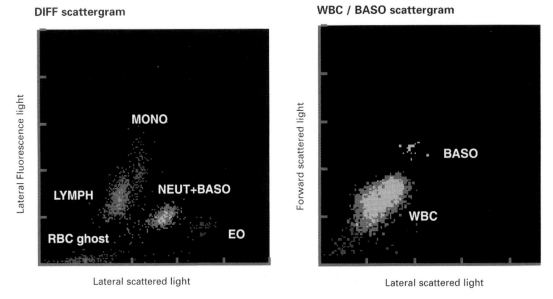

Figure 20.19 Sysmex scatterplot of WBC, lymphs, monocytes, and basophils.

channel is used with a special reagent for detecting the presence of immature cells. This channel is called the IMI channel. This channel also allows for abnormal morphology findings. The last two channels are the EO and the BASO chambers. Eosinophils and basophils are enumerated by impedance after the sample has been treated with specific lysing or buffer reagents[1] (Fig. 20.20).

Cell Dyne Technology

The Cell-Dyne system (Abbott Diagnostics Instrumentation) uses three independent measurement technologies. These measurements include an optical channel for the white count and differential, an impedance channel for the red count and platelets, and a hemoglobin channel for hemoglobin determination.

A unique design of Cell DYNE is the technology of multiangle polarized scatter separation (MAPSS). The WBC count and differential are derived from this patented optical channel. A hydrodynamically focused sample stream is directed through a high-resolution flow cytometer. A cell suspension is prepared with a diluent, which maintains the WBCs in their native state, which is then passed through an air-cooled Argon ion laser light source. Scattered light is measured at multiple angles. Low-angle (1 to 3) forward light scatter represents the cell size. Wide-angle (3 to 11) forward light

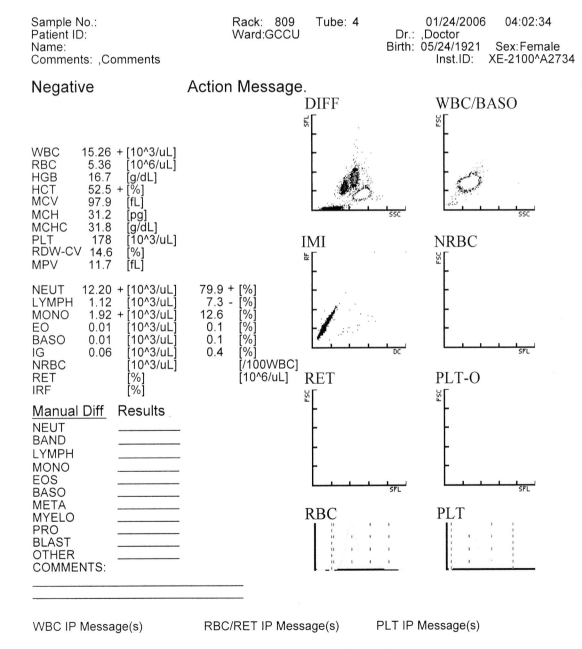

Figure 20.20   Sysmex scatterplot; note that WBC and basos are selected out.

measures the cell complexity. Orthogonal light scatter (90) determines cell lobularity; 90 depolarized (90D) is for the evaluation of cellular granularity. Various combinations of these four angle measurements are used to differentiate the white cell populations. Neutrophils and eosinophils are separated from mononuclear cells by plotting 90 light scatter data, which are on the y-axis, and wide-angle forward light scatter data, on the x-axis. Eosinophils are separated from the neutrophil population by the eosinophils' ability to depolarize the polarized light scatter. The lymphocyte, monocyte, and basophil populations can be separated by plotting low-angle forward light scatter on the y-axis and wide-angle forward light scatter on the x-axis[1] (Fig. 20.21).

Reticulocyte Counting on Automated Instrumentation

Automated reticulocyte counting is quickly becoming the standard for reticulocyte counting in clinical laboratories. For reticulocyte analysis, New Methylene Blue is incubated with whole blood samples. The dye precipi-

tates the basophilic RNA network found in reticulocytes. Hemoglobin and unbound stain are removed by adding a clearing reagent, leaving clear spherical mature RBCs and darkly stained reticulocytes. Stained reticulocytes are differentiated from mature cells and other cell populations by light scatter, direct current measurements, and opacity characteristics. The normal reference range is 0.5% to 1.5%. In comparison to the manual reticulocyte count in which 1000 red cells are counting, the automated reticulocyte procedure counts 32,000 red cells.

FLOW CYTOMETRY: THE BASICS IN HEMATOLOGY INTERPRETATION

The information presented here is purposefully simplistic. An elaborate explanation of flow cytometry is not appropriate for the audience and tone of this text. Flow cytometry is a specialty technique and a recent Google search listed 10 pages of entries referring to certificate programs for this specialty. For additional information, the student is referred to

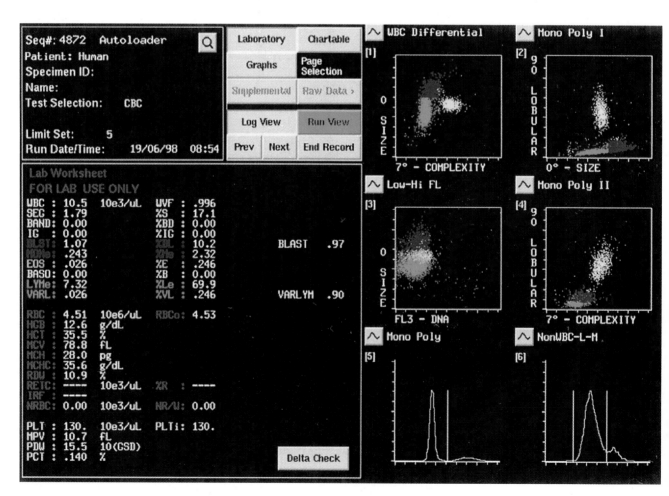

Figure 20.21   Cell Dyne technology.

Table 20.15 ● Applications of Flow Cytometry

- Immunophenotyping
- Diagnosis and staging of leukemia/lymphoma
- Lymphocyte screening panel: AIDS patients
- DNA content analysis
- RNA content
- Enzyme studies
- Fetal cell enumeration

textbooks and websites solely devoted to the principles of flow cytometry and case studies.[†]

Overview

Flow cytometry is a technique that has greatly impacted the diagnosis of hematological malignances. Peripheral blood, bone marrow, lymph nodes, solid tumors, needle aspirates, and splenic tissue are all examined by flow cytometry instruments. Each of these tissues has specific antigen characteristics that can be illuminated through the use of flow cytometry. This technique is usually ancillary to traditional means of diagnosis because of the expense and expertise needed to achieve results. Although flow cytometry has many applications (Table 20.15), its use in immunophenotyping has been particularly beneficial to distinguish hematological neoplasms: lymphomas and leukemias. A flow cytometer can analyze up to 10,000 cells, separating them into subpopulations and then "looking for" particular antigenic or epitope markers. This discovery is accomplished through the use of monoclonal antibodies that determine cell specificity and fluorescent dye that will aid in the detection of the particular antigen-antibody combination on the flow cytometer. Cell suspensions are stained with monoclonal antibodies that contain fluorochromes and then the suspension is analyzed by the flow cytometer. Additionally, flow cytometry analysis is replacing several obscure but long established techniques such as sucrose hemolysis for PNH, Kleihauer-Betke for fetal hemoglobin, and nitroblue tetrazolium test for chronic granulomatous disease.

Principles

Basic analysis of cell preparations includes light scatter and fluorescence.

[†]The author wishes to acknowledge Candace Breen Golightly MS, MT (ASCP) and Mark Golightly, PhD for their assistance with this section.

Light scatter (forward angle light scatter/side scatter) is the angle at which light is scattered depending upon the nuclear and cytoplasmic complexity of the cells and the size of the cells

The intensity of *fluorescence* is related to the antigen density of the markers being investigated; cells are mixed with specific monoclonal antibody probes and the absence or presence of fluorescence provides data relative to the maturational stage and phenotype of cells

The flow cytometer is composed of three distinct systems: the fluid system, the optical system, and the electronic system (Fig. 20.22).

The fluid system handles sampling in a single fluid stream surround by a sheath fluid that produces laminar flow. This fluid within a fluid creates a differential pressure that allows cells to enter into the conical nozzle. Here individual cells are analyzed by laser light sources and fluorescence. After analysis, the cell droplets will fall into the waste collection tubes.

The optical system includes gas ion laser, dioded lasers, and dye lasers. The lasers measure light scatter and emission of fluorescent light. The information gathered from this measurement are directed into the photomultiplier tube (PMT), beam-specific dichromic mirrors, and wavelength selective filters.

The electronic system is driven by a personal computer that has sophisticated data storage capabilities. This data can then be analyzed by a variety of software packages from third party distributors.

Data are generated that will display the intensity of the fluorescence of those cells that possess the antigen marker. Therefore, it is the patterns of the reactive cells rather than the numbers of reactive cells that are important (Fig. 20.23).

Data Interpretation: One Role for the Medical Technologist

Diagnosing a leukemia and lymphoma is a difficult undertaking. Bone marrow aspirate smears, blood smear interpretation, hematology results, patient's symptoms, cytogenetics, and cytochemical staining each plays a role in diagnosis. Flow cytometry adds an additional piece of supporting information to this entire process. Not every laboratory has a flow cytometry instrument used specifically for one of the purposes listed above; yet most laboratory professionals will have

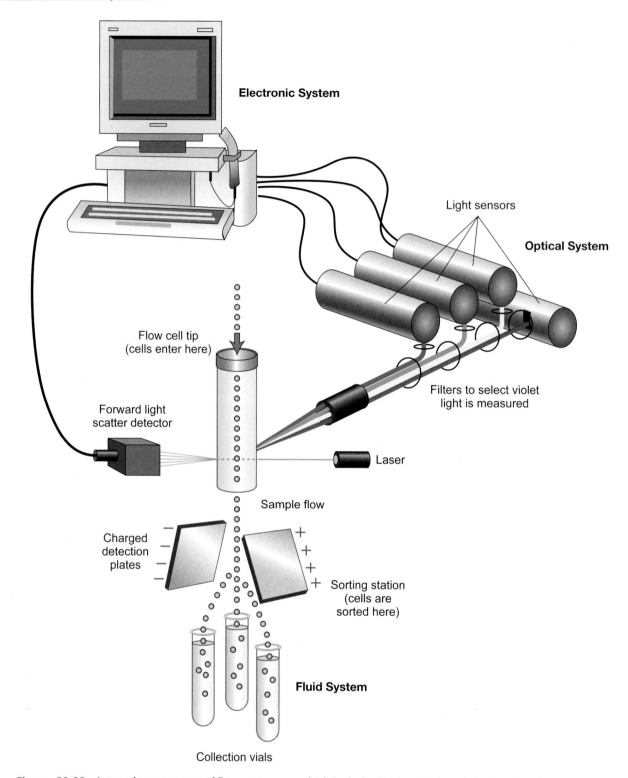

Figure 20.22 Internal components of flow cytometer, which includes fluid, optical, and electronic systems.

some exposure to these data in their laboratory careers. Some will make it their subspecialty. Since this technology is rapidly expanding current lists of CD markers (see Table 20.16), their applications and their interpretation are available in a variety of Internet sources.

Flow Cytometry Case Studies

Case 1

A 67-year-old woman came to her physician's office complaining of flu symptoms. Even though she had

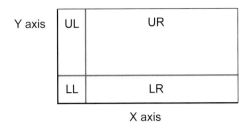

Figure 20.23   How flow cytometry data are graphed. LL, cells negative for both *x*- and *y*-axes. UR, cells positive for both *x*- and *y*-axes. UL, cells positive for *y*-axis and negative for *x*-axis. LR, cells positive for *x*-axis and negative for *y*-axis. Different CD antibodies are placed on the *x*- and *y*-axes.

Table 20.16 ⊙ A Brief List of Useful Hematologic CD Markers	
Cell Type	**Marker**
Hematopoietic progenitor cells	CD34, CD45, CD117
B cells	CD10, CD19, CD20, CD22
T cells	CD3, CD4
Hairy cells	CD103, CD25, CD45
Myelocytic cells	CD33, CD34, CD45
Monocytic cells	CD4, CD14, CD33
Megakaryocytes	CD61, CD41, CD42b

been taking flu medications for 2 weeks, she felt she was not improving. Her CBC revealed increased white cell count, a moderate anemia, and a normal platelet count. Blood smear revealed 90% lymphocytes, most appearing mature. Flow cytometry was performed on a tube of EDTA blood from the patient. The monoclonal antibodies used were CD5, CD19, CD23, and CD2 (Fig. 20.24).

Flow cytometry results show that the patient has CLL with the majority of the cells showing CD19-positive cells.

Case 2

A 43-year-old man presented to his family physician with complaints of feeling weak and fatigued for the past 3 months. He has a low-grade fever. A CBC was drawn and revealed anemia and thrombocytopenia. The patient was admitted for a bone marrow aspirate. Flow cytometry was ordered (Fig. 20.25).

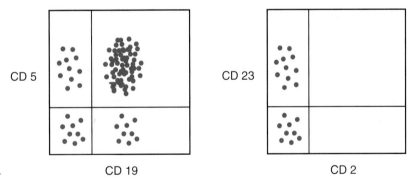

Figure 20.24   Case 1 flow cytometry results.

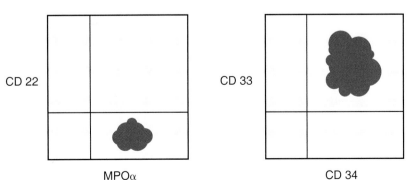

Figure 20.25   Case 2 flow cytometry results.

Flow cytometry results show that the patient's cells were negative for MPO but positive for CD33, CD34. Leukemia was identified as acute myelocytic leukemia (M2).

Reference

1. Ward-Cook C, Lehmann C, Schoeff L, et al. Clinical Diagnostic Technology: The Total Testing Process, Volume 2: The Analytical Phase. Chicago: ASCP Press, 2005: 253–288.

Suggested Reading

Adams C. Autocrit II Centrifuge and Adams Microhematocrit II Centriguge, Becton, Dickinson and Company, 1976.

CAP, 2005 Surveys and Anatomic Pathology Education Programs, Hematology, Clinical Microscopy, and Body Fluids Glossary.

Ciesla BE, Simpson P. Evaluation of cell morphology and evaluation of white cell and platelet morphology. In: Harmening DH, ed. Clinical Hematology Theory and Fundamentals of Hemostasis, 4th ed. Philadelphia: FA Davis, 2002: 95–97.

Davidsohn I, Henry JB. Clinical Diagnosis and Management by Laboratory Methods, 16th ed. Philadelphia: WB Saunders, 1979.

Kjeldsberg C, Knight J. Body Fluids. Chicago: ASCP Press, 1982.

NCCLS. Collection, Transport, and Processing of Blood Specimens for Testing Plasma-Based Coagulation Assays Approved Guideline, 4th ed. Wayne, PA: NCCLS, 2003: NCCLS document H21-A4.

Sysmex Corporation. Sysmex Ca-1500 System Operators Manual. Kobe, Japan: Sysmex Corporation, 2001.

Turgeon ML. Clinical Hematology Theory and Procedures, 3rd ed. Philadelphia: Lippincott, Williams, and Wilkins, 1999.

Wooldridge-King M. Determination of Microhematocrit via Centrifuge. AACN Procedure Manual for Critical Care, 4th ed. Philadelphia: WB Saunders, 2000.

Wyrick GJ, Hughes VC. Routine hematology methods. In: Harmening DH, ed. Clinical Hematology and Fundamentals of Hemostasis, 4th ed. Philadelphia: FA Davis, 2002: 571–573.

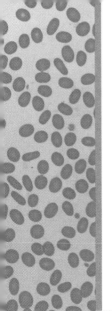
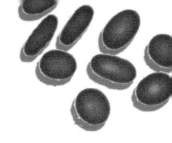

Appendix
Answers To Review Questions

Chapter 1

1. B
2. C
3. A
4. D
5. C
6. D

Chapter 2

1. C
2. A
3. A
4. B
5. B
6. B
7. D
8. B
9. A
10. B

Chapter 3

1. C
2. B
3. D
4. B
5. C
6. B
7. D

Chapter 4

1. B
2. C
3. A
4. C
5. C
6. B
7. B

Chapter 5

1. C
2. B
3. D
4. A
5. C
6. A
7. C
8. D
9. C
10. B

Chapter 6

1. C
2. A
3. B
4. C
5. C
6. D
7. A

Chapter 7

1. D
2. B
3. C
4. C
5. C
6. A
7. B

Chapter 8

1. C
2. D
3. B
4. B
5. A
6. A
7. C

Chapter 9

1. A
2. B
3. C
4. D
5. A

Chapter 10

1. C

2. A

3. B

4. B

5. C

Chapter 11

1. C

2. B

3. A

4. D

5. C

6. A

7. C

Chapter 12

1. D

2. B

3. B

4. C

5. A

6. B

7. C

Chapter 13

1. D

2. A

3. C

4. B

5. C

6. A

7. D

Chapter 14

1. B
2. C
3. A
4. C
5. C

Chapter 15

1. A
2. C
3. A
4. C
5. B
6. B
7. C
8. B
9. D
10. C
11. B

Chapter 16

1. C
2. C
3. B
4. B
5. D
6. D
7. C

Chapter 17

1. C
2. B
3. D
4. A
5. D

Chapter 18

1. C
2. A
3. C
4. B
5. C

Chapter 19

1. A
2. C
3. A
4. D
5. D
6. C
7. A
8. B
9. D
10. A

Index

Note: Page numbers followed by "f" and "t" indicate figures and tables, respectively.

Acanthocytes, 307
Accuracy/precision
  clarification of, 9, 10f
Activated partial thromboplastin time (aPTT), 238
  automated procedure for, 315–318
  in hemophilia A diagnosis, 260
Activated protein C resistance (Factor V Leiden), 285
  laboratory diagnosis, 285–286
  pathway, 285f
Acute basophilic leukemia, 175
Acute erythroid leukemia, 173–174, 173f
Acute hemolytic anemia, 103–104
Acute lymphoblastic leukemia (ALL), 175
  clinical features, 175–176
  epidemiology, 175
  morphological classification, 176, 176t
  precursor B/lymphoblastic lymphoma, 176–178
  precursor T lymphoblastic leukemia/lymphoblastic lymphoma, 178–179
  prognostic factors, 178f, 179–180
Acute megakaryoblastic leukemia, 174, 174f
Acute monoblastic leukemia, 172–173, 172f
Acute monocytic leukemia, 172, 172f
Acute myelofibrosis, 175
Acute myeloid leukemia (AML), 161
  chromosomal alterations in, 168t
  clinical features, 162, 163t
  conditions with increased risk for, 162t
  cytochemical staining, 163–166
  with 11q23, 169, 170f
  epidemiology of, 161–162
  immunophenotypic classification, 166–167, 166t
  with inv(16)(p13q22), 168, 168f
  laboratory features, 163
  with maturation, 171, 171f
  minimally differentiated, 170, 171f
  with myelodysplasia, 170
  not otherwise categorized, 170
  with recurrent genetic abnormalities, 167–168
  with t(8;21)(q22;q22), 168, 168f
  with t(15;17)(q22;q21), 168–169
  with t(16;16)(p13q22), 168
  therapy-related, 170
  WHO classification of, 166–167, 167t
  without maturation, 170–171, 171f
Acute myelomonocytic leukemia (AMML), 171–172, 172f
Acute promyelocytic leukemia, 168–169, 169f
Adenosine diphosphate, 234–235
Adult
  bone marrow formation in, vs. in fetus, 16f
  WBC differential values in, 139t, 307t
Afibrinogenemia, 270
Agglutination
  vs. rouleaux, 213f
AIDS. See HIV-AIDS
Alder's anomaly (Alder-Reilly anomaly), 149, 149f
ALL. See Acute lymphoblastic leukemia
Allosteric changes, in Hgb, 53
Alpha-1-antitrypsin, 273
Alpha-2-antiplasmin, 239, 272–273, 283
Alpha-2-macroglobulin, 239–240, 273
Alpha-naphthyl butyrate/acetate esterase stains, 165–166
AML. See Acute myeloid leukemia
AMML. See Acute myelomonocytic leukemia
Anemias. See also specific types
  acute hemolytic, 103–104
  bone marrow response to, 18
  of chronic disease/inflammation, 71–72
    conditions leading to, 72t
  hemolytic
    classification by intrinsic/extrinsic defects, 58t
    terminology, 58
  iron-deficiency, 68–70
  macrocytic vs. megaloblastic, 86
  morphological classification of, 23–25
  pathophysiology-linked symptoms, 26t
  sickle cell, 115–120
  sideroblastic, 72–74
Anisocytosis, 39
Ankyrin, 38
Antiangiogenic therapies, 223
Anticardiolipin (ACA), 286–287
Anticoagulant drugs, 289
Anticoagulant therapy, 288
Antiglobulin test, direct, 207
Antihemophilic factor (Factor VIII), 236
  complex formation with vWF, 258, 260f
  thrombotic disorder associated with, 286
Antiphospholipid antibodies
  laboratory assays for, 287
Antiphospholipid syndrome, 286–287
Antiplatelet drugs, 288
Antithrombin (AT)
  deficiency of, 284
  effects on serine proteases, 284f
  in thrombosis, 283
Aplastic anemia, 105
Arachidonic acid (AA), 235

Aristotle, 230
Aspirin, 288
  platelet function and, 251
AT. *See* Antithrombin
Auer rods, 163, 168f, 308
Autoimmune hemolytic anemia, 207

Bacteria
  in cerebrospinal fluid, 316f
  extracellular, in peripheral smears, 153f
  intracellular, in segmented neutrophil, 153f
  in peripheral smear, 153
  phagocytosis of, 145
  in precipitated stain, 153f
Baldes, 230
B-ALL. *See* Precursor B lymphoblastic leukemia
Bands, 132f
  hypogranular, 221f
  identification criteria, 132
  toxic granulation in, 308
Barts hydrops fetalis, 76
Basophilic normoblast, 36, 36f
Basophilic normoblast-nucleated, 36f
Basophilic stippling, 45, 46f, 308
Basophils, 133f
  identification criteria, 133
  increase in, conditions associated with, 144
  Sysmex scatterplot of, 324f
B cells, 136
Beckman-Coulter instrumentation, 322–323
Bence Jones protein, 212
Bennett, John, 161
Bernard Soulier syndrome (BSS), 250
Biohazard shield, 7f
Bite cells (helmet cells), 44f, 45f, 103f
  formation, 104f
Bizzozero, 232
Blast crisis
  in CML, 189, 190
Blasts
  excess, refractory anemia with, 222
Bleeding
  evaluation of, 258
  iron deficiency and, 66, 68, 70–71
  open vs. closed, 258
  secondary to chronic disease, 263
B lymphocytes, 137
Bone marrow
  in acute myeloid leukemia, 163
  in chronic lymphocytic leukemia, 206f
  in chronic myelogenous leukemia, 190, 190t
  dysplasia, in MDSs, 220
  formation in fetus, vs. adult, 16f
  Gaucher's cell, 152f
  in hematopoiesis, 16
  incorporation of vitamin B$_{12}$ into, 88
  internal structure, 19t
  in leukemia, 160
  in lipid storage diseases, 152–153

  M:E ratio and, 18
  Niemann-Pick cell, 152f
  responses to anemic stress, 87t
  ringed sideroblasts in, 72f
Bone marrow aspiration, 21, 21f
Bone marrow report, 21–22, 23f
Brodie, 230
Burr cells, 43, 45f, 307

C1 activator, 273
Cabot rings, 308
Calcium, ionized (Factor IV), 235
Calmodulin, 38
Capillary tubes, 299f, 300f
Carboxyhemoglobin, 54, 55
CD. *See* Cluster designation
CD markers, 329t
  in acute leukemias, 174, 175, 177
  in hairy cell leukemia, 208
  of lymphocytes, 134t, 137
  in T-cell development, 179f
CEL. *See* Chronic eosinophilic leukemia
Cell-Dyne technology, 325–326, 326f
Cellular immunity, 19
Centrifuge
  standard microhematocrit, 299f
Cerebrospinal fluid (CSF)
  bacteria in, 316f
  causes of abnormal cells in, 317t
  cell count and differential, 313–315
    normal values of, 317t
    reference factors for calculations, 315t
  color and appearance of, 318t
CFU-GEMM. *See* Committed stem cells
CFU-S. *See* Colony-forming units-spleen
Charache, Samuel, 117
Chediak-Higashi syndrome, 149–150, 149f, 251
Cheilitis, 69
Chemical hazards, 8
Chemotaxis
  in white cell phagocytosis, 145
Cholelithiasis, 99
Christmas disease. *See* Hemophilia B, factor IX
    deficiency
Chronic diseases
  anemia of, 71–72
Chronic eosinophilic leukemia (CEL), 192
Chronic lymphocytic leukemia (CLL)
  bone marrow view in, 206f
  disease progression in, 206–207
  immunological function/treatment options, 207
  modified Rai staging for, 207t
  smudge cells of, 206f
Chronic myelogenous leukemia (CML)
  clinical features/symptoms, 189–190
  diagnosis, 191
  key facts of, 189t
  neutrophilic leukemoid reaction vs., 191t
  overview, 189

pathophysiology of, 189
peripheral blood/bone marrow findings, 190, 190t
prognosis, 191–192
treatment, 191–192
Chronic myeloproliferative disorders (CMPDs). *See also specific disorders*
characteristics of, 189t
differentiation of, 198t–199t
interrelationships of, 188f
terminology of, 188
WHO classification of, 188t
Chronic neutrophilic leukemia (CNL), 192
CLL. *See* Chronic lymphocytic leukemia
Cluster designation (CD), 137. *See also* CD markers
CML. *See* Chronic myelogenous leukemia
CMPDs. *See* Chronic myeloproliferative disorders
CNL. *See* Chronic neutrophilic leukemia
Coagulation, blood
abnormalities in pathogenesis of thrombosis, 283
extrinsic pathway, 237–238
inhibitors of, 240, 240f, 283–284
intrinsic system, 238
laboratory model of, 237
study of, 230
in vitro cascade, 237f
in vivo cascade, 237f
Coagulation factors, 236t
classification of, 235–237
congenital deficiencies of
with absent/mild bleeding, 262
with bleeding manifestations, 262
Coefficient of variation, 9
Cold agglutinin syndrome (CAS), 107–108
Collagen, 231
as aggregating agent, 235
Collagen vascular disease
anemia associated with, 71
Colony-forming units-spleen (CFU-S), 19
Committed stem cells (CFU-GEMM), 19, 20
Complement system, 240
Complete blood count (CBC), 22–23
critical values, 26
in HIV disease, 151
normal values, 25t
sample report, 24f
Congenital nonspherocytic hemolytic anemia, 105
Cooley, Thomas, 74–75
Cooley's anemia, 78–79
Coulter principle, 321, 321f
Coumadin, 238, 264, 289
COX-2 inhibitors
platelet function and, 251
Critical results/values
for CBC, 26
definition of, 11
sample, 139t
for WBC, 22
Cryoprecipitate, 261, 270
CSF. *See* Cerebrospinal fluid

Cubilin, 89
Cytokines, 19–20, 21t
in phagocytosis, 147t
Cytomegalovirus (CMV), 150–151
Cytoplasm
red cell, 43
Cytospin method
in body fluid differentials, 314–315

D-dimers, 273–274
qualitative test for, 318–320
Deleted 5q, 222
Delta checks, 10
Dextran
platelet function and, 251
Diamond-Blackfan anemia, 106
DIC. *See* Disseminated intravascular coagulation
Direct antiglobulin test, 207
Disseminated intravascular coagulation (DIC), 43, 273
acute, mechanism of, 273–274
conditions precipitating, 273f
events triggering, 274t
laboratory profile in, 275t
treatment, 276
DNA synthesis, 87
Döhle bodies, 146f, 148, 148f, 308
Donath-Landsteiner test, 108
Down syndrome, 161, 175
Duckert, F., 230
Dysfibrinogenemia, 271

Ehrlich, Paul, 148, 161
Ehrlichiosis. *See* Human ehrlichiosis
Electrical hazards, 8
Electrophoresis
alkaline, hemoglobin, points in analysis of, 120f
hemoglobin, 119–120
serum protein, 210
patterns in serum of normal vs. multiple myeloma patients, 210f
Elliptocytes, 42–43, 43f, 101f
Elliptocytosis. *See* Hereditary elliptocytosis
Embden-Meyerhof pathway, 40f
in pyruvate kinase deficiency, 105
in RBC metabolism, 38–39
Endothelium, 231
Environmental hazards, 8
Eosinophilia
definition of, 144
Eosinophils, 133f
allergy and, 144
identification criteria, 132
Epinephrine
as aggregating agent, 234
EPO. *See* Erythropoietin
Epstein, 161
Epstein-Barr virus (EBV), 150

Erythrocyte sedimentation rate (ESR), 300
  conditions associated with increase/decrease in, 302
  normal values, 302
  Sediplast ESR rack, 301f
Erythrocytosis
  secondary, causes of, 193
Erythroid hyperplasia, 75f
Erythropoiesis, 34, 34f
  ineffective
    consequences of, 87t
    in megaloblastic anemia, 86–87
Erythropoietin (EPO), 18, 20–21, 34
  increased production of, 27
ESR. *See* Erythrocyte sedimentation rate
Essential thrombocythemia (ET)
  clinical features/symptoms, 196–197
  diagnosis, 197
  diagnostic criteria for, 198t
  key facts for, 196t
  pathophysiology of, 196
  peripheral blood/bone marrow findings, 197
  prognosis, 197
  treatment, 197
Esterase stains, 165–166
ET. *See* Essential thrombocythemia
Extramedullary hematopoiesis, 17
Eye protection, 7f

Factor I. *See* Fibrinogen
Factor II. *See* Prothrombin
Factor III. *See* Thromboplastin
Factor IV. *See* Calcium, ionized
Factor V Leiden, 262
Factor VII. *See* Proconvertin
Factor VIII. *See* Antihemophilic factor
Factor IX. *See* Thromboplastin, plasma component
Factor X. *See* Stuart-Prower factor
Factor XI. *See* Thromboplastin, plasma antecedent
Factor XII. *See* Hageman factor
Factor XIII. *See* Fibrin-stabilizing factor
Fanconi's anemia, 105–106, 161–162
Fauvism, 104
Ferritin, 66, 70–71
Fibrin
  conditions elevating, 273t
  degradation products of, 273f
  formation of, 270
  measurement of, 273–274
Fibrinogen (Factor I), 235
  in clot formation, 231
  disorders of, 270–271
  in hemostasis, 270
  thrombin's activity on, 271f
Fibrinolysis
  abnormalities, in pathogenesis of thrombosis, 283
  in disseminated intravascular coagulation, 275
  natural inhibitors of, 272–273
  physiological activators of, 272
Fibrinolytic system, 239–240

  disorders of, in thrombotic disease, 286
  measurable products of, 273–274
Fibrin-stabilizing factor (Factor XIII), 236
  deficiency of, 263
Fibrometer, 230
Fibronectin receptors, 234
Flagging signals, 10
Flame cells, 211, 211f
Fletcher factor, 237
Flow cytometer
  internal components of, 328f
Flow cytometry, 326–327
  applications of, 327t
  data interpretation, 327–328
  in diagnosis of PNH, 107
  graphing of data from, 329f
Fluids, body
  cell count and differential, 313–315
    normal values of, 317t
    reference factors for calculations, 315t
    worksheet, 315t
Folic acid, 41
  in DNA synthesis, 87
  nutrition requirements of, 87–88
Folic acid deficiency, 89–90
  in megaloblastic anemia, 86

Gaucher's cells, 152f
Gaucher's disease, 152
G-CSF. *See* Granulocyte-colony-stimulating factor
Glanzmann's thrombasthenia, 250–251
Gloves, 6, 7f
Glucose-6-phosphate dehydrogenase (G6PD) deficiency, 102
  agents causing hemolysis in, 104
  clinical manifestations, 103–105
  diagnosis of, 105
  genetics of, 102–103
  genotypes of, 103t
Glutamic acid
  carboxylation of, 264f
GM-CSF. *See* Granulocyte-macrophage colony-stimulating factor
Golhorm, 230
Granulation
  abnormal, platelet, 221f
  toxic, 308
Granulocyte-colony-stimulating factor (G-CSF), 19
Granulocyte-macrophage colony-stimulating factor (GM-CSF), 19
Gray platelet syndrome, 251
Growth factors, 21t
G6PD deficiency. *See* Glucose-6-phosphate dehydrogenase deficiency

Hageman, John, 230
Hageman factor (Factor XII), 236, 237
  deficiency of, 262
Hairy cell leukemia, 207–208, 207f
  CD markers in, 208t

Ham's test, 106, 107f
Handwashing, 7
Hct. *See* Hematocrit
HE. *See* Hereditary elliptocytosis
Heinz bodies, 17, 43, 45, 46f, 104f, 308
    formation, 46f
    in G6PD deficiency, 103
Helmet cells. *See* Bite cells
Hemarthrosis, 260, 260f
Hematocrit (Hct), 22. *See also* Microhematocrit
    normal values, 300
Hematology, 4
    automated data on, interpreting, 320
        Coulter principle, 321, 321f
        flow cells, 322
        hydrodynamic focusing, 321
        instruments, 322–326
        multiple polarized scatter separations, 322
        optical scatter, 321
        radiofrequency resistance, 321
        VSC technology, 321
    automated instruments in, knowledge necessary for
        operator of, 323
Hematopoiesis, 20f
    in acute myeloid leukemia, 162
    definition of, 16
    intramedullary vs. extramedullary, 17
Heme molecule, 52
Hemochromatosis. *See* Hereditary hemochromatosis
Hemoglobin (Hgb), 22
    abnormal, 54–55, 55f
    chromosomes specific to formation of, 53f
    electrophoresis, 119–120, 119f
        alkaline, points in analysis of, 120t
    embryonic, 16
    function, 53–54
    structure of, 52, 52f
    synthesis of, 52–53
        iron in, 39
        in thalassemias, 75
    types of, 52–53
    variants of, in US vs. worldwide, 121f
Hemoglobin A (HgbA)
    gene states of, 76–77, 76f
    normal concentrations, by age, 119t
    postpartum, 16
Hemoglobin Barts (γ4), 76, 77
Hemoglobin C crystals, 308
Hemoglobin C disease, 120–121
Hemoglobin CC (HgbCC), 120f
Hemoglobin D $_{Punjab}$, 122
Hemoglobin E (HgE), 121
Hemoglobin F (HgbF)
    normal concentrations, by age, 119t
    in sickle cell anemia, 114–115, 117
Hemoglobin G $_{phila}$, 122
Hemoglobin H disease, 76–77
    peripheral smear in, 77f
Hemoglobin O $_{Arab}$, 122
Hemoglobin S (HgbS), 42
Hemoglobin S-beta thalassemia, 121

Hemoglobin SC (HgbSC), 120f, 121f
    haplotypes of, 114–115
    solubility screen for, 118, 312, 313f
Hemoglobinemia, 58
Hemoglobinopathies, 114
Hemolysis
    clinical events and, 55t
    extravascular, 56f
    intravascular, 57f
    laboratory evidence of, 56–57
    physiology of, 57–58
    types of, 55–56
Hemolytic uremic syndrome (HUS), 248
    vs. thrombotic thrombocytopenic purpura, 249t
Hemophilia A, factor VIII deficiency, 230
    laboratory diagnosis of, 260
    quality of life issues in, 261–262, 261t
    symptoms of, 258, 259
    treatment for, 261
Hemophilia B, factor IX deficiency
    quality of life issues in, 261t
Hemophilia C, factor X deficiency, 262
Hemorrhage. *See* Bleeding
Hemorrhagic telangiectasia. *See* Hereditary hemorrhagic
    telangiectasia
Hemosiderin, 66
Hemostasis
    basis of, 230
    fibrin in, 271–272, 272f
    fibrinogen in, 270
    normal, 282
    primary system of, 230–231
        platelet aggregation, 234–235
        platelet development, 232–235
        platelet function/kinetics, 233–234
    secondary system of, 231
        coagulation factors, 235–237, 235–241,
            236t
        common pathway, 238
        complement system, 240
        extrinsic pathway, 237–238
        feedback inhibition, 239
        fibrinolysis, 239–240
        interrelationships between systems, 241
        intrinsic pathway, 238
        kinin system, 240
        physiological coagulation, 237
        thrombin formation, 238–239
    vitamin K in, 263
Henoch-Schönlein anemia, 252
Heparin, 289
    low-molecular-weight, 289
Heparin cofactor II
    deficiency of, 284
    in thrombosis, 284
Heparin-induced thrombocytopenia (HIT), 287
    diagnosis, 287–288
    pathophysiology of, 287f
Hepatosplenomegaly, 17
    in leukemia, 160
Hepcidin, 71–72

Hereditary elliptocytosis (HE), 100–101
    variants of, 101t
Hereditary hemochromatosis (HH), 72
    laboratory diagnosis, 73
    symptoms of, 73, 73t
    treatment, 73–74
Hereditary hemorrhagic telangiectasia, 252, 252f
Hereditary pyropoikilocytosis, 101–102, 102f
Hereditary spherocytosis (HS)
    clinical presentation, 98–100
    genetics of, 98
    laboratory diagnosis of, 100
    pathophysiology of, 98
Hereditary stomatocytosis, 102
Hereditary xerocytosis, 102
Hermansky-Pudlak syndrome, 251
Herrick, James B., 117
Hewson, William, 230
Hexosaminidase A, 153
Hexose monophosphate shunt
    in RBC metabolism, 39
Hgb. See Hemoglobin
HH. See Hereditary hemochromatosis
High-molecular-weight kininogen (HMWK), 235
Hippocrates, 230
Histiocytes
    in peritoneal fluid, 316f
HIT. See Heparin-induced thrombocytopenia
HIV-AIDS
    effects on hematology parameters, 151
Hodgkin's lymphoma, 206, 208–209
Homocysteine, 286
Howell-Jolly bodies, 17, 43, 45, 45f, 308
    in megaloblastic anemias, 88f
Human ehrlichiosis, 148, 148f
Humoral immunity, 19
Hypercoagulability, 282
Hypercoagulable states
    conditions requiring evaluation for, 288t
    laboratory screening tests for, 288t
Hyperhomocysteinemia, 286
Hyperviscosity syndrome, 252
Hypochromia, 39, 41, 41f, 308
Hypofibrinogenemia, 270

IDA. See Iron-deficiency anemia (IDA)
Idiopathic thrombocytopenic purpura (ITP), 247
    acute vs. chronic, 247f
Immunity
    cellular, 19
    humoral, 19
Immunoglobulins
    basic structure, 209f
    IgM, 214
    serum protein electrophoresis patterns, 210f
    type and activity range of, 209t
Immunophenotype
    acute myeloid leukemia, 166–167, 166t
    lymphoblastic leukemia, 176–177

precursor B lymphoblastic leukemia, 176–177
    precursor T lymphoblastic leukemia, 178–179
Inclusions, red cell, 17, 43, 45, 45t
    diseases matched to, 310t
    grading, 310t
    recording, 308
Infants/newborns
    jaundice in, 104–105
    red blood cell values in, 25t
    WBC differential values, 138t, 307t
Inflammation
    anemia of, 71–72
Intramedullary hematopoiesis, 17
Iron
    absorption, 66
        enhancers of, 68t
        inhibitors of, 68t
    available recycled, vs. need, 69f
    deficiency, prevention/control recommendations, 71t
    foods high in, 68t
    forms of, 68t
    in hemoglobin formation, 39
    intake, 66
    overload
        anemias related to, 72–74
        organs damaged by, 74f
    storage/recycling, 66, 68
Iron-chelating agents, 74
    rotation of injection sites, 75f
Iron cycle, 67f
Iron-deficiency anemia (IDA)
    causes of, 70–71
    diagnostic tests, 70
    stages of, matched to diagnostic signals, 69t
        causes of, 69t
    treatment, 71
Isoelectric focusing, 120
ITP. See Idiopathic thrombocytopenic purpura

Kasabach-Merritt syndrome, 252
Kidneys. See Renal disease
Kininogen, high-molecular-weight (HMWK), 235, 237
Kinin system, 240
Koilonychia, 69, 70f
Kottman, 230

Labile factor. See Proaccelerin
Lactate dehydrogenase (LDH), 58
LDH. See Lactate dehydrogenase
Lee, Pearl, 74–75
Left shift
    definition of, 144
Leukemia. See also specific types
    acute
        of ambiguous lineage, 175
        vs. chronic, 160, 160t
        clinical findings in, 163t

cytochemical reactions in, 165t
    FAB classification, 166, 167t
definition of, 160
early research on, 160–161
Leukocytes (WBCs), 133f
    agranular cell series, 133
    bands, 132, 132f
    basophils, 133, 133f
    Coulter scatterplots of, 322f
    eosinophils, 132, 133f
    hereditary disorders of, 149–150
    life span of, 130
    lymphocytic series, 133–134
    maturation stages, 130
    metamyelocytes, 131–132, 132f
    myeloblasts, 130–131, 131f
    myelocytes, 131, 131f
    promyelocytes (progranulocyte), 131, 131f
    qualitative defects of, 145–146
    quantitative changes in, 144
        terminology related to, 144–145
    segmented neutrophils, 132, 132f
    terminology of, 130, 146t
    toxic changes in, 146
    toxic granulation in, 146f, 147, 147f
    toxic vacuolization in, 147, 147f
Leukocytosis
    definition of, 144, 146
Leukoerythroblastic picture, 146
    definition of, 144
Leukopoiesis, 130
Lipid storage diseases, 152–153
Liver
    disease, bleeding associated with, 263
    in fetal hematopoiesis, 16
Loeliger, E.A., 230
LSC. *See* Lymphocytic committed cell
Lungs
    in sickle cell disease, 116
Lupus anticoagulant (LA), 286–287
    diagnostic criteria for, 287t
Lymphatic system, 136
    in lymphocyte development/differentiation, 134–135, 135f
Lymph nodes
    in fetal hematopoiesis, 16
Lymphoblastic leukemia (B-LBL), 176
    antigen expression in, 177f
    cytogenetic findings, 178
    immunophenotype, 176–177
    laboratory findings, 176
Lymphoblasts
    identification criteria, 133–134
    morphology, vs. myeloblasts, 164, 164f
Lymphocytes
    antigen markers, 134t
    development of immunocompetency and, 137
    large, 134, 134f
    origins of, 134
    reactive, 151f
        morphology of, vs. resting lymphocyte, 151t
    response to antigenic stimulation, 137

small, 134, 134f
    subpopulations of, 136, 136f
    Sysmex scatterplot of, 324f
    travel path of, 136–137
Lymphocytic committed cell (LSC), 19
Lymphocytosis
    reactive, 150–151
Lymphoid cell lineage, 160
Lymphoproliferative disorders, 206
    overview of, 215t

Macrocytes
    polychromatophilic, 41; *see also* Reticulocytes.
        shape of, pathologies associated with, 92f
    size of, 39
Macrocytic anemias
    categories of, 86
    clinical features of, 88
    erythropoiesis in, 86–87
    hematological features of, 88–89
    laboratory diagnosis of, 90
    non-megaloblastic, 91–92
    red cell precursors in, 86
    treatment, 90–91
Macrocytic normochromic anemia, 24–25
May-Hegglin anomaly, 149
MCH. *See* Mean corpuscular Hgb
MCHC. *See* Mean corpuscular Hgb content
MCV. *See* Mean corpuscular volume
MDSs. *See* Myelodysplastic syndromes
Mean corpuscular Hgb content (MCHC), 22, 25
    normal values, 300
Mean corpuscular Hgb (MCH), 22, 25
    normal values, 300
Mean corpuscular volume (MCV), 22
    conditions related to shifts in, 25t
    in macrocytic anemias, 80f
    normal values, 300
Mediterranean fever, 78–79
Megakaryocytes, 232, 232f
Megaloblastic anemias
    clinical features of, 88
    erythropoiesis in, 86–87
    hematological features of, 88–89
    laboratory diagnosis of, 90
    peripheral blood smear in, 89f
    pernicious anemia, 89
    red cell precursors in, 86, 86f
    treatment, 90
M:E ratio. *See* Myeloid-erythroid ratio
Mercurialis, 230
Metamyelocytes, 132f
    identification criteria, 131–132
Methemoglobin, 54, 55
Methemoglobin reductase pathway, 39
MHA. *See* Microangiopathic hemolytic anemia
Microangiopathic hemolytic anemia (MHA), 248
    after acute DIC, 275

Microcytes, 39, 41
in thalassemia major, 80f
Microcytic disorders
differential diagnosis of, 80
Microcytic hypochromic anemia, 24
Microhematocrit, 298
interpretation, 299–300
procedure, 299
reagents and equipment for, 298
Microscope, 4
care of, 5–6
parts of, 4–5, 5f
Microscopy
innovations in, 6
light, corrective actions in, 6
Miller eye disc, 303, 303f
Minot, George, 89
Modified Westergren sedimentation rate, 300
Monoclonal gammopathy, 211
Monocytes, 133f
identification criteria, 133
increase in, conditions associated with, 144
in phagocytosis, 145
Sysmex scatterplot of, 324f
Morawitz, Paul, 230
Multiple myeloma, 210
chromosomal aberrations in, 210t
disturbed platelet function in, 251, 252
laboratory findings in, 212t
pathophysiology of, 210–212
prognosis/treatment, 212–213
symptoms/screening for, 212
Murphy, William, 89
Myeloblasts, 131f
identification criteria, 130–131
morphology, vs. lymphoblasts, 164, 164f
Myelocytes, 131f
identification criteria, 131
Myelodysplasia
acute myeloid leukemia with, 170
Myelodysplastic syndromes (MDSs), 164, 220
dysplastic changes in, 222t
FAB classification of, 222t
factors indicating progression to leukemia in, 223t
pathophysiology of, 220
prognostic factors/clinical management, 222–223
recognizing, 220–221
therapy-related, 170
unclassifiable, 222
WHO classification of, 221–222, 222t
Myelofibrosis with myeloid metaplasia (MMM), 194
clinical features/symptoms, 195
diagnosis, 195
diagnostic criteria for, 196t
key facts of, 194t
pathophysiology of, 194–195
peripheral blood/bone marrow findings, 195
teardrop RBCs in, 195f
treatment, 195–196
Myeloid cell lineage, 160
Myeloid-erythroid ratio (M:E ratio), 18, 21, 130

Myeloperoxidase, 165
Myelosuppressive therapy
in CML, 191

Naegeli, 161
Naphthol AS-D chloroacetate esterase, 165
Neonatal jaundice, 104–105
Neumann, Ernst, 161
Neutrophilia, 146
definition of, 144
Neutrophils
alterations in, in peripheral smears, 147t
hypersegmentation of, 148, 148f
increase in, conditions associated with, 144
maturation spectrum, in CML, 190f
in phagocytosis, 145
segmented
bacteria in, 153f
identification criteria, 132, 132f
toxic granulation in, 146f, 147, 308
Niemann-Pick cell, 152f
Niemann-Pick disease, 152
NK cells, 137
Non-Hodgkin's lymphoma, 206, 209
Normoblastic erythropoiesis, 86f
Normoblasts
polychromatic, 86f
Normocytic normochromic anemia, 24
NSAIDs
platelet function and, 246–247
Nucleus:cytoplasm ratio (N:C ratio), 34
in leukocytes, 130
red cell maturation and, 35
Nygaard, 230

OD curve. *See* Oxygen dissociation curve
Opsonization
in white cell phagocytosis, 145
Orthochromic normoblast, 36f
Orthochromic normoblast-nucleated (nRBC), 36
Osler-Weber-Rendu disease, 252
Osmotic fragility curve, 100f
Ovalocytes, 42–43, 307
Ovalocytosis, Southeast Asian, 101, 101f
Overwhelming postsplenectomy infections (OPSIs), 17
Owren, Paul, 230
Oxygen dissociation curve (OD curve), 53–54, 54f

Pappenheimer bodies, 17, 45, 72f, 308
Paroxysmal cold hemoglobinuria (PCH), 107–108
Paroxysmal nocturnal hemoglobinuria (PNH), 106–107
Pauling, Linus, 114
Pavlosky, 230
PCH. *See* Paroxysmal cold hemoglobinuria
Pelger-Huët anomaly, 149, 149f

Pentose-phosphate shunt, 40f
Peritoneal fluid
　cell count and differential, 313–315
　histiocyte in, 316f
Pernicious anemia, 89
Personal protective equipment (PPE), 6–7, 8t
Phagocytosis, white cell
　essential elements leading to, 147t
　mechanism of, 145, 145f
Philadelphia chromosome
　in CML, 189, 191, 192
Pica, 69
PK deficiency. *See* Pyruvate kinase deficiency
Plasma cell leukemia, 214, 214f
Plasma cells, 210f, 211
　with inclusion, 211f
　sheets of, 211f
　structure/function of, 209–210
Plasmin, 239, 272, 273
　in disseminated intravascular coagulation, 275
　inhibitors of, 283
Plasminogen activator inhibitor 1 (PAI-1), 272–273
Plasminogen activator system, 239
Platelet(s)
　abnormalities
　　in myelodysplastic syndromes, 220
　　in pathogenesis of thrombosis, 282
　aggregation, 234f
　　principle of, 234–235
　Coulter scatterplots of, 322f
　count, 22
　　estimate, from peripheral smear, 306t
　　Unopette system for, 309–311
　　　normal values in, 312
　development of, 232
　dysfunction of, due to vascular disorders, 252
　function
　　acquired defects in, 251–252
　　drugs affecting, 252t
　　kinetics and, 233–234
　　zones of, 233t
　giant, 221f
　　abnormal granulation of, 221f
　inherited qualitative disorders of
　　adhesion disorders, 249–251
　　release defects, 251
　quantitative disorders of, 246–249
　response of, to vascular injury, 232f
　satellitism, 153–154, 153f
　　formation, 154f
　structure of, 232–233, 233f
Pleural fluid
　cell count and differential, 313–315
　mesothelial cell in, 316f
PLL. *See* Prolymphocytic leukemia
PNH. *See* Paroxysmal nocturnal hemoglobinuria
Poikilocytosis, 39, 307–308
Polychromasia, 18, 41, 308
Polychromatophilic macrocytes, 41f
Polychromatophilic normoblasts, 36, 36f
Polycythemia vera (PV), 192

clinical features/symptoms, 192
　diagnosis, 193
　diagnostic criteria for, 194t
　increased RBCs in, 193f
　key facts of, 192t
　pathophysiology of, 192t
　peripheral blood/bone marrow findings, 192–193
　treatment, 193–194
Postanalytic variables, 10, 11t
Preanalytic variables, 10, 10f
　thrombocytopenia related to, 246
Precursor B lymphoblastic leukemia (B-ALL), 176, 177f
　antigen expression in, 177f
　cytogenetic findings, 178
　immunophenotype, 176–177
　laboratory findings, 176
Precursor T lymphoblastic leukemia (T-ALL), 179f
　antigen expression in, 179f
　cytogenetic findings, 179
　immunophenotype, 178–179
　laboratory findings, 178
Prekallikrein, 235, 237
Priapism
　in sickle cell disease, 116–117
Proaccelerin (labile factor, Factor V), 235–236
Proconvertin (stable factor, Factor VII), 236, 237
　deficiency of, 262
Prolymphocytes, 134
Prolymphocytic leukemia (PLL), 208
Promonocytes
　identification criteria, 133
Promyelocytes (progranulocyte), 131f
　abnormal, 169f
　identification criteria, 131
Protein C, 284f
　deficiency of, 284–285
　pathway, 284f
Protein S, 284
　deficiency of, 285
Prothrombin (Factor II), 235
　deficiency of, 262
　mutation, 286
Prothrombin time (PT), 238, 270
　automated procedure for, 315–318
　procedure, 318f
Protonormoblast, 35, 35f
Punnett square, 114f
Purpura, 252, 252f
Pyknosis, 153–154
Pyropoikilocytosis. *See* Hereditary pyropoikilocytosis
Pyruvate kinase (PK) deficiency, 105

Quality assurance
　indicators of, 9t
　monitoring, 9–10
　normal (reference) values, 9–10
　plans, basic concepts of, 8–9
　　monitoring, 7

RA. *See* Refractory anemia
Radioactive hazards, 8
RAEB. *See* Refractory anemia with excess blasts
RARS. *See* Refractory anemia with ringed sideroblasts
RBCs. *See* Red blood cells
RCDW. *See* Red cell distribution width
RCM. *See* Red cell mass
Red blood cell indices. *See also* Mean corpuscular Hgb; Mean corpuscular Hgb content; Mean corpuscular volume
  calculating, 300
Red blood cells (RBCs), 37f
  abnormal morphologies, 39
    clinical conditions matched to, 309t
    color variations, 41
    qualitative grading of, 309t
    recording, 307–308
    shape variations, 41–43
    size variations, 39–41
  bone marrow production of, 16
  Coulter scatterplots of, 322f
  elliptocytes, 42–43
  fragmented, 43
  hypochromic, 41f, 70f
    dimorphism in, 72f
  inclusions, 17, 43, 45, 45t
    recording, 308
  life span of, 17
  macrocytic, 221f
  maturation, 34
    key features of, 35t
    terminology, 35t
  metabolism, 38–39
  microcytic, 66, 70f
  in microcytic anemias, 66
  normal values, in newborn, 25t
  nucleated
    in chronic lymphocytic leukemia, 206f
    observing/recording, 307
  ovalocytes, 42–43
  polychromatophilic macrocyte, 41f
  in polycythemia vera, 193, 193f
  precursors
    in megaloblastic anemia, 86, 86f
  sickle cell, 42, 42f
  spherocytes, 42, 42f
Red cell distribution width (RCDW), 22
  value of, 25–26
Red cell mass (RCM)
  in polycythemia vera, 192, 193
Red cell membrane, 37f
  cytoskeleton, 38
  development and function, 37
  disorders of
    role of spleen in, 98
  lipid composition, 37–38
  protein composition in lipid bilayers, 38
Reed-Sternberg cells, 208
Reference intervals, 9
Reflex testing, 10
Refractory anemia (RA), 221
Refractory anemia with excess blasts (RAEB), 222
Refractory anemia with multilineage dysplasia, 221–222

Refractory anemia with ringed sideroblasts (RARS), 221
Renal disease
  anemia associated with, 71
  bleeding associated with, 263
  disturbed platelet function in, 252–253
Reticulocyte count
  with automated instrumentation, 326
  conditions associated with increase/decrease in, 304
  manual, procedure, 302
  with Miller eye disc procedure, 302
  normal values, 304
  value of, 26–27
Reticulocytes, 36, 36f
  definition of, 26
Reticuloendothelial system (RES), 17, 66
  in leukemia, 160
  in lipid storage diseases, 152
Retinopathy
  in sickle cell disease, 117
Ringed sideroblasts, 72, 72f
Ristocetin co-factor assay, 250
Rouleaux, 212, 212f
  vs. agglutination, 213f
Russell bodies, 211f

Safety precautions, 6–9
Scatterplots/scattergrams, 322, 322f
  Coulter
    of leukocytes, 322f
    of platelets, 322f
    of RBCs, 322f
  Sysmex, 324f, 325f
Schilling, 161
Schilling test, 90, 91f
Schistocytes, 43, 248f, 308
  in microangiopathic hemolytic anemia after acute DIC, 275
Sedimentation rate, modified Westergren, 300
Sediplast ESR rack, 301f
Serine protease, effects of antithrombin on, 284f
Serine protease inhibitors, 240f
Serous fluids
  causes of abnormal cells in, 318t
  cell count and differential, 313–315
    normal values of, 317t
    reference factors for calculations, 315t
Sézary cells, 208f
Sézary syndrome, 208
SH. *See* Hereditary spherocytosis
Sickle cell anemia
  clinical considerations, 115–117
  genetics/incidence of, 114–115
  laboratory diagnosis, 117–120
  management, 117, 118t
  pathophysiology of sickling process, 115
  prognosis, 117
Sickle cell gene
  haplotypes of, 114–115
Sickle cells, 42, 42f, 118f, 308
Sickle cell screen, 309–311

Sickle cell trait, 120
Sickle solubility test, 119f
Sideroblastic anemias, 72–74
Sideroblasts
  ringed, 220, 222f
    refractory anemia with, 221
Siderotic granules, 45, 45f
Smears
  wedge-type
    preparation of, 304, 305f
    three zones of, 306f
    zigzag method for differential, 306f
Southeast Asian ovalocytosis, 101f
Spectrin, 38
Spherocytes, 42, 42f, 98f, 308
  formation mechanisms, 99f
  treatment/management of, 100
Spherocytosis. *See* Hereditary spherocytosis
Spleen
  in fetal hematopoiesis, 16
  functions of, 17, 18t
  role in red cell membrane disorders, 98
  in sickle cell disease, 116
  in thrombocytopenia, 246
Splenectomy
  in hereditary spherocytosis, 100
  Howell-Jolly bodies observed following, 43, 45
  overwhelming infections following, 17
  in thalassemia major, 79
Stable factor. *See* Proconvertin
Standard deviation, 9
Statistical quality control, 9–11
Stem cells, 18–19
Stomatocytes, 102f, 308
Stomatocytosis. *See* Hereditary stomatocytosis
Streptokinase, 272, 290
Stroke
  in sickle cell disease, 117
Stuart-Prower factor (Factor X), 236
  deficiency of, 262
Sudan black B, 165
Sugar water test, 106
Sulfhemoglobin, 54, 55
Synovial fluid
  causes of abnormal cells in, 318t
  cell count and differential, 313–315
    normal values of, 317t
    reference factors for calculations, 315t
Sysmex instrumentation, 324f

T-ALL. *See* Precursor T lymphoblastic leukemia
Target cells, 42–43, 44f, 308
  formation of, 44f
Tay-Sachs disease, 152, 153
T-cell lymphomas, 208
T cells, 19, 136, 137
  development, CD markers in, 179f
  in lymphoproliferative disorders, 206
T cytotoxic/suppressor cells (CD8), 137
  in HIV disease, 151

Teardrop cells, 308
  in myelofibrosis with myeloid metaplasia, 195f
Telangiectasia, 252, 252f
Terminal deoxynucleotidyl transferase, 165–166
TFPI. *See* Tissue factor pathway inhibitor
Thalassemia gene
  alpha, 75
  beta, 75
    expression in population, 76t
  lineage of, from Queen Victoria, 259f
Thalassemia syndromes, 74–75, 75f
  alpha, 76–77
    clinical states of, 76f
  beta major, 78
    treatment/management of, 79
  beta thalassemia trait, 78–79
  diagnosis, 76
  diagnostic clues for, 80t
  microcytic cells in, 39–40
  minor
    microcytic hypochromic blood smear, 80f
  pathophysiology of, 75–76
  RBC morphology in, 39
  thalassemia intermedia, 78
  treatment, 76
Thalidomide, 213
T helper cells (CD4), 137
  in HIV disease, 151
Thrombin
  activity on fibrinogen, 271f
  role in hemostasis, 271–272, 272f
Thrombocythemia, 196t. *See* Essential thrombocythemia
Thrombocytopenia
  drug-induced, 246–247
  related to altered platelet distribution, 246
  related to decreased platelet production, 246
  related to sample integrity/ preanalytic variables, 246
Thrombocytopenia with absent radii (TAR), 251
Thrombocytosis, 249
  relative, causes of, 197t
Thrombolytic drugs, 289–290
Thrombolytic therapy, 272
Thromboplastin, plasma antecedent (Factor XI), 236
Thromboplastin, plasma component (Factor IX), 236
Thromboplastin (Factor III), 235
Thrombosis
  acquired, conditions associated with, 283t
  anticoagulant therapy in, 288–290
  arterial vs. venous, 282
  definition of, 282
  inherited, conditions associated with, 283t
  pathogenesis of, 282
    antithrombotic factors, 283–284
    coagulation abnormalities, 283
    fibrinolytic abnormalities, 283
    platelet abnormalities, 282
    vascular injury, 282
  risk factors for, 283f
Thrombotic disorders
  acquired, 286–288
  inherited, 284–286
  laboratory diagnosis, 288

Thrombotic thrombocytopenic purpura, 43
Thrombotic thrombocytopenic purpura (ITP), 248
    vs. hemolytic uremic syndrome, 249t
Thromboxane A₂, 234, 252, 288
Thymidine triphosphate (TTP), 87
Thymus
    in fetal hematopoiesis, 16
TIBC. *See* Total iron-binding capacity
Tissue factor pathway inhibitor (TFPI), 237
    deficiency, 286
T-LBL. *See* T lymphoblastic lymphoma
T lymphoblastic lymphoma (T-LBL)
    laboratory findings, 178
Total iron-binding capacity (TIBC), 70
Toxic granulation, 146f, 147, 147f
TPA. *See* Tissue-plasminogen activator
    in fibrinolysis, 272
Transferrin, 66
TTP. *See* Thymidine triphosphate
2,3-Diphosphoglycerate (2,3-DPG), 52, 53, 54

Unopette white blood cell/platelet count, 309
Uremia
    disturbed platelet function in, 251, 252
Urokinase, 272, 290

Variables
    postanalytic, 10–11, 11t
    preanalytic, 10, 10f
Vascular system
    injury
        events following, 231–232
        in pathogenesis of thrombosis, 282
    overview, 231
Vasoconstriction
    mechanism of, 231
Vaso-occlusive conditions
    in sickle cell disease, 116
VCS technology, 321
    in Beckman-Coulter instrumentation, 322, 324f
    results from, verifying and sending, 323
Victoria (Queen), 258
    lineage of thalassemia gene from, 259f
Virchow, Rudolph, 161
Vitamin B₁₂, 41
    absorption and transport, 88f

in DNA synthesis, 87
    nutrition requirements of, 87–88
    sources of, 87t
Vitamin B₁₂ deficiency, 89–90
    in megaloblastic anemia, 86
Vitamin K
    coagulation factors dependent on, 233–237
    deficiency of, 264
    dependent proteins, 284
    drugs interfering with activity of, 264t
Von Willebrand factor (vWF), 249
    in clot formation, 231
    Factor X and, 258
    large multimers, 248
Von Willebrand's disease, 249–250
    basic test profile for, 250t
    primary derivatives of, 250t

Waldenström's macroglobulinemia, 214
    disturbed platelet function in, 251, 252
Warfarin, 238, 264
    in acute thrombosis, 288
    associated skin necrosis, in protein C deficiency, 285
WBC. *See* White blood cell count
WBCs. *See* Leukocytes
White blood cell count (WBC), 22, 137, 144
    differential, 138
        absolute values
            adult, reference range for, 139t
            vs. relative values, 139
        manual
            principle, 305
            procedure, 306–307
            reference ranges for adults and infants, 138t
            vs. scan, 138–139
        normal values in adults/infants, 307t
    from peripheral smear, 306t
    Unopette system for, 309–311
        normal values in, 309–311
    values
        critical, 22, 139t
        at different ages, 138t
    zigzag method of, 306f
Wiskott-Aldrich syndrome, 251

Xerocytosis. *See* Hereditary xerocytosis